THE
VSITE
REVIEW
MANUAL

THE
VSITE
REVIEW
MANUAL

Michael D. Sgroi, MD | Guillermo A. Escobar, MD

Associate Clinical Professor of Surgery
Associate Program Director
Vascular Surgery Residency and Fellowship Program
Stanford University
Stanford, California

Associate Professor of Surgery
Vascular Surgery Program Director
Emory University School of Medicine
Atlanta, Georgia

ELSEVIER

Elsevier
3251 Riverport Lane
St. Louis, Missouri 63043

THE VSITE REVIEW MANUAL   ISBN: 978-0-323-87588-2

Content Strategist: Jessica L. McCool
Content Development Specialist: Shweta Pant
Senior Content Development Specialist: Himanshi Chauhan
Publishing Services Manager: Deepthi Unni
Senior Project Manager: Manchu Mohan
Senior Book Designer: Amy L. Buxton

Printed in India

Last digit is the print number: 9   8   7   6   5   4   3   2   1

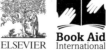

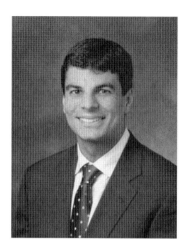

Dr. Weesam Al-Khatib

The *VSITE Review Manual* is dedicated to the memory of Dr. Weesam Al-Khatib. Dr. Al-Khatib was a graduate of the University of Kansas Medical School and General Surgery Residency. He then went to Stanford University for a vascular surgery fellowship, and eventually became a clinical instructor at Stanford University and Palo Alto VA Medical Center. Sadly, he passed away from a rare form of cancer in 2012. Prior to his passing, Dr. Al-Khatib was devoted to medical education. He started writing a Stanford Vascular Surgery Review, determined to help the trainees with their education. His tireless work ethic and passion for teaching influenced many, including myself when I was a medical student and worked with him. It was his initial efforts that influenced me to write this book for all of you. It was an honor to know him and I hope he would be proud of this book designed to help the next generation of vascular surgeons.

—**Michael D. Sgroi**

I wish to dedicate this book to my parents who laid the foundations for me as an educator who strives to excel and learn as much as I can so as to teach it to others. To my wife who is a constant source of happiness and inspiration; repeatedly showing me how we can overcome anything together. To my tenacious and inquisitive son who continuously reminds me of the joy of teaching and learning.

—**Guillermo A. Escobar**

About the Editor

Dr. Michael D. Sgroi is a Clinical Associate Professor of Surgery, as well as the Associate Program Director for the Vascular Surgery Residency and Fellowship Program at Stanford University. After completing a general surgery residency at University of California, Irvine, he then performed a fellowship in vascular surgery at Stanford University. Upon completion of the fellowship in 2018, Dr. Sgroi was asked to join the faculty as an assistant professor where he has taken over responsibility of vascular surgery simulation, become clerkship director for vascular surgery, and is also the assistant director of surgical education for the division. Most recently, he took over as Section Chief for the division of vascular surgery at Santa Clara Valley Medical Center. In addition to roles at Stanford University, he is an active member of SVS, SCVS, and APDVS. Dr. Sgroi is on the editorial board for VSCORE, he is a committee member for the Ad Hoc research committee for APDVS, and director of Stanford's VSIG.

Dr. Escobar is the Program Director for the vascular surgery training programs at Emory University and also a co-founder of its integrated residency. He is a passionate educator who has won skills and teaching awards throughout his career as a trainee and as a faculty member. He has collaborated as a question writer for the Vascular Education and Self-Assessment Program (VESAP), as well as for the American Board of Surgery's Vascular Surgery Qualifying Exam and is an examiner for the American Board of Surgery's Vascular Surgery Certifying Exam.

Contributors

Olamide Alabi, MD
Assistant Professor of Surgery
Division of Vascular and Endovascular Surgery
Emory University
Atlanta, Georgia

Shipra Arya, MD, SM
Professor of Surgery
Division of Vascular Surgery
Stanford University School of Medicine
Stanford, California
Section Chief
Vascular Surgery
VA Palo Alto Healthcare System
Palo Alto, California

Barath Badrinathan, MD, RPVI
Assistant Professor
Division of Vascular and Endovascular Surgery
Emory University
Atlanta, Georgia

Adam Baraka, BS
Morehouse School of Medicine
Atlanta, Georgia

Jaime Benarroch-Gampel, MD, MS
Associate Professor
Division of Vascular and Endovascular Surgery
Emory University
Atlanta, Georgia

Karthik Bhat, MD
Vascular Surgery Resident
Division of Vascular and Endovascular Surgery
Emory University
Atlanta, Georgia

Jack S. Bontekoe, MD
Integrated Vascular Surgery Resident
Division of Vascular Surgery
University of Wisconsin Hospitals and Clinics
Madison, Wisconsin

Saideep Bose, MD, MPH
Assistant Professor
Surgery
Saint Louis University
St. Louis, Missouri

Luke Brewster, MD, PhD
Associate Professor Surgery
Division of Vascular and Endovascular Surgery
Emory University
Section Chief, Vascular Surgery
Department of Surgery
Atlanta VA Medical Center
Atlanta, Georgia

Middleton Chang, MD
Assistant Professor of Surgery
Division of Vascular and Endovascular Surgery
Emory University
Atlanta, Georgia

Shernaz S. Dossabhoy, MD, MBA
Resident
Division of Vascular Surgery, Department of Surgery
Stanford University School of Medicine
Stanford, California

Guillermo A. Escobar, MD
Program Director
Division of Vascular and Endovascular Surgery
Emory University
Atlanta, Georgia

Monserrat P. Escobar, MD
Resident
Universidad Nacional Autonoma de Mexico, Mexico

Arash Fereydooni, MD, MHS
Vascular Surgery Resident
Division of Vascular and Endovascular Surgery
Department of Surgery
Stanford University Medical Center
Stanford, California

Amanda Fobare, MD
Vascular Surgeon
Department of Surgery
Kaiser Permanent
Clackamas, Oregon

Katherine Gallagher, MD
Professor of Surgery
Department of Surgery, Section of Vascular Surgery
University of Michigan
Ann Arbor, Michigan

Manuel Garcia-Toca, MD, MS
Chief
Grady Memorial Hospital
Associate Professor
Division of Vascular and Endovascular Surgery
Emory University
Atlanta, Georgia

Theodore G. Hart, MD
Vascular Surgeon
Department of Surgery
San Antonio Uniformed Services Health Education
    Consortium
Fort Sam Houston, Texas

Joel Harding, DO
Vascular Surgeon
Department of Surgery
University of Maryland Medical Center
Baltimore, Maryland

Kai W. Hata, MD
Assistant Professor
Department of Vascular Surgery
Uniformed Services University of Health Sciences
Bethesda, Maryland

William Jordan, MD
Department Chair and Professor
Department of Surgery
Medical College of Georgia, Augusta University
Augusta, Georgia

Loay Kabbani, MD, MPH
Program Director
Department of Vascular Surgery
Henry Ford Hospital
Detroit, Michigan

Nii-Kabu Kabutey, MD
Associate Professor of Surgery
Department of Surgery
University of California, Irvine
Irvine, California

Karthikeshwar Kasirajan, MD
Clinical Professor
Department of Surgery
Stanford Health Care
Palo Alto, California
Section Chief
Department of Vascular Surgery
Stanford TriValley
Pleasanton, California

Isabella Kuo, MD
Associate Professor
Department of Surgery/Division of Vascular and
    Endovascular Surgery
University of California
Irvine, California

Yahya Madian, MD
Surgical Intensivist
Department of Trauma Surgery/Surgical Critical Care
Geisinger Medical Center
Danville, Pennsylvania

Kevin Mangum, MD, PhD
Vascular Surgery Resident
Department of Surgery, Section of Vascular Surgery
University of Michigan
Ann Arbor, Michigan

Charles Marquardt, MD
Department of Surgery, Division of Vascular and
    Endovascular Surgery
Saint Louis University, School of Medicine
St. Louis, Missouri

Krishna Martinez-Singh, MD
Resident
Department of Vascular Surgery
Stanford University
Stanford, California

Katharine L. McGinigle, MD, MPH
Department of Surgery, Division of Vascular Surgery
University of North Carolina at Chapel Hill
Chapel Hill, North Carolina

Richard A. Meena, MD
Resident Physician
Division of Vascular and Endovascular Surgery
Emory University
Atlanta, Georgia

Brandi M. Mize, MD
Resident Physician
Division of Vascular and Endovascular Surgery
Emory University
Atlanta, Georgia

Naiem Nassiri, MD
Associate Professor of Surgery (Vascular)
Department of Surgery
Yale University School of Medicine
New Haven, Connecticut
Chief, Vascular and Endovascular Surgery
Department of Surgery
VA Connecticut Healthcare System
West Haven, Connecticut
Director, Vascular Malformations Program
Yale New Haven Hospital
Member
The Aortic Institute
Yale New Haven Hospital
New Haven, Connecticut

Andrea T. Obi, MD
Assistant Professor of Surgery
Department of Vascular Surgery
University of Michigan
Ann Arbor, Michigan

Kevin Onofrey, MD
Fellow
Department of Vascular Surgery
Henry Ford Hospital
Detroit, Michigan

Benjamin Jay Pearce, MD, FACS
Associate Professor
Department of Surgery
Division of Vascular Surgery and Endovascular Therapy
University of Alabama at Birmingham
Birmingham, Alabama

Pranavi Ravichandran, MD
Assistant Professor
Division of Vascular and Endovascular Surgery
Emory University
Atlanta, Georgia

John E. Rectenwald, MD, MS
Professor of Surgery, Chair Division of Vascular Surgery
Department of Surgery
University of Wisconsin
Madison, Wisconsin

Morris Sasson, MD
Associate Staff
Department of Vascular Surgery
Cleveland Clinic Florida
Weston, Florida

Michael D. Sgroi, MD
Associate Clinical Professor of Surgery
Associate Program Director
Vascular Surgery Residency and Fellowship Program
Stanford University
Stanford, California

Brian M. Sheehan, MD
Fellow
Division of Vascular and Endovascular Surgery
Stanford University School of Medicine
Stanford, California
Vascular Surgery Specialist
Intermountain Medical Center
Salt Lake City, Utah

Matthew R. Smeds, MD
Professor of Surgery
Department of Surgery, Division of Vascular and
    Endovascular Surgery
Saint Louis University
St. Louis, Missouri

Brigitte Smith, MD, MHPE, FACS, FSVS
Associate Professor of Vascular Surgery
Department of Surgery
University of Utah
Salt Lake City, Utah

Jordan R. Stern, MD
Associate Professor of Surgery
Department of Surgery
Stanford University
Stanford, California

Vivek Sreeram, MD
Resident Physician
Department of Surgery
Case Western Reserve University
Cleveland, Ohio

Victoria J. Teodorescu, MD, MBA, RVT
Associate Professor
Division of Vascular and Endovascular Surgery
Emory University
Atlanta, Georgia

Steven Tohmasi, MD
General Surgery Resident
Department of Surgery
Washington University in St. Louis
St. Louis, Missouri

Jacob Weber, MD
Anesthesiology Resident
Department of Anesthesiology
University of Alabama at Birmingham
Birmingham, Alabama

Anudeep Yekula, MBBS
Division of Vascular and Endovascular Surgery
Department of Surgery
Yale University School of Medicine
New Haven, Connecticut

Foreword

Vascular surgery is an evolving specialty that embraces medicine, critical care, and open surgical and endovascular techniques. In the past 3 decades, the introduction of endovascular techniques dramatically improved treatment for many patients with peripheral occlusive disease, aneurysms, dissections, and traumatic injuries. More recently the ever-continuing development of endovascular methods to treat complex diseases has been an equally dramatic sea change in the way vascular pathology can be effectively managed.

The VSITE Review Manual by Sgroi and Escobar is a must-have for anyone preparing for the American Board of Surgery In-Training Examination (ABSITE) board certification, and for those participating in continued education of faculty and trainees. Clearly described chapters emphasize in bullet points the most relevant data and findings from landmark studies, as well as basic science concepts on all topics of vascular medicine and surgery. The chapters are comprehensive yet easy to go through for all levels of training, from medical students to senior staff seeking to have access to updated information on the latest clinical trials.

The chapters deal with all possible related issues, including variations in normal aortic anatomy, mechanisms and natural history of aortic disease, analysis of imaging techniques, and how to prevent and manage complications, extending in a systematic fashion across 27 areas. Thus this jewel of a text provides the most relevant updated and flash-type information on everything one needs to know to master the most important vascular certification tests, yet also provides a great source for regular reading and education. It covers what vascular medicine, surgery, and endovascular surgery are about in a most thorough, up-to-date, and unbiased way. This volume is not only a must have for all vascular trainees and students but also will be an often-used reference source for faculty.

Gustavo S. Oderich, MD, FACS
John P. and Kathrine G. McGovern Professor of
Surgery and Distinguished Chair
Vascular and Endovascular Surgery
Director
Aortic Center and Advanced Endovascular
Aortic Program

Preface

Each year, hundreds of vascular surgery residents and fellows across the country prepare for the American Board of Surgery Vascular Surgery In-Training Examination (VSITE). The exam is furnished to programs as an evaluation instrument to assess the knowledge and progress attained by the trainees on the many topics in vascular surgery, as well as some key topics in general surgery. Ever since we were trainees, we remember being dismayed that there were no study resources that were specifically designed to review topics succinctly and efficiently in vascular surgery (unlike general surgery and so many other specialties).

During a spontaneous discussion, we discovered that both of us had independently been crafting the data and structure of a book that would both cover *all* of vascular surgery, *and* be specifically designed to prepare for exams like the VSITE. We joined forces as Editors and vowed to ensure the text would be written by true experts in the topic, yet worded so a student could read, review, and retain high-yield information. We also wanted it to be easily accessible throughout the day to facilitate study/review on demand.

With this blueprint, we crafted the first edition of *The VSITE Review Manual* to contain high-yield information on all aspects of vascular surgery, written in a way to easily gain and retain core principles. Our book allows access at any time of the day either through the textbook itself or the included mobile-friendly version.

This textbook's outline format makes it easy to find the essential points on each topic, without needing to read the extraneous information found in many textbooks. It helps promote memorization, which does not always come with question and answer books. At the same time, our chosen expert writers have created original tables, images, and included PubMed references that the reader can use to learn more, or just to discover the source for the topic.

The VSITE Review Manual was proudly designed by two passionate learners for *anyone* studying vascular surgery, no matter their age or stage of career! While our goal is for it to be the landmark study guide for the VSITE, we hope this easy-to-read book will be sought after by medical students who want to be prepared for their rotation, as well as residents, fellows, and practicing physicians preparing for certification and recertification. We hope you will find it not only the best resource to review things you need to remember in vascular surgery, but also learn something new in every chapter.

Michael D. Sgroi
Guillermo A. Escobar

Contents

CHAPTER 1

Medical Management of Vascular Disease

VIVEK SREERAM, MD and SAIDEEP BOSE, MD, MPH

It is fitting that this book starts with a topic that is the least exciting to vascular surgeons but perhaps the most important when it comes to improving the quality and quantity of life of most patients with vascular disease.

OVERVIEW OF PERIPHERAL ARTERIAL DISEASE

When dealing with peripheral arterial disease (PAD), it is first important to figure out where on the spectrum a patient is.

- Asymptomatic PAD: generally, stays asymptomatic
- Claudication: rarely progress to rest pain or tissue loss, mortality from other causes[1]
  - Progression over 5 years: 70%–80% with stable claudication, 10%–20% with worsening claudication, 1%–2% with chronic limb-threatening ischemia (CLTI)[2]
  - 5-year major amputation rate is <5% (<1% per year)
  - Mortality is still 30% at 5 years and 50% at 10 years
- Chronic limb-threatening ischemia: often will progress toward amputation before mortality[3]
  - 1-year major amputation rate is 30%
  - Mortality is 25% at 1 year and 60% at 5 years

Both claudicants and patients with CLTI have high 5-year mortality, but the risk of limb loss is significantly higher in the CLTI group.

Management of Claudication

Claudicants who undergo intervention have a hazard ratio (HR) 2.9 of progressing to CLTI and HR 4.5 of requiring a major amputation compared with claudicants who are medically managed.
- Supervised exercise therapy (SET):
  - More effective than unsupervised therapy programs
  - Generally, 2–3 times per week, 30 minutes–1 hour, 3–6 month durations
  - CLEVER trial: SET and endovascular intervention equivalent improvement in functional status and quality of life at 18 months
- Cilostazol: phosphodiesterase (PDE) inhibitor; suppresses platelet aggregation
  - Increases pain-free and maximal walking distance by 50% when compared with placebo or pentoxifylline (Trental); benefits can be seen after 4 weeks
  - Should not be prescribed in patients with heart failure

Smoking Cessation

Smoking is associated with multiple risk factors associated with vascular disease—aneurysm expansion, increased risk of progression to CLTI, need for unplanned revascularization, risk of major amputation, and risk of major adverse cardiovascular events (MACE).

Quit rate with various interventions:
- Minimal intervention versus intensive counseling: 6.8% vs. 21.3% (6 months)
- Varenicline (Chantix) versus placebo: odds ratio (OR) 3.61 (12 months)
- Varenicline versus bupropion: OR 1.68
- Varenicline versus nicotine patch: OR 1.75

All patients who are current smokers should be advised to quit. Varenicline with or without nicotine replacement therapy should be first-line therapy.

Antilipid Therapy

Most data from antilipid therapy for vascular patients come from trials looking at coronary artery disease. In addition to decreasing MACE, there is some evidence it reduces adverse limb events as well.

- Simvastatin (Heart Protection Study): 16% decrease in first peripheral event regardless of baseline low-density lipoprotein (LDL) levels, decreased mortality, no decrease in major amputations
- Statins (REACH): HR 0.82 of major adverse limb events (MALEs)
- High-intensity statins (Veterans Study): HR 0.67 of major amputations
- Ezetimibe (IMPROVE-IT): LDL reduction 24%, HR 0.94 of MACE; peripheral events not reported
- PCSK9 inhibitors
  - (FOURIER): HR 0.73 for MACE, decrease in MALE in overall group but not in PAD patients
  - (ODYSSEY): HR 0.69 for composite endpoint (CLTI, major amputation, revascularization)

All patients with PAD should be on high intensity statin (atorvastatin 80 mg or rosuvastatin 20–40 mg). US guidelines aim for a reduction in LDL >50% and European guidelines aim for a target <70 mg/dL.

Antiplatelet Therapy

While almost all patients with PAD are on some degree of antiplatelet therapy for mortality benefit, there is inconsistent evidence on benefits specifically related to limb events.

- Aspirin (POPADAD): no difference in cardiovascular (CV) events in patients with DM and PAD (18.2%)
- Aspirin (ASA): no difference in CV events or claudication in patients with PAD
- Clopidogrel (CAPRIE): decreased MACE vs. acetylsalicylic acid (ASA) in PAD (risk reduction 23.8%), similar bleeding
- Ticagrelor (EUCLID):
  - P2Y12 receptor inhibitor but is not a prodrug (unlike clopidogrel)
  - Compared with clopidogrel, equivalent MACE, acute limb ischemia, and unplanned revascularization
- Dual antiplatelet therapy
  - CHARISMA: no decrease in MACE in PAD compared with ASA only
  - CASPAR: no decrease in mortality; benefit in decreasing prosthetic graft occlusions

Antithrombotic Therapy

Historically, there has been very little role for antithrombotic therapy in PAD. Newer data regarding direct oral anticoagulants (DOACs) are changing this paradigm.

- Warfarin (WAVE): no reduction in MACE compared with ASA, increase in life-threatening bleeding
- Rivaroxaban (VOYAGER): PAD patients who had undergone revascularization (claudicants/CLTI)
  - Decrease in combined primary outcome (MACE, ALI, major amputation) vs. ASA: HR 0.85
  - Benefit seen in both endovascular and surgical patients
  - Overall bleeding increased (5.9% vs. 4.1%) but not life-threatening or intracranial hemorrhage

MEDICAL MANAGEMENT OF OTHER SPECIFIC VASCULAR PATHOLOGIES

Deep Venous Thrombosis Prophylaxis (DVT)

Hospitalized patients are at a much higher risk of developing a DVT and having a subsequent pulmonary embolism (PE) than their age- and sex-matched peers in the community.

- Higher-risk populations: surgical patients, intensive care unit (ICU) patients, cancer patients, stroke patients
- Mortality is higher in patients who received delayed DVT prophylaxis (within 24 hours) versus immediately upon admission (8% vs. 6% ICU mortality)[3,4]
  - Mechanical thromboprophylaxis: reserved for patients with contraindication to anticoagulation
- Intermittent pneumatic compression (IPC): multimodal— reduces venous stasis, increases endogenous fibrinolytic activity (plasminogen activator inhibitor-1)
  - CLOTS3 (immobile patients with stroke): lower venous thromboembolism (VTE) at 30 days with IPC (8.5% vs. 12%)
  - PREVENT: no additional benefit of IPC in patients already on low-molecular-weight heparin (LMWH) (3.0% vs. 4.2%)
- Graduated compression stockings: no robust evidence for prevention of DVT

Pharmacologic thromboprophylaxis: mainstay of therapy for most patients

- Unfractionated heparin (UFH): 5000 units subcutaneously three times a day
  - TID dosing may reduce VTE risk compared with BID dosing; inconclusive studies
  - Obese patients may need dose increased to 7500 units
- LMWH: enoxaparin/Lovenox 40 mg subcutaneously daily
  - Should be avoided (or dose reduced) in patients with renal insufficiency

- UFH versus LMWH: both do an excellent job of reducing DVT and PE
  - General medical population the relative risk with UFH or LMWH, respectively, for DVT (0.33 vs. 0.56) and PE (0.64 vs. 0.37)[5]
    - LMWH is more effective in preventing DVT (risk ratio [RR] 0.68) but no difference in mortality
  - In the critically ill, compared with UFH, LMWH was better at preventing symptomatic PE (RR 0.58) but not symptomatic or asymptomatic DVT (RR 0.90)[6]
- In general, pharmacologic prophylaxis is given until the patient returns to their baseline functional status or is discharged from the hospital
  - Cancer patients may benefit from prolonged VTE prophylaxis based on their Khorana score (LMWH or DOAC preferred to warfarin (Coumadin))

Cerebrovascular Disease

The primary prevention for ischemic stroke is similar to that of all CV disease, 90% of stroke burden is attributable to modifiable risk factors:
- Smoking, obesity, unhealthy diet, physical inactivity, dyslipidemia, hypertension, diabetes
- Risk factors are at least additive and may be synergistic
- Polypills, multiple drugs in one pill (atorvastatin, amlodipine, losartan, and hydrochlorothiazide) had a significantly better reduction in blood pressure (BP) and LDL as well as compliance at 1 year compared with controls[7]

Secondary prevention of ischemic stroke: treatment of all risk factors, reduces risk of recurrent stroke by 80% compared with no intervention[8]
- **Hypertension:** goal is office measurement of <130/80 mm Hg
  - Permissive hypertension in the first 48 hours of an ischemic stroke
  - Patients with fluctuating deficits may benefit from delayed BP control
  - Angiotensin-converting enzyme/angiotensin receptor blocker (ACE/ARB) rather than beta-blocker if a single agent; ACE/ARB + calcium channel blocker (CCB) for two agents
- **Hyperlipidemia:** goal is LDL cholesterol <70 mg/dL
  - SPARCL trial: 5-year absolute risk reduction of stroke with atorvastatin is 2.2%
  - TST trial: HR 0.78 for CV or cerebrovascular events with LDL control
- **Diabetes:** twice the risk of stroke; goal is HbA_{1C} <7
  - No evidence however, that diabetes mellitus (DM) *control* leads to decreased stroke or death in type 2 DM[9]
- **Smoking:** 39% of strokes may be attributable to smoking; elevated risk declines 5 years after quitting

Antithrombotic/antiplatelet therapy: the highest risk of a subsequent event is within the first 2 weeks after a transient ischemic attack (TIA) or stroke

- In TIA: the $ABCD^2$ score can be used to predict risk of ischemic stroke within 2 days
  - All patients should be immediately started on ASA
  - For high-risk TIA ($ABCD^2 \geq 4$): ASA and clopidogrel for 21 days
  - If patients were already on a single antiplatelet during their TIA, then dual antiplatelet therapy (DAPT) for 21 days
  - If patients are already on anticoagulation, a single antiplatelet agent can be added
    - Triple therapy is associated with significantly increased hemorrhagic risks
- In stroke: National Institutes of Health Stroke Scale (NIHSS) score used to guide therapy similar to TIA algorithm; high risk is NIHSS ≥ 5
  - CHANCE trial: significant reduction in stroke for DAPT for 90 days (8.2% vs. 11.7%)
- Lifelong single agent antiplatelet therapy after the acute treatment phase
- Extracranial carotid disease
  - ASA reduces the risk of stroke of any cause in patients undergoing carotid endarterectomy (CEA)
  - ACE trial: patients on ASA 81 mg after CEA had lower MACE than high dose ASA at 3 months
  - DAPT at the time of CEA reduces neurologic events but increases bleeding risk[10]
  - After carotid stenting, DAPT is recommended for at least 30 days, but many continue for 90 days. There is both a protective CV effect and also an increased bleeding risk with prolonged therapy. There are no guidelines as to the optimal agents, dose, or duration
- No good evidence for early parenteral anticoagulation unless patient has cardioembolic source

MEDICAL MANAGEMENT OF ABDOMINAL AORTIC ANEURYSM (AAA) AND THORACIC AORTIC ANEURYSM (TAA)

The goal of the management of aortic aneurysm disease is the prevention of rupture, which carries significant morbidity and mortality. Although the prevalence of AAA is 4% in screening studies focusing on males, only 0.4%–0.6% will have AAA >5.5 cm.[11]

The yearly risk of rupture in AAA is strongly related to diameter:[12]
- 3–3.9 cm   <1%
- 4–4.9 cm   1%
- 5–5.9 cm   1%–11%
- 6–6.9 cm   10%–22%
- >7 cm   30%–33%

Medical management: almost any mortality benefit seen generally comes from reducing overall CV risk and mortality, rather than aneurysm-related mortality.

- Metformin: diabetic patients in ADAM trial had 25%–40% the expansion rate[13]
  - Large VA Cohort study ($N = 13,834$) demonstrated that metformin use was an independent predictor of decreased AAA enlargement[14]
  - Ongoing randomized trials—MAAGI, LIMIT, MAT will hopefully answer the question
- Statins: no randomized trial data. A metaanalysis demonstrates no impact on AAA expansion, but a significant benefit for overall mortality, likely secondary to CV protection[15]

- Antiplatelet therapy: theoretically may reduce aortic wall inflammation and reduce thrombus formation
  - Subgroup analysis of UK Small Aneurysm trial found no benefit[16]
- Antiinflammatory: attractive target as many AAA walls have high levels of inflammatory cells; suppressing these in animal models with antineoplastic agents suppresses AAA development
  - AORTA trial: no benefit of pemirolast in reducing AAA enlargement[17]
- Beta-blockers: (propranolol trial)—poorly tolerated and no effect on the growth of small AAAs[18]

- Doxycycline: antiinflammatory properties and preventing secondary infection of aortic wall
  - PHAST trial: no benefit in AAA expansion with doxycycline[19]
  - N-TA³CT trial: no benefit, growth of 0.36 cm over 2 years in both arms[20]
- Fluroquinolones: US Food and Drug Administration (FDA) black box warning to patients who have a history of AAA
  - Increased incidence of AAA formation in US adults (HR 1.31)[21]
  - Similar findings in cohort study in Taiwan (RR 2.43)[22]
- ARB/ACE: no consistent trend shown in trials or animal models
  - TEDY trial: telmisartan had no effect on small AAA expansion[23]
  - AARDVARK trial: no effect of perindopril or amlodipine on AAA expansion[24]

Genetic disorders: generally associated with thoracoabdominal aneurysms/dissections
- Marfan syndrome (fibrillin-1 defect)
  - Beta-blocker: propranolol leads to significantly slower rate of aortic dilation[25]
  - ARB: losartan monotherapy leads to similar outcomes as propranolol[26]

- There may be synergistic effect in using both a beta-blocker and an ARB
- CCBs and fluoroquinolones should be avoided
- Loeys Dietz syndrome (*TGFBR, TBFB2, SMAD* mutations)
  - More aggressive than Marfan in terms of aneurysmal degeneration
  - Need full body imaging on diagnosis (50% have extraaortic aneurysms) and within 6 months–1 year, with repeat lifelong imaging depending on aneurysms found

Management of Anemia

Anemia is defined as a decrease in red blood cell (RBC) mass, which we generally use surrogate measures to detect in our patients—hemoglobin (Hb), hematocrit, and RBC count.

Microcytic anemia: mean corpuscular volume (MCV) <80; decreased *production* of Hb, main constituent of RBCs[27]
- Cells are smaller because they undergo an extra cellular division before the Hb concentration required to arrest mitosis is achieved
- Iron absorption occurs in duodenum → DMT1 transporter on enterocytes → transferrin takes iron to liver and bone marrow for storage → stored as ferritin
- Iron deficiency anemia: most common anemia
  - Lack in diet, gastric ulcers, menorrhagia, pregnancy, gastrointestinal (GI) bleeding
- Thalassemia: diseases of hemoglobin synthesis
  - Beta thalassemia common in Mediterranean and Southeast Asia
  - Thalassemia major–transfusion dependent, thalassemia minor–microcytic anemia
- Anemia of chronic disease: seen in chronic inflammation states, cancer
  - Renal production of erythropoietin is suppressed by inflammatory cytokines
  - Hepcidin is an acute phase reactant that leads to reduced iron absorption and reduced release of iron from body stores
- Diagnosis

Test	Measurement
Total iron-binding capacity (TIBC)	Measures transferrin
% Saturation	% Transferrin bound to iron (about 33%)
Serum ferritin	Iron stores in macrophages and liver

Type	Serum Ferritin	Iron	TIBC	% Saturation
Iron deficiency	↓	↓	↑	↓
Sideroblastic	↑	↑	↓	↑
Anemic of chronic disease	↑	↓	↓	↓

- Treatment
  - Thalassemia: chronic transfusions, chelation, and stem cell transplantation
  - Anemia of chronic disease: erythropoietin stimulating agents
  - Iron deficiency
  - Oral therapy: limitation is enterocyte iron absorption is saturable; maximum of ~15–25 mg of elemental iron daily
    - Causes intense GI issues in many patients (30%–40%); every other day dosing may be better tolerated and absorbed better
    - Certain foods may inhibit iron absorption; tea is potent inhibitor
    - May take 6–8 weeks to improve anemia, and 6 months to replete iron stores
  - Intravenous iron: faster replacement (1–2 infusions), may lead to less blood transfusion and be more cost-effective overall

Macrocytic anemia: MCV >100 fL; folate or vitamin B_{12} deficiency from diet

- Folate deficiency: folate inhibitors (numerous drugs), pregnancy
  - Absorbed in jejunum; clinically may manifest as glossitis
  - Labs: low serum folate, increased serum homocysteine, *normal* methylmalonic acid
- Vitamin B_{12} deficiency: caused by dietary deficiency, pancreatic insufficiency, or parietal cell destruction → intrinsic factor deficiency (pernicious anemia)
  - Absorbed in ileum; clinically manifests itself as paresthesia and neuropathy
  - Binder in saliva carries B_{12} to stomach, binds to intrinsic factor in stomach fundus (parietal cells) → pancreatic protease liberates B_{12}
  - Labs: low B_{12} increased serum homocysteine, *increased* methylmalonic acid
- Treatment: folate/B_{12} supplementation
  - Intravenous (IV) supplementation for patients who are symptomatic or who have issues with absorption

Normocytic anemia: destruction of normal RBCs or decreased production

- Reticulocyte count = immature RBCs; low count means low production and high count means peripheral destruction
- Hemolysis
  - Intravascular: complement autoantibody, mechanical destruction/shearing
    - Increase in free hemoglobin, hemosiderin (in urine) and decreased free haptoglobin (since bound to free hemoglobin)
  - Extravascular: destruction in spleen, lymph nodes, liver
    - Jaundice (increase in indirect bilirubin), black gallstones, splenomegaly

- Treatment involves addressing underlying cause (antiinflammatory if autoimmune, splenectomy if related to splenic sequestration)

MEDICAL THERAPY AFTER LOWER EXTREMITY BYPASS SURGERY

As the proportion of patients who are undergoing endovascular revascularization has increased, patients undergoing bypass are generally sicker, with longer-segment occlusions. It has become even more critical to optimize medical therapy perioperatively to ensure long-term patency of the bypass.

Figs. 1.1 and 1.2, from data pooled from metaanalysis, demonstrate that the primary patency for veins is far better than that of any other conduit, especially in infrageniculate bypasses.[28]

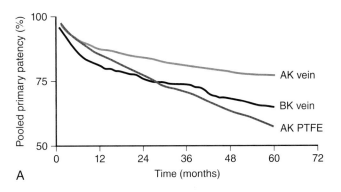

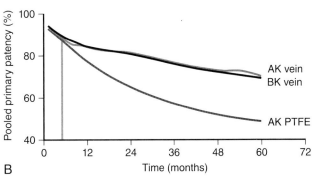

FIGURE 1.1 (A) Metaanalysis of primary patency in claudicants for above-knee femoropopliteal polytetrafluoroethylene *(PTFE)* bypass grafts *(green line)*, above-knee femoropopliteal saphenous vein bypass grafts *(red line)*, and below-knee saphenous vein bypass grafts *(blue line)*. (B) Metaanalysis of primary patency in patients with critical ischemia for above-knee femoropopliteal PTFE bypass grafts *(green line)*, above-knee femoropopliteal saphenous vein bypass grafts *(red line)*, and below-knee saphenous vein bypass grafts *(blue line)*. The *vertical line* indicates when above-knee saphenous vein grafts surpassed PTFE grafts. *AK,* Above knee; *BK,* below knee.

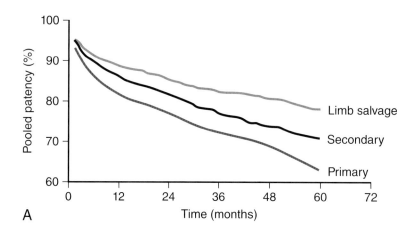

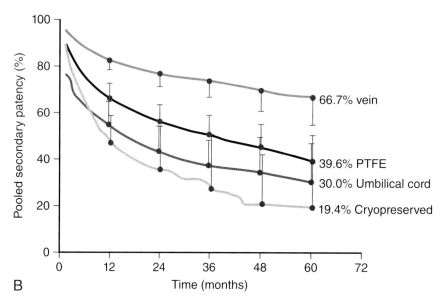

FIGURE 1.2   Patency of infrageniculate bypass grafts. (A) Random effects meta-analysis of popliteodistal bypass grafts for primary patency *(green line)*, secondary patency *(blue line)*, and foot preservation *(red line)*. (B) Metaanalysis survival curve of secondary patency for alternative autologous vein *(red line)*, polytetrafluoroethylene *(blue line)*, umbilical cord vein *(green line)*, and cryopreserved vein *(yellow line)*. Bars are half the amplitude of 95% confidence intervals. *PTFE,* Polytetrafluoroethylene.

ANTITHROMBOTIC THERAPY

- All patients with PAD should be on at least an antiplatelet at baseline
- Statins improve secondary patency at 2 years regardless of cholesterol levels[29]
- Given the heterogeneity of conduit (vein, spliced, compositive, polytetrafluoroethylene [PTFE], cryo, etc.), origin, and target in any lower revascularization procedure, there is no consensus on what the optimal antithrombotic therapy should be after bypass

- DAPT (ASA/Plavix)
  - CASPAR trial: composite outcome of graft occlusion/revascularization, major amputation, or death similar in overall cohort undergoing-knee bypasses[30]
    - In subgroup analysis, the prosthetic bypass cohort had a lower event rate (HR 0.65, $P = .025$) on DAPT, while the vein cohort did not (HR 1.25)
  - VQI (2020): no benefit of DAPT in overall cohort[31]
    - In subgroup analysis, benefit seen in the prosthetic cohort in terms of primary patency (HR 0.81) and secondary patency (HR 0.6)

- Anticoagulation
  - VA trial (warfarin): primary patency improvement in 6-mm prosthetic bypass[32]
    - No patency improvement in 8-mm prosthetic bypass or vein bypasses
    - Significantly increased major bleeding events with anticoagulation
  - Dutch trial (warfarin): overall, no difference in primary patency ($N = 2690$)[33]
    - In subgroup analysis, anticoagulation improved patency in vein grafts (HR 0.69)
    - Significantly more bleeding with anticoagulation (HR 1.96)
  - VQI: no difference in primary patency in below-knee bypasses; however, improved secondary patency seen in prosthetic below-knee bypasses (HR 0.77)[34]
    - Increased wound complications on anticoagulation
  - VOYAGER-PAD: rivaroxaban 2.5 mg BID after revascularization either surgically (35%) or endovascularly/hybrid (66%) in patients with claudication (77%) or CLTI (23%)[35]
    - In surgical patients, the combined endpoint of acute limb ischemia, major amputation, myocardial infarction, stroke, or CV death was significantly lower in the rivaroxaban group (18.4% vs. 22.0%, $P = .026$)
    - Similar trend in the overall cohort at 3 years (17.3% vs. 19.9%, HR 0.85)
    - Composite endpoint mainly driven by significant reduction of acute limb ischemia (HR 0.67)

Other Therapies

- Prevent III trial (edifoligide): no benefit treating vein grafts ex-vivo in terms of graft reintervention or limb salvage[36]
- Cilostazol (PDE3 inhibitor)
  - Iidia et al. trial (2008): improved freedom from target lesion revascularization and amputation when compared with ticlopidine in femoropopliteal endovascular intervention[37]
  - STOP-IC trial: improved 3-year primary patency after femoropopliteal endo intervention[38]
  - Unclear whether the results from these trials can be generalized to open bypass or arterial segments outside of the femoropopliteal

MEDICAL MANAGEMENT OF TYPE B AORTIC DISSECTIONS

In the widely used Stanford classification, any dissection that involves the ascending aorta is a type A dissection; the rest are type B. Patients who have uncomplicated type B dissections can be managed, at least initially, with medical therapy.

Impulse control therapy: the goal is to decrease shear stress on the aortic wall, prevent propagation of the dissection, and to prevent development of complications (aneurysmal degeneration and rupture)

- Most patients (71%) present with a SBP >150 mmHg[39]
- Goal heart rate <60 beats/min and BP <120/80 mmHg
  - No good trial data, but based on expert consensus and case series[40] that show reduced rates of aortic degeneration and rupture
- Need arterial line for adequate hemodynamic monitoring; pain control with IV opioids
- Beta-blocker infusion as first line therapy to allow rapid and precise titration[41]
  - Esmolol: beta-1–selective blockade
    - 500-mcg/kg loading dose, 50-mcg/kg per minute infusion; titrate up to 300 mcg/kg per minute
    - Onset: 1–2 minutes; duration: 10–30 minutes
  - Labetalol: alpha-1–selective blockade, nonselective beta blockade
    - 20-mg bolus loading dose, 2-mg/min infusion; titrate up to 10 mg/minute
    - Onset: 2–5 minutes; duration: 2–6 hours
    - May allow heart rate/BP control with one agent
- CCB: use if patient cannot tolerate a beta-blocker
  - Diltiazem: nondihydropyridine CCB
    - 0.35-mg/kg loading dose, 5-mg/h infusion; titrate up to 20 mg/h
    - Onset: 1–3 minutes; duration: 1–10 hours
- Vasodilators: start *after* heart rate control has been achieved with beta-blocker or CCB, if BP goals not met
  - Nitroprusside: direct relaxation of smooth muscle in arterioles and venules
    - 0.5 mcg/kg per minute; titrate up to 10 mcg/kg per minute
    - Onset: immediate; duration: 1–10 minutes
    - Concerns about cyanide toxicity at high/prolonged doses
  - Nicardipine: CCB
    - 5 mg/h; titrate up to 15 mg/h
    - Onset: 5–15 minutes; duration: 1–8 minutes
  - Clevidipine: CCB
    - 1 mg/h; titrate up to 16 mg/h (most patients respond to <6 mg/h)
    - Onset: 2–4 minutes; duration: 5–15 minutes
    - Rapidly cleared by plasma esterase; not dependent on renal/hepatic clearance
    - Very useful for resistant hypertension
- Once the patient's BP and heart rate have stabilized for at least 24 hours and their symptoms have resolved, they can be transitioned to oral medications for sustained heart rate and BP control

Repeat imaging is usually obtained if the patient's pain persists to ensure that there is no progression of the dissection. Imaging is then usually obtained at 3 months, 6 months, and 1 year. Patients need close follow-up with their primary care physician or cardiologist to ensure adequate outpatient BP control.

REFERENCES

1. Dormandy J, Heeck L, Vig, S. The natural history of claudication: risk to life and limb. *Semin Vasc Surg*. 1999;12(2):123-137.
2. Gerhard-Herman MD, Gornik HL, Barrett C, et al. 2016 AHA/ACC guideline on the management of patients with lower extremity peripheral artery disease: a report of the American College of Cardiology/American Heart Association Task Force on Clinical Practice Guidelines. *J Am Coll Cardiol*. 2017;69(11):e71-e126.
3. Benoit E, O'Donnell Jr TF, Kitsios GD, Iafrati MD. Improved amputation-free survival in unreconstructable critical limb ischemia and its implications for clinical trial design and quality measurement. *J Vasc Surg*. 2012;55(3):781-789.
4. Ho KM, Chavan S, Pilcher D. Omission of early thromboprophylaxis and mortality in critically ill patients: a multicenter registry study. *Chest*. 2011;140(6):1436-1446.
5. Wein L, Wein S, Haas SJ, Shaw J, Krum H. Pharmacological venous thromboembolism prophylaxis in hospitalized medical patients: a meta-analysis of randomized controlled trials. *Arch Intern Med*. 2007;167(14):1476-1486.
6. Alhazzani W, Lim W, Jaeschke RZ, Murad MH, Cade J, Cook DJ. Heparin thromboprophylaxis in medical-surgical critically ill patients: a systematic review and meta-analysis of randomized trials. *Crit Care Med*. 2013;41(9):2088-2098.
7. Muñoz D, Uzoije P, Reynolds C, et al. Polypill for cardiovascular disease prevention in an underserved population. *N Engl J Med*. 2019;381(12):1114-1123.
8. Hackam DG, Spence JD. Combining multiple approaches for the secondary prevention of vascular events after stroke: a quantitative modeling study. *Stroke*. 2007;38(6):1881-1885.
9. Kleindorfer DO, Towfighi A, Chaturvedi S, et al. 2021 guideline for the prevention of stroke in patients with stroke and transient ischemic attack: a guideline from the American Heart Association/American Stroke Association. *Stroke*. 2021;52(7):e364-e467.
10. Jones DW, Goodney PP, Conrad MF, et al. Dual antiplatelet therapy reduces stroke but increases bleeding at the time of carotid endarterectomy. *J Vasc Surg*. 2016;63(5):1262-1270.
11. Von Allmen RS, Powell JT. The management of ruptured abdominal aortic aneurysms: screening for abdominal aortic aneurysm and incidence of rupture. *J Cardiovasc Surg*. 2012;53(1):69-76.
12. Chaikof EL, Dalman RL, Eskandari MK, et al. The Society for Vascular Surgery practice guidelines on the care of patients with an abdominal aortic aneurysm. *J Vasc Surg*. 2018;67(1):2-77.
13. Bhak RH, Wininger M, Johnson GR, et al. Factors associated with small abdominal aortic aneurysm expansion rate. *JAMA Surg*. 2015;150(1):44-50.
14. Itoga NK, Rothenberg KA, Suarez P, et al. Metformin prescription status and abdominal aortic aneurysm disease progression in the US veteran population. *J Vasc Surg*. 2019;69(3):710-716.
15. Twine CP, Williams IM. Systematic review and meta-analysis of the effects of statin therapy on abdominal aortic aneurysms. *Br J Surg*. 2011;98(3):346-353.
16. Sweeting MJ, Thompson SG, Brown LC, Greenhalgh RM, Powell JT. Use of angiotensin converting enzyme inhibitors is associated with increased growth rate of abdominal aortic aneurysms. *J Vasc Surg*. 2010;52(1):1-4.
17. Sillesen H, Eldrup N, Hultgren R, et al. Randomized clinical trial of mast cell inhibition in patients with a medium-sized abdominal aortic aneurysm. *Br J Surg*. 2015;102(8):894-901.
18. Propranolol Aneurysm Trial Investigators. Propranolol for small abdominal aortic aneurysms: results of a randomized trial. *J Vasc Surg*. 2002;35(1):72-79.
19. Meijer CA, Stigmen T. Doxycycline for stabilization of abdominal aortic aneurysms: a randomized trial. *J Vasc Surg*. 2014;59(4):1175-1176.
20. Baxter BT, Matsumura J, Curci JA, et al. Effect of doxycycline on aneurysm growth among patients with small infrarenal abdominal aortic aneurysms: a randomized clinical trial. *JAMA*. 2020;323(20):2029-2038.
21. Newton ER, Akerman AW, Strassle PD, Kibbe MR. Association of fluoroquinolone use with short-term risk of development of aortic aneurysm. *JAMA Surg*. 2021;156(3):264-272.
22. Lee CC, Lee MTG, Chen YS, et al. Risk of aortic dissection and aortic aneurysm in patients taking oral fluoroquinolone. *JAMA Intern Med*. 2015;175(11):1839-1847.
23. Golledge J, Pinchbeck J, Tomee SM, et al. Efficacy of telmisartan to slow growth of small abdominal aortic aneurysms: a randomized clinical trial. *JAMA Cardiol*. 2020;5(12):1374-1381.
24. Bicknell CD, Kiru G, Falaschetti E, Powell JT, Poulter NR; AARDVARK Collaborators and AARDVARK Collaborators. An evaluation of the effect of an angiotensin-converting enzyme inhibitor on the growth rate of small abdominal aortic aneurysms: a randomized placebo-controlled trial (AARDVARK). *Eur Heart J*. 2016;37(42):3213-3221.
25. Shores J, Berger KR, Murphy EA, Pyeritz RE. Progression of aortic dilatation and the benefit of long-term β-adrenergic blockade in Marfan's syndrome. *N Engl J Med*. 1994;330(19):1335-1341.
26. Lacro RV, Dietz HC, Sleeper LA, et al. Atenolol versus losartan in children and young adults with Marfan's syndrome. *N Engl J Med*. 2014;371(22):2061-2071.
27. DeLoughery TG. Microcytic anemia. *N Engl J Med*. 2014;371(14):1324-1331.
28. Mills JL. Infrainguinal disease: surgical treatment. In: *Rutherford's Vascular Surgery*. Elsevier; 2014:1768.
29. Abbruzzese TA, Havens J, Belkin M, et al. Statin therapy is associated with improved patency of autogenous infrainguinal bypass grafts. *J Vasc Surg*. 2004;39(6):1178-1185.
30. Belch JJ, Dormandy J; CASPAR Writing Committee. Results of the randomized, placebo-controlled clopidogrel and acetylsalicylic acid in bypass surgery for peripheral arterial disease (CASPAR) trial. *J Vasc Surg*. 2010;52(4):825-833.
31. Belkin N, Stoecker JB, Jackson BM, et al. Effects of dual antiplatelet therapy on graft patency after lower extremity bypass. *J Vasc Surg*. 2021;73(3):930-939.
32. Johnson WC, Williford WO. Benefits, morbidity, and mortality associated with long-term administration of oral anticoagulant therapy to patients with peripheral arterial bypass procedures: a prospective randomized study. *J Vasc Surg*. 2002;35(3):413-421.
33. Dutch Bypass Oral Anticoagulants or Aspirin (BOA) Study Group. Efficacy of oral anticoagulants compared with aspirin after infrainguinal bypass surgery (The Dutch Bypass Oral Anticoagulants or Aspirin Study): a randomised trial. *Lancet*. 2000;355(9201):346-351.
34. Liang NL, Baril DT, Avgerinos ED, Leers SA, Makaroun MS, Chaer RA. Comparative effectiveness of anticoagulation on

midterm infrainguinal bypass graft patency. *J Vasc Surg.* 2017; 66(2):499-505.

35. Bonaca MP, Bauersachs RM, Anand SS, et al. Rivaroxaban in peripheral artery disease after revascularization. *N Engl J Med.* 2020;382(21):1994-2004

36. Conte MS, Bandyk DF, Clowes AW, et al. Results of PREVENT III: a multicenter, randomized trial of edifoligide for the prevention of vein graft failure in lower extremity bypass surgery. *J Vasc Surg.* 2006;43(4):742-751.

37. Iida O, Nanto S, Uematsu M, Morozumi T, Kitakaze M, Nagata S. Cilostazol reduces restenosis after endovascular therapy in patients with femoropopliteal lesions. *J Vasc Surg.* 2008;48(1):144-149.

38. Soga Y, Hamasaki T, Edahiro R, et al. Sustained effectiveness of cilostazol after endovascular treatment of femoropopliteal lesions: midterm follow-up from the sufficient treatment of peripheral intervention by cilostazol (STOP-IC) study. *J Endovasc Ther.* 2018;25(3):306-312.

39. American College of Cardiology Foundation, American Heart Association Task Force on Practice Guidelines, American Association for Thoracic Surgery, American College of Radiology, American Stroke Association, Society of Cardiovascular Anesthesiologists, Society for Cardiovascular Angiography and Interventions, Society of Interventional Radiology, Society of Thoracic Surgeons, Society for Vascular Medicine, and North American Society for Cardiovascular Imaging. 2010 ACCF/AHA/AATS/ACR/ASA/SCA/SCAI/SIR/STS/SVM guidelines for the diagnosis and management of patients with thoracic aortic disease. *J Am Coll Cardiol.* 2010;55(14):e27-e129.

40. Van Bogerijen GH, Tolenaar JL, Rampoldi V, et al. Predictors of aortic growth in uncomplicated type B aortic dissection. *J Vasc Surg.* 2014;59(4):1134-1143.

41. Hiratzka LF, Bakris GL, Beckman JA, et al. 2010 ACCF/AHA/AATS/ACR/ASA/SCA/SCAI/SIR/STS/SVM guidelines for the diagnosis and management of patients with Thoracic Aortic Disease: a report of the American College of Cardiology Foundation/American Heart Association Task Force on Practice Guidelines, American Association for Thoracic Surgery, American College of Radiology, American Stroke Association, Society of Cardiovascular Anesthesiologists, Society for Cardiovascular Angiography and Interventions, Society of Interventional Radiology, Society of Thoracic Surgeons, and Society for Vascular Medicine. *Circulation.* 2010;121:e266.

CHAPTER 2

Hemostasis and Coagulation

ANDREA T. OBI, MD, KAI W. HATA, MD, and KEVIN MANGUM, MD, PHD

THROMBOSIS

Normal Coagulation

- Phases of coagulation: vasoconstriction, platelet activation/adhesion, thrombin generation, fibrinolysis
- Overall goal of the coagulation cascade is creation of fibrin polymers to create clot for hemostasis
- Ionized calcium is critical for *all* clotting, originally known as factor IV
  - Scenarios with low ionized calcium (citrate after mass transfusion of packed red blood cell [pRBC], high magnesium, high use of cell saver, etc.) will *always* lead to more bleeding if not checked/corrected
- Platelets
  - Fragments of megakaryocytes full of secretory bodies
  - When activated express surface glycoproteins (GPs)
  - GPs either bind platelets to each other via fibrinogen bridges (aggregation) or anchor them to the subendothelial matrix (adhesion)
    - Fibrinogen (via GP IIb/IIIa)
    - von Willebrand factor (vWF) (via GP 1b)
    - Collagen (via GP VI)
    - Fibronectin and others
  - Secrete adenosine diphosphate (ADP) for positive-loop activation (by binding to the P2Y$_{12}$ platelet receptor—inhibited by celecoxib [Celebrex], inhibited by "Thienopyridines like clopidogrel, prasugrel etc. and ticagrelor" etc.)
  - Secrete thromboxane A2 (TXA2) for vasoconstriction and activation (via cyclooxygenase [COX] prostaglandin pathways—hence COX inhibitors block aggregation)

Clotting Cascade

All clotting factors are inherently inactivated zymogens with a prefix of "X-gen," which is lost when in an activated form. Many clotting factors are enzymes that cleave and activate the next zymogen as an apparent positive-feedback loop, but simultaneously activate anticoagulation or fibrinolysis zymogens to downregulate themselves.

- Extrinsic pathway:
  - Clotting pathway triggered by exposure to extravascular *"tissue factor" (factor III);* common etiology is trauma/extravasation
  - IIIa activates VII to complete the extrinsic cascade
    - *Pneumonic:* remember that for extrinsic, *III + VII will get you to X* (common pathway) and is tested by prothrombin time (PT)/international normalized ratio (INR)
- Intrinsic pathway: initially described as it occurred even without being exposed to extravascular components
  - Primarily activated by endothelial damage
  - Also activated when the ratio of activators vs. anticoagulants is disproportionate
  - *Pneumonic:* all the other factors (except extrinsic's III + VII) are in the intrinsic pathway and are tested by the partial thromboplastin time (PTT) (more initials in it than a PT)

Common Pathway

- Factor X is the conversion point for both pathways and it activates factor II
- Activated prothrombin (factor IIa—thrombin) forms a complex with X, V, iCa^{2+}, platelet factor 3 to activate more clotting proteins
  - Derivatives of hirudin (from leech saliva) are *"direct thrombin inhibitors"* and include the intravenous argatroban (Acova) and bivalirudin, (Angiomax, Angiox), and the oral agent dabigatran (Pradaxa). The latter is reversed with idarucizumab
- Fibrin (factor Ia)—forms long polymeric fibers that ultimately interlock with platelets
- Fibrin-stabilizing factor (XIII)—forms crosslinking between fibrin strands to produce a mature web of fibrin

Clotting Factors

- Factor II—longest half-life
- Factor VII—produced in the liver and has shortest half-life (3–6 h) of all clotting factors
  - Factor V (proaccelerin) and VIII (from hemophilia A) are "labile" factors as they are heat sensitive and if improperly handled will yield falsely low values
  - Factor VIII is an acute-phase factor that can elevate 2–4 times in inflammatory states and is suspected to be related to acute, "provoked" deep venous thrombosis (DVT) (especially in children and older patients)
- Factor IX (hemophilia B—Christmas disease thanks to Stephen Christmas in 1952)
- Factor XI (hemophilia C—Rosenthal syndrome)
- Factor XII (Hageman factor [named after the patient] binds to fibronectin) is activated by negative charges (intrinsic pathway) and activates XI
- Vitamin K–dependent factors: II, VII, IX, X, and proteins C and S
  - If you remember that II + VII = IX, you will get X on your exam (and not a C or an S)!

ENDOGENOUS ANTICOAGULATION

- Endogenous heparin
  - In secretory granules in mast cells—unclear physiological role!
  - Named after being extracted and purified from a dog liver (second-year medical student McLean in 1916 and his principal investigator, Dr. Howell)
- Antithrombin III (AT III)
  - Serine protease inhibitor
  - Inhibits factors IIa and Xa (and XIa) by binding to their active sites and changing/inactivating them
  - Activity increased by heparin (which binds to both AT III and Xa)
- Proteins C and S (vitamin K–dependent and activated by thrombin)
  - Protein C—serine protease degrades factors Va and VIIIa
  - Protein S—cofactor for protein C
- Fibrinolysis
  - Plasminogen activates to plasmin (active form) by tissue plasminogen activator (tPA) or urinary plasminogen activator (uPA)
  - Plasminogen is maintained inactive by plasminogen activator inhibitor-1 (PAI-1), which inhibits binding by tPA and uPA
  - tPA is stored in the endothelium and released by shear stress, thrombin, histamine, or bradykinins
  - Plasmin breaks fibrin polymers to D-dimers and fibrin split/degradation products in any thrombus—thus when elevated is *not* specific to disseminated intravascular coagulation (DIC)

LABORATORY MEASUREMENTS OF COAGULATION

- PT (INR) measures the extrinsic pathway by adding III (thromboplastin) and Ca^{2+} to decalcified blood (thus needs VII in the sample)
  - Most sensitive for low II, V, VII, X, and I
  - An indicator of liver function (especially vitamin K–dependent factors synthesized in the liver)
  - *INR was created in 1983* via World Health Organization (WHO) to standardize times and reagents for safe anticoagulation with warfarin!
- Activated PTT (aPTT) evaluates intrinsic pathway and common pathway
  - Used to detect congenital deficiencies
    - Used for monitoring of unfractionated heparin therapy
- Anti-Xa levels measure heparin-mediated inhibition
- Activated clotting time (ACT)—point-of-care test that measures function of the intrinsic pathway and common pathways (heparin and thrombin inhibitors)
  - Used to evaluate the effects of heparin or other direct thrombin inhibitors
- Thromboelastogram (TEG) (Table 2.1)—oscillating viscometer that evaluates clotting performance of platelets, intrinsic pathway, AND fibrinolysis
- Platelet function
  - Platelet function assay-100 (PFA-100)—measurement of time for platelet aggregation when exposed to collagen/epinephrine or collagen/ADP
  - *Platelet factor 4 (PF4)–heparin antibody enzyme-linked-immunosorbent assay (ELISA)* screens immunoglobulin G (IgG) vs. PF4 to detect heparin-induced thrombocytopenia (HIT) (has nearly perfect sensitivity = false negatives are almost impossible) but is not SPECIFIC (false positive possible) for HIT

TABLE 2.1   **Normal Values of a Thromboelastogram**

Value	Definition	Measure
R (reaction time)	Reaction to fibrin formation	Intrinsic pathway
K (kinetic time)	Fibrin crosslinking time	Fibrinogen, platelet number
Alpha angle	Angle from baseline to top of tracing, measures clot formation	Fibrinogen, platelet number
MA	Maximum amplitude of tracing	Platelet number and function
G	Clot strength	Coagulation cascade
Ly30		Clot lysis, fibrinolysis

- *"Functional"* platelet activation studies (like serotonin release, or membrane activation flow cytometry) confirm heparin-mediated platelet activation and are SPECIFIC (>95%) but may miss HIT (not as sensitive)

MEDICATIONS

Anticoagulation

- **Heparin**—potentiates the actions of AT III by acting as a template for binding thrombin and antithrombin simultaneously
  - Half-life 60–90 minutes
  - Bolus dosing of 70–100 U/kg and then infusion rate depending on indication
  - Monitor response with aPTT or anti-Xa level <u>or</u> ACT for point of care
  - Consider *heparin-induced thrombocytopenia and thrombosis (HITT)* if platelet count drops below 50% of baseline
  - **Protamine sulfate**—*positively charged* protein derived from sturgeon (salmon) sperm nuclei that binds and inactivates heparin. Dose is traditionally 1 mg/100 units of heparin to reverse
    - Protamine always lowers blood pressure in a dose-dependent way (benign—thought to be related to its charge)
    - Protamine anaphylactoid reaction—immune-mediated sustained and severe hypotension, pulmonary hypertension, cardiogenic shock with bradycardia
      - High suspicion in prior protamine exposure, neutral protamine hagedorn (NPH) insulin, fish allergy, *or history of prostate/vasectomy procedure*
- **Low-molecular-weight heparin (LMWH, dalteparin, enoxaparin, tinzaparin, ardeparin)**—activates antithrombin by the same mechanism as heparin
  - Dosing is subcutaneous (SC) and dependent on indication
  - Half-life of 4.5 hours
  - Monitor with anti-Xa levels; minimal effect on PTT
    - Draw levels 4–6 hours after third dose
    - Anti-Xa levels should be 1–2 with 24-hour dosing; 0.5–1 units/mL with 12-hour dosing
  - Renally cleared (dose adjustment for creatinine clearance <30)
- **Argatroban**—parenteral direct thrombin inhibitor
  - Hepatically cleared with LONGER half-life of 45 minutes (dose adjustment if hepatic impairment)
  - Monitor with aPTT 1.5–3 times baseline
    - Will prolong INR
    - When bridging to warfarin, wait until INR >4 during infusion, hold 4–6 hours, and repeat INR for "real" warfarin-mediated INR

- **Bivalirudin**—parenteral direct thrombin inhibitor
  - Half-life of 25 minutes (shorter so better for procedures)
  - Monitor anticoagulation effect with aPTT or ACT
  - *Renally excreted*
- **Fondaparinux**—subcutaneous analog of heparin and LMWH that potentiates factor Xa inhibition but does not bridge thrombin to antithrombin
  - 2.5 mg daily for venous thromboembolism (VTE) prophylaxis, 7.5 mg daily for treatment of VTE. Need dose adjustments for weight
- **Vitamin K agonist (VKA); Coumadin (warfarin)**—oral, inhibits the synthesis of factors II, VII, IX, and X (and proteins C + S)
  - Monitor with PT or INR
    - INR for treatment of VTE: 2.0–3.0
    - INR for mechanical mitral valve: 2.5–3.5
    - INR for antiphospholipid antibody syndrome: 2.0–3.0
  - Reverse with fresh frozen plasma (FFP), prothrombin complex concentrate (PCC), or vitamin K
    - *PCC is first line and lower volume to infuse*
    - FFP if heparin allergy (PCC contains heparin)
    - Oral (PO) vitamin K if reversal can occur in ≥ 24 hours, IV/SC vitamin K if urgent reversal is necessary ~24 hours
  - Contraindicated during pregnancy—saddle nose, pelvis agenesis
  - Warfarin-induced skin necrosis—localized thrombosis of the fatty tissues and skin from transient hypercoagulable state secondary to initiation of warfarin and inhibition of proteins C or S
    - Commonly with congenital or acquired deficiencies of proteins C or S
    - Prevent with bridging with heparin or LMWH

Direct Oral Anticoagulants (DOACs)

- Direct thrombin inhibitors
  - **Dabigatran (Pradaxa)**—oral thrombin inhibitor
    - Half-life of 14–17 hours
    - Predominantly renal excretion
    - Reversal through Praxbind (idarucizumab), a monoclonal antibody to active site
- Direct Xa inhibitors
  - **Rivaroxaban** (Xarelto)
    - Half-life of 7–11 hours, renally cleared
    - **COMPASS trial**—low dose (2.5 mg twice daily [BID]) + aspirin 81 mg had lower major adverse limb events (MALE) and lower major adverse cardiac events (MACE) vs. rivaroxaban or aspirin (ASA) alone
    - **VOYAGER trial**— randomized controlled trial (RCT) low-dose rivaroxaban + aspirin 81 mg following revascularization had lower rates of MALE compared with ASA/placebo

- Good outcomes in DOACs for cancer-related VTE compared with LMWH. *BUT RISK FOR gastrointestinal (GI) BLEEDING (avoid in GI malignancy)*
- **Apixaban** (Eliquis)
  - Plasma half-life of 8–14 hours and cleared via multiple pathways
- Reversal agent for apixaban and rivaroxaban is *andexanet alfa (Andexxa)*—recombinant, soluble Xa to bind Xa Inhibitors

Product and Miscellaneous Medications

- FFP
  - Acellular portion of blood
  - Contains all coagulation factors (lower labile factors)
  - Rapid onset/effect
  - INR of FFP is ~1.1, *but* giving it will not go below 1.6, so do not transfuse for INR ~1.7. Reversal effect is proportional to initial INR (Holland et al.)
- Cryoprecipitate
  - *Fibrinogen*, factor VII, vWF, factor XIII, and fibronectin
- Platelets (PLTs)
  - *Pooled* PLTs from multiple (4–6) blood donors
    - The *most* immunogenic/dose for transfusion-related acute lung injury (TRALI) (although FFP is more commonly reported likely from more administrations but lower incidence TRALI/dose)
  - General thresholds: prophylactically <10,000 PLTs or planned surgery target PLTs >50,000
- PCC
  - Contains factors II, VII, IX, X, and proteins C and S (vitamin K–dependent factors)
  - Used to reverse coagulopathy in emergent cases
    - Dosing based on weight and INR
    - Administer with 10 mg vitamin K intravenously
  - Contains heparin to prevent clotting, ensure no heparin allergy prior to administration
- Desmopressin (DDAVP)
  - Increases vWF, factor VIII, and tPA
  - Bleeding from dysfunctional platelets (type 1 von Willebrand disease, uremia, *patients with end-stage renal disease*)
    - Can be given to patients with hemophilia A preoperatively if VIII is >5%

Antiplatelets

- Cyclooxygenase-1 (COX-1) inhibitors
  - **Aspirin**—*irreversibly* binds COX-1, which inhibits production of thromboxane (TXA2)
    - Normally dosed at 81 mg or 325 mg (no evidence that higher dose is more effective)
    - Contraindication—history of allergy/reaction resulting in bronchospasm

- P2Y$_{12}$ inhibitors (thienopyridines)—blocks binding of ADP
  - **Clopidogrel** (Plavix)—*irreversible* inhibitor
    - Normally dosed at 75 mg daily, loading dose is 300 mg
  - **Ticagrelor** (Brilinta)—*reversible*
    - Normally dosed at 90 mg BID with a loading dose of 180 mg
    - Does not require metabolic activation (faster on/off)
    - *Preferred for neurological indications*
  - **Prasugrel** (Effient)—*irreversible*
    - *Contraindicated for neurological indications*
- **Dipyridamole**
  - Inhibits phosphodiesterase, increasing cylicic adenosine monophosphate and reducing intracellular potassium, inhibiting platelet activation

Thrombolytics

- **tPA**
  - Alteplase—recombinant form identical to tissue plasminogen factor
  - Dosing based on indication and delivery (catheter-based delivery, pharmacomechanical thrombectomy, systemic thrombolysis). Typically 0.5–1 mg/h
  - Half-life 5 minutes
  - tPA attaches to fibrin and activates fibrin-bound plasminogen
  - Check fibrinogen levels when giving tPA
  - Do not therapeutically anticoagulate during infusion due to increased bleeding

DISORDERS OF COAGULATION

Coagulopathies

- **von Willebrand disease**—disorder of platelet adherence from lack of functional vWF
  - Most common inherited bleeding disorder
  - Three main types with mixed somatic inheritance patterns
  - Type I and III quantitative; III more severe
  - Type II qualitative
  - Type I: Treat with DDAVP
  - Type II and III: Treat with factor VIII vWF concentrate
- **Hemophilia A**
  - X-linked deficiency of factor VII
  - Prolonged PT and normal PTT
  - Inability to stabilize platelet plug with fibrin
  - Rule out von Willebrand disease with vWF assay
  - DDAVP for mild disease, factor VIII concentrates for more significant disease
- **Hemophilia B** (Christmas disease)
  - X-linked deficiency of factor IX
  - Prolonged PT and normal PTT
  - Concentrated factor IX prior to surgery or for management of spontaneous bleeding complications

TABLE 2.2 Scoring System for Diagnosis of Heparin-Induced Thrombocytopenia and Thrombosis (HITT)

| Variable | POINTS | | |
	2	1	0
Thrombocytopenia	Platelet count decrease of >50% and nadir of ≥20,000	Platelet count decrease of 30%–50% or nadir of 10,000–19,000	Platelet count decrease of <30% or nadir ≤10,000
Timing of onset after heparin exposure	Days 5–10, or day 1 if recent heparin exposure	>Day 10 or unclear exposure	≤Day 4 without recent heparin exposure
Thrombosis	New thrombosis or anaphylaxis after heparin bolus	Progressive or recurrent thrombus	None
Other causes of thrombocytopenia	None	Possible	Definite
Total score and result	6–8, high pretest probability of HITT	4 or 5, intermediate pretest probability of HITT	0–3, low pretest probability of HITT

- **HITT** (Table 2.2)—antibody creation against PF4-heparin complex → platelet activation → thrombosis
  - Consumptive coagulopathy—platelets <100 or drop >50% of admission levels
  - Usually venous thrombosis, but arterial can develop (stroke, renal failure, extremity, etc.)
  - Diagnose with PF4/heparin ELISA or serotonin release assay
  - Stop heparin and start a direct thrombin inhibitor
  - No warfarin monotherapy, bridge with parenteral anticoagulation
  - The 4Ts scoring (PMID: 20403090—Table II) has almost perfect negative predictive value (NPV). Each scores 0–2 points:
    - Magnitude of **T**hrombocytopenia
    - **T**iming of fall in platelet count or complication
    - **T**hrombosis (or other HIT complication)
    - no o**T**her explanation for thrombocytopenia
      - Scores of 0–3 = low probability for HIT, 4–5 intermediate, and 6–8 high probability
- **DIC**—systemic activation of clotting cascade that causes hemorrhage and thrombosis
  - Uncontrolled production of thrombin → fibrin production → microvascular thrombosis → end-organ damage
  - Consumptive coagulopathy
  - Prolonged PT, PTT, low fibrin
  - Supportive therapy (cryoprecipitate, FFP, blood) and treat underlying disorder
  - Most commonly caused by sepsis, extensive tissue injury, cancer, and amniotic fluid embolism
- Dilutional coagulopathy in massive transfusion
  - Avoid with 1:1:1 resuscitation
  - **Acidosis** and **hypothermia** exacerbate coagulopathy

Hypercoagulability Disorders (Tables 2.3 and 2.4)

- Hypercoagulable states: increased age, oral contraceptive use, hormone replacement therapy, malignancy, pregnancy, infection, trauma, surgery
- Thrombophilia/hypercoagulability workup
  - Do not test if provoked by strong risk factors (major trauma, major surgery, immobility, major illness)

TABLE 2.3 Inherited and Acquired Hypercoagulable Disorders With Associated Thrombophilic Defect and Type of Thrombus

Arterial Thrombosis	Venous Thrombosis
Lupus anticoagulant	Factor V Leiden deficiency
Cardiolipin antibodies	Prothrombin G20210A
Beta-2–glycoprotein I antibodies	Antithrombin deficiency
Lipoprotein (a)	Protein C deficiency
Sticky platelet syndrome	Protein S deficiency
	Elevated factor VIII, IX, and XI levels
	Dysfibrinogenemia
	Hyperhomocysteinemia
	Lupus anticoagulant
	Cardiolipin antibodies
	Beta-2–glycoprotein I antibodies

TABLE 2.4   **Thrombophilia Presentation, Diagnosis, and Treatment**

Disorder	Clinical Presentation	Diagnosis and Treatment
High Risk for Thrombosis		
Antithrombin deficiency	• Venous >>> arterial • Unusual sites of thrombosis • Inherited cases present by age 50 • Can be acquired (liver or kidney disease, sepsis, DIC, or malnutrition)	• Suspect if ineffective anticoagulation with heparin • Treatment: direct thrombin inhibitors, FFP with heparin; lifelong anticoagulation after first VTE
Protein C deficiency	• Venous >>> arterial • Age of presentation of VTE 15–30 years old • Homozygous death in utero (purpura fulminans) • Can be acquired (liver failure, DIC, nephrotic syndrome)	• Suspect in patient with warfarin-induced skin necrosis • Treatment: prophylactic anticoagulation in heterozygotes in perioperative period; lifelong anticoagulation after first VTE
Protein S deficiency	• Venous >>> arterial • Similar presentation to protein C deficiency • Can be acquired (liver disease, nephrotic syndrome, OCP use, pregnancy, and during breastfeeding)	• Same as protein C deficiency
APLS	• Venous > arterial • Thrombosis, miscarriages, stroke, MI, visceral thrombosis, graft thrombosis, gangrene • May be provoked by medications, cancer, and infections	• Treatment: warfarin followed by heparin • Higher thrombosis risk with DOACs • LMWH for recurrent fetal loss
Low Risk for Thrombosis		
FVL	• Venous >> arterial • Most common cause of heritable venous thrombosis	• Diagnose with clot-based assay and genetic analysis • Treatment: long-term anticoagulation for recurrent thrombosis
Prothrombin G20210A	• Venous >> arterial • Higher prevalence in White population	• Treatment: long-term anticoagulation for recurrent thrombosis if patient also has FVL

APLS, Antiphospholipid antibody syndrome *DIC,* disseminated intravascular coagulation; *DOAC,* direct oral anticoagulant; *FFP,* fresh frozen plasma; *FVL,* factor V Leiden; *LMWH,* low-molecular-weight heparin; *MI,* myocardial infarction; *OCP,* oral contraceptive; *VTE,* venous thromboembolism.

- Do not test at time of VTE event and do not test while on anticoagulant therapy
- Consider testing with recurrent VTE or young patients with weak provoking factors or strong family history
- Test for antiphospholipid, factor V Leiden, protein C or S deficiency, AT III deficiency, and prothrombin gene mutation

VENOUS THROMBOEMBOLISM/ DEEP VENOUS THROMBOSIS

Virchow Triad: Hypercoagulability, Stasis, Endothelial Damage

DVT Risk Factors

- Hospitalization, higher if recent surgery
- Malignancy
- Prior central line
- Prior history of superficial vein thrombosis
- Immobility
- Varicose veins
  - 4 times risk: age 45 years
  - 2 times risk: age 60 years
- Congestive heart failure
- Anatomic—iliac vein compression (e.g., nonthrombotic iliac vein lesion [NIVL], formerly May-Thurner syndrome), upper/lower extremity compression, popliteal vein entrapment

Diagnostic Workup

- Duplex ultrasound—diagnostic test of choice
  - Increased intraluminal echogenicity, increased venous diameter, inability to compress with transducer, absence of spontaneous flow, absence of flow augmentation with distal compression
  - Characteristics of thrombus on ultrasound

- Acute—hypoechoic, free floating, soft, smooth edges, homogenous
- Chronic—partial occlusion, stationary, firm, irregular edges, echogenic, heterogenous

Phlegmasia—Acute Threatened Limb From Venous Hypertension

- Phlegmasia cerulea dolens (blue limb)—edematous, blue limb, usually with associated compartment syndrome
- Phlegmasia alba dolens (white limb)—arterial compromise secondary to venous hypertension

CHEST VTE Guidelines

- DVT/pulmonary embolism (PE) without cancer—long-term (3 months) DOAC > VKA > LMWH
- DVT/PE + cancer—LMWH > VKA = DOAC
- Subsegmental PE without proximal DVT—clinical surveillance > anticoagulant (AC) if low risk of recurrence; AC > surveillance if high risk of recurrence
- PE with hypotension—aggressive therapies— catheter-directed thrombolysis (CDT), thrombolysis, mechanical thrombectomy
- recurrent DVT/PE—indefinite AC

Indications for Thrombolysis

- First episode of acute (<14 days) iliofemoral DVT
- NOT indicated for isolated femoropopliteal DVT
- Must not have contraindications for anticoagulation; low bleeding risk; ambulatory

Complications of DVT

- PE
  - Most devastating complication of acute DVT
  - Majority are clinically silent, 50%–80% of symptomatic DVT have asymptomatic PE
  - Consider pulmonary vein thrombolysis if hemodynamic instability or significant right heart strain
  - Initial presentation for 25% of patients with PE is sudden death
  - Inferior vena cava (IVC) filter if:
    - Acute DVT present and anticoagulation is contraindicated
    - Continued thrombosis despite anticoagulation
    - Decreased cardiopulmonary reserve that will not tolerate additional PEs
  - Thrombolysis (systemic or catheter-based) if hemodynamic instability or new pulmonary hypertension present
- Postthrombotic syndrome (PTS)
  - Long-term consequence after acute DVT, develops in 20%–50% of patients
  - Pain, heaviness, edema, and/or hyperpigmentation due to venous hypertension after DVT
  - Combination of venous reflux from destroyed valves and venous stenosis from fibrosis
- Mortality—up to 19% at 3 months after acute DVT (PMID: 17171594); 21% at 1 year (PMID: 19630818)
- Calf vein thrombosis
  - Higher rate of recanalization than in proximal deep veins
  - Lower rate of DVT recurrence than proximal deep veins

SUGGESTED READINGS

Connors JM. Thrombophilia testing and venous thrombosis. *N Engl J Med.* 2017;377(12):1177-1187.

Cuker A, Arepally GM, Chong BH, et al. American Society of Hematology 2018 guidelines for management of venous thromboembolism: heparin-induced thrombocytopenia. *Blood Adv.* 2018;2(22):3360-3392.

Holland LL, Brooks JP. Toward rational fresh frozen plasma transfusion: the effect of plasma transfusion on coagulation test results. *Am J Clin Pathol.* 2006;126(1):133-139.

Obi AT, Alvarez R, Diaz JA, Myers DD, Henke PK, Wakefield TW. Chapter 16: Pathophysiology of Thrombosis. In: Farber A, ed. *Vascular Imaging and Endovascular Interventions.* Ashland OH: 44805, USA. Jaypee Brothers Medical Publishers; 2017.

Kearon C, Akl EA, Ornelas J, et al. Antithrombotic therapy for VTE disease: CHEST guideline and expert panel report. *Chest.* 2016;149(2):315-352. Erratum in: *Chest.* 2016;150(4): 988.

VSITE QUESTIONS

1. Which coagulation factor is not intravascular?
   a. Factor II
   b. Factor III
   c. Factor V
   d. Factor IV
   e. Factor XIII

2. Heparin inhibits thrombosis by neutralizing the effect of:
   a. Thrombin
   b. Factor VIII
   c. Factor XI
   d. Tissue factor
   e. Calcium

3. Inability to achieve therapeutic anticoagulation intraoperatively with intravenous heparin may be improved with which of the following?
   a. Platelets
   b. Fresh plasma
   c. Calcium
   d. Cryoprecipitate
   e. Factor VIII-vWF concentrate
4. The substance that is active in degrading fibrin is:
   a. Thrombin
   b. Heparin
   c. Urokinase
   d. Thrombomodulin
   e. Plasmin

5. After open repair of a ruptured AAA, the patient will not stop bleeding around the repair and in the retroperitoneum. Transfusions with packed red blood cells and plasma (ratio 1:1) were administered throughout, in addition to 10 U of cell saver, 3 packs of platelets and protamine. Using which of the following is most likely to achieve hemostasis?
   a. Topical thrombin
   b. Factor VII concentrate
   c. Calcium chloride
   d. Activated factor VII
   e. F8-vWF concentrate

CHAPTER 3

Pharmacology

MIDDLETON CHANG, MD and KARTHIK BHAT, MD

ANTICOAGULANTS

Unfractionated Heparin

- Discovered in 1916 in dog livers by medical student, Jay McLean, and attributed to his mentor, William Howell, who presented it in 1922. Named after "hepar"—Latin name for liver
- Sulfated polysaccharide isolated from mammalian mast cells. Clearance is not renal and has a half-life of 1 hour
- Precautions: bleeding, heparin-induced thrombocytopenia (HIT incidence: 3%–5% most after cardiac bypass), osteoporosis, elevated transaminases, lack of efficacy in antithrombin III (AT III) deficiency (may need fresh frozen plasma [FFP] transfusions or switch anticoagulant). Indicated during pregnancy (infusion)
- Indications
  - Deep vein thrombosis (DVT) prophylaxis, venous thromboembolism (VTE)/pulmonary embolism (PE), acute coronary syndromes, prophylaxis and treatment of arterial/venous thrombosis, cardiogenic emboli such as atrial fibrillation or left ventricular thrombus
- Mechanism of action
  - Activates AT III, which binds to IIa, and factor Xa
- Dosing
  - 5000 U subcutaneously q12h or q8h for DVT prophylaxis
  - Initial 60–80 U/kg bolus depending on indication
  - 12–15 U/kg per hour to 18 U/kg per hour continuous infusion depending on indication
- Monitoring
  - Xa levels, activated partial thromboplastin time (aPTT), or activated clotting time (ACT)
- Reversal agent
  - Protamine sulfate, made up of positively charged polypeptides isolated from salmon (sturgeon) sperm, binds to heparin with high affinity: 1 mg/100 U heparin

Low-Molecular-Weight Heparin (LMWH)

- Prepared from unfractionated heparin by enzymatic breakdown of unfractionated heparin. Half-life is 2–4 hours depending on formula
- Precautions: less risk of getting HIT (NOT FOR heparin-induced thrombocytopenia [HITT] TREATMENT), osteoporosis, and bleeding. Renally cleared and can accumulate in patients with renal failure. Lack of efficacy in AT III deficiency (may need FFP transfusions or switch anticoagulant)
- Indications
  - Similar to heparin, preferred in patients with *malignancy* and agent indicated during pregnancy
- Mechanism of action
  - Activates antithrombin, which accelerates the rate of inhibition of clotting enzymes, particularly factor Xa
- Dosing
  - 1 mg/kg subcutaneously q12h or 1.5 mg/kg every day for therapeutic treatment
  - 30 mg q12h or 40 mg q24h for DVT prophylaxis
- Monitoring
  - Infusions: PTT or Xa levels 4–6 hours after infusion started
  - Intraprocedure boluses: ACT 1–2 minutes afterward (with normal cardiac output)
- Precautions: bleeding, thrombocytopenia, *osteoporosis*
- Reversal agent
  - Incompletely neutralized by protamine sulfate (~1 mg protamine:1 mg enoxaparin)

Fondaparinux

- Synthetic pentasaccharide of the antithrombin binding sequence. *Very low risk of HIT* and MAY be used in treatment for HITT (not first-line agent). Half-life of 17 hours
- Indication
  - Alternative to unfractionated heparin and LMWH for initial treatment of established VTE
- Mechanism of action
  - Activates antithrombin, which inhibits Xa
- Dosing
  - 2.5 mg daily for prevention of VTE
  - 7.5 mg daily for established VTE and can be adjusted based on weight
  - 2.5 mg daily for acute coronary syndromes
- Monitoring
  - Xa levels
- Precautions: bleeding, can cause HIT (rare)
- Reversal agent: none (recombinant factor VIIa)

HEPARIN-INDUCED THROMBOCYTOPENIA AND THROMBOSIS SYNDROME

- Antibody-mediated response against neoantigens on platelet factor 4 (PF4) formed on first exposure to heparin (immunoglobulin M [IgM]), 5–14 days later IgG (causative to HIT)
- PF4 is released from the alpha-granules of activated platelets, which binds to heparin. IgG binds to PF4-heparin complex and cross-reacts with FcγIIa (IgG) receptors on platelets
- IgG-platelet Fc activates platelets = prothrombotic platelet aggregates
- HITT is associated with venous (most common) or arterial thrombosis (most common HITT event after cardiac surgery)
- Highest risk after unfractionated heparin, cardiopulmonary bypass, and orthopedic surgery
- Suspect it after platelet drops of 50% or more or platelet count of <100,000/µL
- Management: stop heparin, *start argatroban (normal liver), bivalirudin (normal kidneys and/or for procedures),* or fondaparinux and *start warfarin when platelets begin to rise.* Do NOT give platelets—worsens thrombosis
  - Goal PTT >50 sec
  - Goal international normalized ratio (INR) 2–3 (argatroban will elevate INR, so do not stop infusion until INR is >4
- Diagnosis: IgG vs. antibodies against PF4-heparin complex has sensitivity >98%—no IgG = no HIT!
  - Confirmation via platelet activation testing such as serotonin release assay. Addition of HIT antibodies induces platelet activation and serotonin release

VACCINE-INDUCED IMMUNE THROMBOTIC THROMBOCYTOPENIA (VITT)

Antibodies against PF4 WITHOUT heparin reported after vaccination (especially with virus vector). Most notably: Oxford–AstraZeneca and Janssen COVID-19 vaccines.

Parenteral Direct Thrombin Inhibitors

Bivalirudin and Desirudin

- Derivatives of hirudin. *Bivalirudin cleared renally*
- Indications
  - Desirudin (administered subcutaneously): VTE prophylaxis after elective hip surgery
  - Bivalirudin (continuous intravenous [IV] infusion): heparin alternative for patients undergoing vascular interventions usually with HIT (has shortest half-life: 30 min. Bolus: 0.75 mg/kg, infusion for ACT >250 s, 0.75–1.75 mg/kg per hour)
- Mechanism of action
  - Bind and interact with 3 sites on thrombin, which inhibits thrombin
- Monitoring
  - aPTT, ACT, or direct thrombin inhibitor assay
- Side effects
  - Bleeding

Argatroban

- Small-molecule direct thrombin inhibitor. *Metabolized hepatically.* Half-life of 45 minutes
- Indications
  - First-line agent for treatment/anticoagulation in HIT or history of HIT
- Mechanism of action
  - Targets the active site of thrombin
- Monitoring
  - aPTT, ACT
- Side effects
  - Bleeding. Increases INR, which can complicate transition to warfarin

Anticoagulants (Oral)

Warfarin

- Water-soluble coumarin derivative initially created as a rodenticide
- Indications (Food and Drug Administration [FDA] website)
  - Prophylaxis and/or treatment of VTE/PE
  - Prophylaxis and/or treatment of atrial fibrillation (AFib per AMA and Dorland's) and/or cardiac valve replacement thromboembolic complications

- Reduction in risk of death, recurrent myocardial infarction (MI), and thromboembolic events (stroke, systemic embolization) after an MI
- Mechanism of action
  - Inhibits vitamin K epoxide reductase, thereby inhibiting the synthesis of vitamin K–dependent factors (II, VII, IX, and X) and vitamin K–dependent anticoagulant proteins (C and S)
- Dosing
  - Start at 5–10 mg and titrate to achieve INR goal
- Monitoring
  - Prothrombin time (PT)/INR
- Side effects
  - Bleeding (reversed with PO/IV vitamin K and/or prothrombin complex concentrate [PCC] depending on the INR level and presence of active bleeding)
  - *Skin necrosis* (proteins C and S have shorter half-lives than factors with a significant decrease in levels leading to a hypercoagulable state). Typically seen 2–5 days after warfarin initiation. Presents as well-demarcated, erythematous lesions on thighs, buttocks, breast, or toes. The center of lesion progressively becomes necrotic. This complication is prevented with administration of unfractionated heparin or LMWH to prevent the hypercoagulable state
  - Fetal abnormalities. However, it can be administered in nursing mothers
- Reversal
  - Vitamin K
  - PCC (preferred)
  - FFP

Direct Oral Anticoagulants

- Dabigatran, rivaroxaban, apixaban
- Indications (FDA)
  - Stroke and systemic embolization risk reduction in patients with nonvalvular AFib (dabigatran, apixaban, and rivaroxaban)
  - Treatment of DVT/PE and risk reduction of recurrent DVT/PE (rivaroxaban)
  - DVT prophylaxis, especially in patients undergoing elective hip or knee replacement surgery (rivaroxaban)
- Mechanism of action
  - Dabigatran: direct thrombin inhibitor
  - Rivaroxaban/apixaban: direct factor Xa inhibitor
- Dosing for FDA indications
  - Dabigatran: 150 mg BID
  - Apixaban: 5 mg BID
  - Rivaroxaban: 20 mg qday (nonvalvular AFib). 15 mg BID for 21 days and then 20 mg qday (VTE/PE). 10 mg qday (VTE/PE prophylaxis for knee/hip surgery). 2.5 mg BID with aspirin 100 mg for patients with chronic vascular disease reduces risk of major adverse cardiovascular events

- Monitoring
  - Not necessary in most situations. PT for factor Xa inhibitors and aPTT for dabigatran
- Side effects
  - Bleeding (reversal agents for dabigatran and rivaroxaban/apixaban include idarucizumab and andexanet alfa, respectively). Uncontrolled and/or life-threatening bleeding in setting of direct factor Xa inhibitors are primarily treated with PCC in the absence of an appropriate reversal agent
  - Dyspepsia with dabigatran

Contraindications to Anticoagulants

- Absolute contraindications
  - Active bleeding
  - Severe bleeding diathesis or platelet count $\leq$20,000/mm^3
  - Neurosurgery, ocular surgery, or intracranial bleeding within the past 10 days
- Relative contraindications
  - Mild to moderate bleeding diathesis or thrombocytopenia
  - Brain metastases
  - Recent major trauma
  - Major abdominal surgery within the past 2 days
  - Gastrointestinal or genitourinary bleeding within the past 14 days
  - Endocarditis
  - Severe hypertension (systolic blood pressure >200 mm Hg and/or diastolic blood pressure >120 mm Hg)

THROMBOLYTIC AGENTS

Alteplase

- Recombinant plasminogen activator and most used in the United States
- Indication
  - Acute ischemic stroke
  - Acute MI
  - Acute massive PE for lysis
  - Catheter directed arterial or venous thrombolysis
- Mechanism
  - Assist in the conversion of plasminogen into active plasmin, which then cleaves cross-linked fibrin
- Monitoring
  - Fibrin levels
  - D-dimer
  - aPTT
- Side effects
  - Bleeding
  - Spontaneous intracranial hemorrhage
  - Distal embolization in catheter-directed lysis

- Contraindications (Rutherford, Chapter 101, Box 101.1)
  - Absolute
    - Active bleeding disorder
    - Active internal bleeding
    - Gastrointestinal bleeding within 10 days
    - Cerebrovascular event within 6 months
    - Intracranial or spinal surgery within 3 months
    - Head injury within 3 months
    - Prior severe allergic reaction
  - Relative
    - Major surgeries, recent eye surgery, trauma, or cardiopulmonary resuscitation (within the past 10 days)
    - Hypertension (systolic >180 mm Hg or diastolic >110 mm Hg)
    - Puncture of noncompressible vessel
    - Intracranial tumor
    - Bacterial endocarditis
    - Severe liver or kidney disease
    - Diabetic hemorrhagic retinopathy
    - Acute pancreatitis
    - Pregnancy
    - Noncompressible vessel
    - Condition where bleeding would be a significant hazard or be difficult to manage because of its anatomic location
- Reversal
  - Aminocaproic acid
    - Aminocaproic acid binds reversibly to the kringle domain of plasminogen and blocks the binding of plasminogen to fibrin and its activation to plasmin

ANTIPLATELET AGENTS

Aspirin

- Indications
  - Prevention of cardiovascular events in patients with established coronary artery disease, peripheral arterial disease (PAD), or cerebrovascular occlusive disease
- Mechanism of action
  - Nonselective irreversible inhibitor of cyclooxygenase (COX) 1 and 2, which inhibits production of thromboxane A2. Inhibits COX2 at higher doses, leading to antiinflammatory effect
- Dosing
  - 75–325 mg/d depending on indication
- Monitoring
  - No monitoring necessary
- Side effects
  - Gastrointestinal (dyspepsia, gastritis, ulcers)
  - Bleeding
  - Aspirin intolerance/allergy, especially in patients with asthma, urticaria, nasal polyps, or chronic rhinosinusitis

Clopidogrel

- Indications
  - Patients with unstable angina/non–ST-segment–elevated MI, ST-segment–elevated MI, recent MI, recent cerebrovascular accident (CVA), established PAD
  - Off-label indications include adjunctive therapy to percutaneous coronary intervention (PCI), coronary artery bypass graft (CABG) surgery, peripheral arterial transluminal balloon angioplasty/stent placement
  - Intolerance/allergy to aspirin
- Mechanism of action
  - Prodrug activated hepatically (CYP450 enzyme system) and irreversibly inhibits the $P2Y_{12}$ component of the adenosine diphosphate (ADP) receptor on the platelet surface
- Dosing
  - 75 mg qday
  - 300–600-mg bolus dose depending on indication
- Monitoring
  - Not necessary
- Side effects
  - Bleeding
  - Pruritus
- Resistance
  - Variable $P2Y_{12}$ resistance in the population, uncertain clinical effect but it is a topic to be aware of and possibly a reason to switch to a different agent

Ticagrelor

- Indications
  - Reduces the risk of cardiovascular death, MI, and stroke in patients with acute coronary syndromes
- Mechanism of action
  - Noncompetitive, reversible inhibitor of the ADP P2Y12 receptor, which prevents platelet aggregation
- Dose
  - Loading dose of 180 mg. Maintenance dose of 60–90 mg BID
- Monitoring
  - Not necessary
- Side effects
  - Bleeding
  - Elevated uric acid levels
  - Transient dyspnea

Prasugrel

- Indications
  - Acute coronary syndrome managed by PCI
- Mechanism of action
  - Prodrug that is activated by the CYP450 enzyme system. Irreversibly blocks the $P2Y_{12}$ component of the ADP receptor

- Dose
  - Loading dose of 60 mg. Maintenance dose of 10 mg/qd
- Monitoring
  - Not necessary
- Side effects
  - Bleeding, hypertension, hyperlipidemia, and thrombotic thrombocytopenic purpura
- Contraindications
  - Patients with history of transient ischemic attack or stroke

HEMORRHEOLOGIC AGENTS

Cilostazol

- Indication
  - Treatment of intermittent claudication
- Mechanism of action
  - Inhibitor of phosphodiesterase III, which increases levels of cyclic adenosine monophosphate (cAMP) and results in inhibition of smooth muscle contraction and platelet aggregation
- Dosing
  - 100 mg BID
  - Dosage can be reduced to 50 mg BID when taking CYP3A4 inhibitors (ketoconazole, itraconazole, erythromycin, and diltiazem) or CYPC19 inhibitors (fluconazole and omeprazole)
- Monitoring
  - Not necessary
- Side effects
  - Headaches
  - Gastrointestinal (diarrhea and pain)
- Contraindications
  - Congestive heart failure

Pentoxifylline

- Indication
  - Treatment of intermittent claudication
- Mechanism
  - Improves blood flow by decreasing viscosity
- Dosing
  - 400 mg BID
- Monitoring
  - Not necessary
- Side effects
  - Impairs normal coagulation, especially when taken in combination with warfarin

BRIEF REVIEW OF ACLS MEDICATIONS

Epinephrine

- Alpha- and beta-receptor agonist

- Indications
  - Ventricular fibrillation/pulseless ventricular tachycardia (VF/pVT)
  - Pulseless electrical activity (PEA) arrest and/or asystole
  - Persistent symptomatic bradycardia when atropine is ineffective
- Dose (IV)
  - 1 mg every 3–5 minutes (VF/pVT/PEA/asystole)
  - 2–10 mcg/min IV infusion. Titrate to patient response (bradycardia)

Atropine

- Anticholinergic agent
- Indications
  - Persistent bradycardia with symptoms (hypotension, altered mental status, signs of shock, ischemic chest discomfort, and/or acute heart failure)
- Dose (IV)
  - 0.5-mg bolus (repeat every 3–5 min. Maximum dose of 3 mg)

Adenosine

- Adenosine receptor agonist (blocks conduction through atrioventricular [AV] node)
- Indications
  - Persistent tachyarrhythmia (regular, narrow complex) with significant symptoms (hypotension, altered mental status, signs of shock, ischemic chest discomfort, and/or acute heart failure)
  - Persistent tachyarrhythmia (regular, narrow complex) with a QRS ≥0.12 seconds without significant symptoms (hypotension, altered mental status, signs of shock, ischemic chest discomfort, and/or acute heart failure)
  - Persistent tachyarrhythmia (regular complex) with a QRS <0.12 seconds without significant symptoms (hypotension, altered mental status, signs of shock, ischemic chest discomfort, and/or acute heart failure)
- Dose (IV)
  - First dose: 6-mg bolus. Second dose: 12-mg bolus, if necessary, must be administered *quickly* as the drug is metabolized rapidly

Metoprolol

- Beta-blocker (blocks conduction through AV node)
- Indications
  - Persistent tachyarrhythmia with a QRS <0.12 seconds without significant symptoms (hypotension, altered mental status, signs of shock, ischemic chest discomfort, and/or acute heart failure)

- Dose (IV)
  - 5 mg over 5 minutes for a total of 15 mg

Amiodarone

- Potassium channel blocker (has effects on all antiarrhythmic classes)
- Indications
  - Persistent tachyarrhythmia (regular, narrow complex) with a QRS ≥0.12 seconds without significant symptoms (hypotension, altered mental status, signs of shock, ischemic chest discomfort, and/or acute heart failure)
  - ventricular fibrillation/pulseless ventricular tachycardia (VF/pVT)
- Dose (IV)
  - 150 mg over 10 minutes. Followed by maintenance infusion of 1 mg/min for first 6 hours (tachyarrhythmia with a pulse)
  - First dose: 300-mg bolus. Second dose: 150-mg bolus

ANESTHETICS

Local

- Aminoester (duration of action)
  - Chloroprocaine (30–50 min)
- Aminoamides (duration of action)
  - Lidocaine (60–180 min), mepivacaine (60–180 min), bupivacaine (180–360 min), ropivacaine (180–360 min)
- Mechanism of action
  - Blocks sodium channels by binding to receptors on the inner portion of the channel. Most effective in rapid-firing neurons
  - Concurrently given with epinephrine, which decreases bleeding and increases the local anesthetic effect by decreasing systemic concentration
  - Efficacy decreased in acidic tissue, as alkaline nature is charged and cannot penetrate tissue. More anesthetic needed
- Side effects
  - Central nervous system excitation (benzodiazepine if seizure does not terminate spontaneously), cardiovascular toxicity (bupivacaine). The American Society of Regional Anesthesia and Pain Medicine recommends lipid emulsion therapy (bolus injection and infusion) to rescue patients from severe local anesthetic toxicity. Mechanism of action not known

Intravenous Anesthetics

- Propofol
  - Gamma-aminobutyric acid (GABA)-mediated inhibition. Short acting and nausea-free emergence
  - Indications

- Short procedures
- Asthmatic patients requiring IV anesthetics
- Side effects
  - Burns on administration
- Ketamine
  - Inhibits glutamate receptors of the N-methyl-D-aspartate (NMDA) subtype
  - Indications (dissociative anesthetic)
    - Brief, superficial procedures (does not provide skeletal muscular relaxation)
    - IV anesthetic in patients with severe hypovolemia
  - Side effects
    - Hypertension and tachycardia
    - Avoid in coronary artery disease (tachycardia), traumatic brain injury (increases cerebral blood flow)
    - Delirium
- Etomidate
  - GABA-mediated inhibition
  - Indications
    - Preserves blood pressure and is an alternative for patients with cardiovascular disease or severe hypovolemia
  - Side effects
    - Burning on administration
    - Myoclonus
    - Adrenal suppression in critically ill patients
- Fentanyl
  - Synthetic drug that is an opioid receptor agonist, short acting
  - Indications
    - Maintenance of anesthesia
    - Added to intrathecal and epidural blocks to improve analgesia
  - Side effects
    - Respiratory depression
    - Inconsistent hypnosis and amnesia
- Midazolam
  - GABA-mediated inhibition
  - Indications
    - Induces profound amnesia for painful or anxiety-producing events
    - Premedication component of a multidrug anesthetic
    - Synergistic with opioids in patients with cardiac contractility dysfunction
  - Side effects
    - Respiratory depression with opioid administration

Inhaled Anesthetics

- Nitric oxide, desflurane, isoflurane, sevoflurane, halothane
- Lipid-soluble, nontoxic drugs that facilitate rapid induction and emergence. Typically used in a multidrug anesthetic
- Important characteristics include blood/gas solubility coefficient (B/G) and mean alveolar concentration (MAC). B/G measures solubility in blood. A high solubility means slower induction and emergence (halothane), and low solubility

means more rapid induction and emergence (nitric oxide and desflurane). Isoflurane and sevoflurane have intermediate B/G solubility coefficients. MAC is a measure of drug potency. It is defined as the concentration of inhaled anesthetic agent that is required to prevent 50% of patients from moving in response to noxious stimuli (skin incision). A higher MAC translates to a lower potency

- Side effect
  - Malignant hyperthermia
    - Inherited disorder, autosomal dominant
    - Gene responsible: ryanodine receptor (*RYR1*)
    - Triggering agents include inhaled anesthetics and/or succinylcholine, resulting in uncontrolled release of free calcium from the sarcoplasmic reticulum
    - Signs and symptoms include unexplained increase in end-tidal carbon dioxide (most sensitive indicator), unexplained tachycardia, skeletal muscle rigidity/masseter muscle spasm, temperature elevation, and laboratory abnormalities
    - Treatment involves stopping offending agents, administering *dantrolene*, and beginning supportive therapy/cooling measures

REVIEW OF STANDARD ANTIBIOTICS

Beta-lactam antibiotics are inhibitors of cell wall synthesis. They are structural analogs of D-Ala-D-Ala and bind to penicillin-binding proteins (transpeptidases). They block cross-linking of peptidoglycan in cell walls. Antibiotics in this class include penicillin G (IV and intramuscular [IM] form)/penicillin V (oral), amoxicillin (oral)/ampicillin (IV), nafcillin/dicloxacillin/oxacillin, ampicillin-sulbactam/amoxicillin-clavulanic acid/piperacillin-tazobactam, cephalosporins, carbapenems, monobactams, and lipoglycopeptides. Adverse reactions include hypersensitivity reactions and interstitial nephritis. However, cephalosporins, carbapenems, and monobactams have less cross-reactivity with penicillins. Resistance is developed by bacterial penicillinase, which is a type of beta-lactamase. Addition of a beta-lactamase inhibitor (sulbactam, clavulanic acid, tazobactam) protects antibiotic against penicillinase.

Carbapenems have a five-carbon ring structure attached to their core beta-lactam structure. Their alkyl groups are oriented in a *cis* vs. *trans* configuration (characteristic of other beta-lactam agents). This provides the resistance to beta-lactamases. Carbapenems have a risk of neurotoxicity (seizures). Meropenem is administered with cilastatin (inhibitor of renal dehydropeptidase), which prevents inactivation in renal tubules. Monobactams bind to penicillin-binding protein 3 and are less susceptible to beta-lactamases, but drug resistance is widespread. Indicated in situations where organism is susceptible and in patients with penicillin allergy.

Lipoglycopeptides include vancomycin and daptomycin. Vancomycin is associated with nephrotoxicity, ototoxicity, and thrombophlebitis. Another adverse effect is red man

syndrome, which presents as diffuse flushing. This can be prevented by pretreatment with antihistamine and a slow infusion rate. Mechanism of resistance develops in bacteria (*Enterococcus*) through an amino acid modification of D-Ala-D-Ala to D-Ala-D-Lac. Daptomycin disrupts cell membranes by creating a channel in the membrane. Side effects include myopathy and rhabdomyolysis in severe cases. It is not used in pneumonia because the surfactant binds and inactivates daptomycin.

Protein synthesis inhibitors include aminoglycosides, tetracyclines, clindamycin, macrolides, and oxazolidinones. Aminoglycosides (gentamicin, neomycin, amikacin, and tobramycin) are bactericidal and work by irreversibly inhibiting initiation of protein synthesis by binding of the 30S subunit. Aminoglycosides require O_2 for uptake and are infective against anaerobes. Side effects include nephrotoxicity, neuromuscular blockade, and ototoxicity, and they are teratogenic. Resistance is developed through bacterial transferase inactivation.

Tetracyclines (doxycycline) have a similar mechanism of action to aminoglycosides but are bacteriostatic. Contraindicated during pregnancy and <8 years of age due to dental toxicity. Patients being treated with tetracyclines can have photosensitivity as well.

Oxazolidinones (linezolid) bind to the 50S ribosomal subunit. Gram-negative bacteria are resistant due to efflux pumps that excrete oxazolidinones. They are one of the few options available for oral antibiotic treatment of methicillin-resistant *Staphylococcus aureus* (MRSA).

Clindamycin also binds to the 50S ribosome subunit. It is associated with development of *Clostridium difficile* infection. Given its mechanism of action, inhibition of protein synthesis, this antibiotic is frequently added to necrotizing soft tissue infections to inhibit toxin synthesis.

Fluoroquinolones (ciprofloxacin and levofloxacin) inhibit DNA gyrase (DNA folding protein in preparation for replication), which inhibits bacterial DNA synthesis. Side effects include QTc prolongation and interaction with warfarin (increasing INR). A positive association between fluoroquinolones and the development of an aortic aneurysm has been found.

Trimethoprim-sulfamethoxazole is a cytotoxic agent that has 2 active agents. Trimethoprim is bacteriostatic by interfering with bacterial folic acid synthesis. Sulfamethoxazole inhibits dihydrofolate reductase, which converts dihydrofolic acid to tetrahydrofolic acid, which has a bactericidal effect. Adverse effects include hemolysis (patients with glucose-6-phosphate dehydrogenase deficiency), photosensitivity, Stevens-Johnson syndrome, displacement of other drugs from albumin (warfarin), and bone marrow suppression.

Metronidazole is a cytotoxic, bactericidal agent that forms free radicals after intracellular reduction that damages bacterial DNA. Side effects include a disulfiram-like reaction (severe flushing, tachycardia, and hypotension with alcohol use), headaches, and a metallic taste.

The antibiotic coverage chart is included in Fig. 3.1.

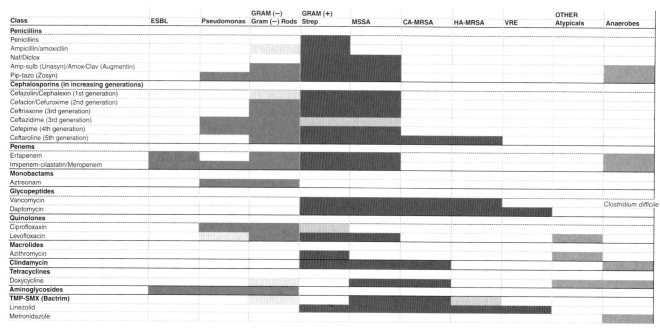

FIG. 3.1 **Antibiotic Coverage Chart.** *Dark shades* represent full coverage and *light shades* represent partial coverage. *Amox/Clav,* amoxicillin/clavulanate; *Amp-sulb,* ampicillin-sulbactam; *CA-MRSA,* community-associated methicillin-resistant *Staphylococcus areus*; *ESBL,* Extended-spectrum beta-lactamase organism; *HA-MRS,* hospital-acquired methicillin-resistant *Staphylococcus areus*; *MRSA,* methicillin-resistant *Staphylococcus aureus*; *MSSA,* methicillin-sensitive *Staphylococcus aureus*; *Naf/Diclox,* nafcillin/dicloxacillin; *Pip-Tazo,* piperacillin-tazobactam; *TMP-SMX,* trimethoprim-sulfamethoxazole; *VRE,* vancomycin-resistant enterococcus. Modified from initial version created by Trevor Steinbock, MD (Department of Medicine, University of Washington School of Medicine) and Elizabeth Chang, MD (Department of Medicine, Emory University School of Medicine).

SUGGESTED READINGS

Anticoagulants/Thrombolytics/Antiplatelet/Claudication

Bates SM, Ginsberg JS. Clinical practice. Treatment of deep-vein thrombosis. *N Engl J Med.* 2004;351(3):268-277.

Sidawy AN, Bruce PA. *Rutherford's Vascular Surgery and Endovascular Therapy.* 9th ed. Elsevier; 2019.

ACLS Medications

ECC Committee, Subcommittees and Task Forces of the American Heart Association. 2005 American Heart Association guidelines for cardiopulmonary resuscitation and emergency cardiovascular care. *Circulation.* 2005;112(suppl 24):IV1-IV203.

Anesthetics

Ali SZ, Taguchi A, Rosenberg H. Malignant hyperthermia. *Best Pract Res Clin Anaesthesiol.* 2003;17(4):519-533.

Berg-Johnsen J. Virkningsmekanismer for intravenøse anestesimidler [Action mechanisms of intravenous anesthetics]. *Tidsskr Nor Laegeforen.* 1993;113(5):565-568.

Townsend CM, Beauchamp RD, Evers BM, Mattox KL. *Sabiston Textbook of Surgery: The Biological Basis of Modern Surgical Practice.* 20th ed. Elsevier; 2017.

Review of Standard Antibiotics

Rawla P, El Helou ML, Vellipuram AR. Fluoroquinolones and the risk of aortic aneurysm or aortic dissection: a systematic review and meta-analysis. *Cardiovasc Hematol Agents Med Chem.* 2019;17(1):3-10.

Townsend CM, Beauchamp RD, Evers BM, Mattox KL. *Sabiston Textbook of Surgery: The Biological Basis of Modern Surgical Practice.* 20th ed. Elsevier; 2017.

Vaccine-Induced Immune Thrombotic Thrombocytopenia

Greinacher A, Thiele T, Warkentin TE, Weisser K, Kyrle PA, Eichinger S. Thrombotic thrombocytopenia after ChAdOx1 nCov-19 vaccination. *N Engl J Med.* 2021;384(22):2092-2101.

Schultz NH, Sørvoll IH, Michelsen AE, et al. Thrombosis and thrombocytopenia after ChAdOx1 nCoV-19 vaccination. *N Engl J Med.* 2021;384(22):2124-2130.

CHAPTER 4

Thrombolytic Therapy

CHARLES MARQUARDT, MD and MATTHEW R. SMEDS, MD

BACKGROUND AND TECHNIQUE

- Federal Drug Administration (FDA)–approved lytic agents
  - Streptokinase
  - Urokinase
  - Alteplase
  - Reteplase
  - Tenecteplase
- Mechanism of action of lytic agents
  - Tissue plasminogen activators (tPAs) that convert plasminogen to plasmin, a proteolytic enzyme that degrades fibrin, the primary adhesive component of clots, into soluble fibrin degradation products
- Catheter-directed thrombolysis (CDT)
  - Can be performed as an alternative to open bypass or thromboembolectomy in both the venous and arterial systems
  - Shown to be effective in acute (<14 days) cases
  - Technique:
    - An appropriate-sized sheath is placed proximal to thrombosed vessel for support
    - A thrombotic lesion is crossed with a wire over which a side-hole infusion catheter is placed. These catheters come in various treatment lengths, which are used depending on the length of the lesion
      - Ideally with the side holes oriented within the thrombus
      - A central stylette forces fluid out the side holes directly into the thrombus
      - Side holes should be within the thrombus. tPA will release in the area of least resistance. If catheter

chosen is too long, it will not treat the area of need as well
  - Continuous infusion of the lytic agent through the catheter for 12–24 hours. Thrombolysis beyond 48 hours has shown no benefit (and increased risks)
- Heparin is infused via the sheath (and around the catheter) to prevent thrombus formation and often systemically to maintain an activated prothrombin time of 1.5 times control
- Patients should be monitored in the intensive care unit (ICU) with serial extremity examination
- Monitoring—lysis results in dissolution of clot in response to which the body attempts to reform clot. Fibrinogen, the precursor to fibrin, can be monitored to follow this consumption of coagulation factors. Activated partial thromboplastin time (aPTT) can be followed to monitor anticoagulation. Both should be followed q4–6 hours
- Fibrinogen levels <100 mg/dL should trigger a decrease in tPA rate or cessation of therapy[1]
- aPTT >100 seconds should trigger decrease in heparin rate
- Efficacy and patency
  - Patency and limb salvage after CDT variable by study[2-5]
  - Chronicity, anatomic location, and native vessel vs. bypass conduit all variables affecting patency

LANDMARK TRIALS

Rochester Trial[6]

- 114 Patients with acute limb ischemia (ALI) (<7 days duration) randomized to thrombolysis with urokinase vs. surgery
  - Mortality higher in surgical group (58% vs. 84%) due to cardiopulmonary complications
  - Rate of limb salvage identical (80%)

Surgery Versus Thrombolysis for the Ischemic Lower Extremity (STILE) Trial[7]

- 393 Patients with ALI randomized to thrombolysis with alteplase, thrombolysis with urokinase, or surgery

- A 30-day follow-up demonstrated identical mortality rates (4% for lysis, 5% for surgery) and amputation rates (5% for lysis, 6% for surgery)
- At 6 months, major amputation was 11% for CDT vs. 30% for surgical intervention for patients with symptoms <14 days. In those with symptoms >14 days, there was a 12% major amputation rate with CDT compared to 3% with surgery
- *This trial demonstrated that the use of lysis within 14 days of ALI is superior while surgery is superior for chronic disease >14 days' duration*

Thrombolysis or Peripheral Arterial Surgery (TOPAS) Trial[8]

- 544 Patients with ALI randomized to thrombolysis with recombinant urokinase vs. surgery
  - No difference in overall amputation-free survival (72% CDT vs. 75% surgery)
  - Patients with native artery occlusion treated with lysis had lower 1-year amputation-free survival as compared to those with surgery (61% vs. 71%) while patients with prosthetic grafts had identical rates (68%)
  - Increased requirement for transfusion in CDT group (12.5% vs. 5.5%)

INDICATIONS FOR LYSIS

- Acute arterial thromboembolism (ALI <14 days' symptom duration)
  - Patient should have minimal sensory impairment and no motor impairment (Rutherford IIa or less ischemia)
  - Those with more profound symptoms should warrant quicker treatment (surgery vs. mechanical thrombectomy)
  - May consider in chronic occlusion if patient is a poor open surgical candidate
- Deep vein thrombosis (DVT)
- Pulmonary embolism
- Arteriovenous graft occlusion

CONTRAINDICATIONS

Absolute	Relative
Active bleeding	Operation/obstetric procedure, or biopsy in a noncompressible location within 10 days
Stroke, head or spinal trauma, intracranial or intraspinal surgery within 2 months	Gastrointestinal bleed, trauma, cardiopulmonary resuscitation within 10 days

Absolute	Relative
Known intracranial neoplasm	Left heart thrombus
Severe, uncontrolled hypertension	Subacute bacterial endocarditis
Clotting disorders	Severe liver or kidney disease
Allergy to tPA	Diabetic hemorrhagic retinopathy
Allergy to heparin	Pregnancy
Rutherford III ischemia	Rutherford IIb ischemia

RISKS AND COMPLICATIONS

- Bleeding
  - For ALI lysis, major hemorrhage risk of 8.8% and intracranial hemorrhage risk of 1.6%[9]
  - Significant drop in hemoglobin should precipitate investigation into possible source of bleeding
  - Higher risk of bleeding for arterial lysis compared to venous lysis
- Allergic reactions—rare; can be treated with steroids and antihistamines
- Embolism of lysed fragments may occur during lysis. These fragments may be treated with continued lysis, suction embolectomy, mechanical thrombectomy, or open embolectomy
  - High risk of bleeding when performing open surgery after thrombolysis

COMBINATION THROMBOLYTICS AND MECHANICAL THROMBECTOMY

- Rheolytic/pharmacomechanical thrombectomy (PMT)
  - Mechanically removes clot along with the disintegration caused by the thrombolytic therapy given just prior, to "soften" the clot
- Inconsistent findings; however, combination therapy may have an advantage over CDT alone[10]
  - PMT only has been shown to have worse amputation and survival outcomes[11]

EKOS ENDOVASCULAR SYSTEM

- Lytic catheter with ultrasonic core
- Ultrasound vibrations increase the uptake of tPA into the thrombus
- Created initially for pulmonary embolism and has been found safe in ALI; however, studies have not yet demonstrated increased efficacy over CDT alone[11]

REFERENCES

1. Ouriel K, Kandarpa K, Schuerr DM, Hultquist M, Hodkinson G, Wallin B. Prourokinase versus urokinase for recanalization of peripheral occlusions, safety and efficacy: the PURPOSE trial. *J Vasc Interv Radiol.* 1999;10(8):1083-1091.

2. Schrijver AM, de Vries JP, van den Heuvel DA, Moll FL. Long-term outcomes of catheter-directed thrombolysis for acute lower extremity occlusions of native arteries and prosthetic bypass grafts. *Ann Vasc Surg.* 2016;31:134-142.

3. Nehler MR, Mueller RJ, McLafferty RB, et al. Outcome of catheter-directed thrombolysis for lower extremity arterial bypass occlusion. *J Vasc Surg.* 2003;37(1):72-78.

4. Koraen L, Kuoppala M, Acosta S, Wahlgren CM. Thrombolysis for lower extremity bypass graft occlusion. *J Vasc Surg.* 2011; 54(5):1339-1344.

5. Lian WS, Das SK, Hu XX, Zhang XJ, Xie XY, Li MQ. Efficacy of intra-arterial catheter-directed thrombolysis for popliteal and infrapopliteal acute limb ischemia. *J Vasc Surg.* 2020;71(1): 141-148.

6. Ouriel K, Shortell CK, DeWeese JA, et al. A comparison of thrombolytic therapy with operative revascularization in the initial treatment of acute peripheral arterial ischemia. *J Vasc Surg.* 1994;19(6):1021-1030.

7. Results of a prospective randomized trial evaluating surgery versus thrombolysis for ischemia of the lower extremity. The STILE trial. *Ann Surg.* 1994;220(3):251-266; discussion 266-268.

8. Ouriel K, Veith FJ, Sasahara AA. A comparison of recombinant urokinase with vascular surgery as initial treatment for acute arterial occlusion of the legs. Thrombolysis or Peripheral Arterial Surgery (TOPAS) Investigators. *N Engl J Med.* 1998;338(16):1105-1111.

9. Darwood R, Berridge DC, Kessel DO, Robertson I, Forster R. Surgery versus thrombolysis for initial management of acute limb ischaemia. *Cochrane Database Syst Rev.* 2018;8(8):CD002784.

10. Gandhi SS, Ewing JA, Cooper E, Chaves JM, Gray BH. Comparison of low-dose catheter-directed thrombolysis with and without pharmacomechanical thrombectomy for acute lower extremity ischemia. *Ann Vasc Surg.* 2018;46:178-186.

11. Chait J, Aurshina A, Marks N, Hingorani A, Ascher E. Comparison of ultrasound-accelerated versus multi-hole infusion catheter-directed thrombolysis for the treatment of acute limb ischemia. *Vasc Endovascular Surg.* 2019;53(7):558-562.

CHAPTER 5

Surgical Critical Care for Vascular Surgery

KEVIN ONOFREY, MD, YAHYA MADIAN, MD, and LOAY KABBANI, MD, MPH

SHOCK

There are primarily four types of shock that are outlined in Fig. 5.1.

Pathophysiology

All four types lead to end-organ hypoxia and resultant disfunction.

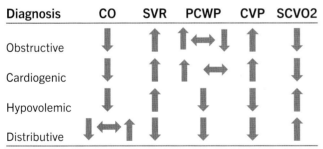

Diagnosis	CO	SVR	PCWP	CVP	SCVO2
Obstructive	↓	↑	↑↔↓	↑	↓
Cardiogenic	↓	↑	↑	↔	↓
Hypovolemic	↓	↑	↓	↓	↑
Distributive	↓↔↑	↓	↓	↓	↑

CO, Cardiac output; *CVP*, central venous pressure; *PCWP*, pulmonary capillary wedge pressure; *SCVO2*, central venous oxygen saturation; *SVR*, systemic vascular resistance.

Obstructive Shock

Extrinsic compression or obstruction of the cardiac inflow, outflow, or both leads to a significant reduction in CO.

Tension pneumothorax, hemothorax, cardiac tamponade, pulmonary embolism (PE)

Diagnosis

- Jugular venous distention (JVD)
- Chest x-ray (CXR), echocardiogram (Echo)/focused assessment with sonography in trauma (FAST), computed tomography angiography (CTA)

Cardiac Tamponade

- Early Echo sign is impaired diastolic filling of right atrium (RA)
- Treatment. Fluid resuscitation until pericardial fluid is drained. Pericardial blood does not clot. Cardiopulmonary resuscitation (CPR) helps when needed

Pulmonary Embolism

- Tachypnea, chest pain, hypoxia, hypocarbia with respiratory alkalosis (from hyperventilation)
- Most common source: iliofemoral deep vein thrombosis (DVT) (1/3 have negative lower extremity [LE] DVT scan)
- Diagnosis is CTA or transesophageal echocardiogram (TEE)
- Treatment: Anticoagulation and volume resuscitation
- PE can be classified into massive (5%–10% of cases), submassive (20%–25% of cases), and low risk (70% of cases)
- Massive PE (shock hypotension >15 min on pressors, severe bradycardia), right heart strain (Echo, CTA reflux of contrast to inferior vena cava [IVC] and/or troponins), consider thrombolysis/thromboembolectomy
- Submassive PE (hemodynamic normal with right heart strain or myocardial necrosis), there is potential to undergo a cycle of progressive right ventricular (RV) failure. A submassive PE requires continuous intensive care unit (ICU) monitoring. Thromboembolectomy or catheter-directed thrombolysis usually improves cardiac and pulmonary hemodynamics but consensus not obtained due to conflicting data in randomized controlled trial (RCT) (mortality high or no long-term difference)
- In low-risk PE, only dyspnea and/or hypoxemia not needing intubation. No hypotension or ventricular dysfunction/necrosis

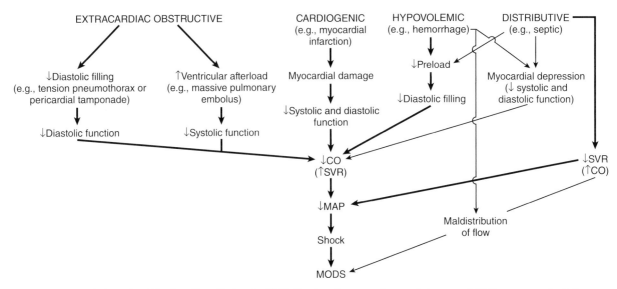

FIG. 5.1   Types of Shock. *CO,* Cardiac Output; *SVR,* Systemic vascular resistance; *MAP,* mean arterial pressure; *MODS,* Multiorgan Dysfunction Syndrome

Air Embolus

- Most common cause is sucking air through large central line
- Treatment
  - Trendelenburg + *left lateral decubitus to keep air in RV and RA (not in pulmonary artery* [PA])
  - Suck air out of central line
  - 100% O_2/hyperventilation; helps resorb air embolus faster

Cardiogenic Shock

Insufficient oxygen delivery leads to end-organ dysfunction and ischemia. Myocardial infarction (MI), congestive heart failure (CHF) exacerbation, severe valvular dysfunction, severe cardiomyopathy.

Diagnosis

- Monitor central venous pressure (CVP), lactic acidosis, and SCVO2
- Normal SCVO2 >70%. However, coronary sinus oxygen saturation is <30% in a normal individual
- Echo—helps delineate grade of shock and etiology
- PA catheter—pulmonary capillary wedge pressure (PCWP), PA pressure, and transpulmonary gradient can help with titration of diuresis, inotropic support, and pulmonary vasodilatory medications

Treatment Principles

Steps: (1) Achieve euvolemia (preload), (2) afterload reduction, and (3) inotropy

- Rule out PE and MI in acute cardiogenic shock
- Achieve euvolemia:
  - Hypervolemia should be treated aggressively with diuresis or dialysis

- Hypovolemia (especially in mixed septic and cardiogenic shock) should be treated with volume to assure euvolemia. Inotropy in hypovolemia will lead to cardiac ischemia
- *Afterload reduction:* a goal *mean arterial blood pressure* (MAP) of 65–75 mmHg will assure adequate coronary perfusion while limiting myocardial oxygen consumption
- Surgical therapy:
  - Intraaortic balloon pump (IABP): inflates on T wave (diastole) and deflates on P wave (systole)—increases coronary perfusion in diastole and decreases afterload via Venturi effect in systole
  - Ventricular assist devices (VADs): implanted impeller pumps used as bridge to transplant. Not indicated if transplant cannot be performed
  - Venoarterial extracorporeal membrane oxygenation (VA ECMO): used in acute cardiogenic shock as a bridge to resolution of the primary cause or bridge to surgery

Hypovolemic Shock

The initial physiologic response is tachypnea and a decreased pulse pressure.

First response in hypovolemic shock is increase in diastolic blood pressure (BP).

	Class I	Class II	Class III	Class IV
Blood loss (%)	0–15	15–30	30–40	>40
Central nervous system	Slightly anxious	Mildly anxious	Anxious or confused	Confused or lethargic
Pulse (beats/ min)	<100	>100	>120	>140

	Class I	Class II	Class III	Class IV
Blood pressure	Normal	Normal	Decreased	Decreased
Pulse pressure	Normal	Decreased	Decreased	Decreased
Respiratory rate	14–20/min	20–30/min	30–40/min	>35/min
Urine (mL/h)	>30	20–30	5–15	Negligible
Fluid	Crystalloid	Crystalloid	Crystalloid + blood	Crystalloid + blood

Treatment Principles

- Replace the volume losses with equivalent fluid. If bleeding whole blood if is best. Transfuse universal red blood cell (RBC) and plasma in a ratio between 1:1 and 1:2 (plasma to RBC). Transfuse one single donor apheresis or random donor platelet pool for each six units of RBC
- Use balanced electrolyte solutions for insensible, gastrointestinal (GI), and genitourinary losses
- Treat the underlying cause: hemorrhage control, abdominal closure, skin grafting, motility agents, etc.

Distributive Shock

(*Fluid is in the body, but not effective.*) Three main types of shock: neurogenic, septic, and anaphylactic. *All cause decreased* systemic vascular resistance (SVR).

Neurogenic Shock

Vasodilation due to sudden loss of sympathetic nervous tone due to dysfunction or injury of the *proximal* central nervous system, classically the spinal cord. Not to be confused with spinal shock which is muscle flaccidity caused by spinal cord injury.
- Hypotension, commonly bradycardia, decreased inotropy, and temperature dysregulation (warm LE despite hypothermia)
- Loss of sympathetic tone, with preserved parasympathetic function, leading to autonomic vasodilation and instability

- Hypotension mainly from venodilation → increased venous capacitance and lack of venous return (but also arteriolar tone may also be affected)
- Injury to the descending sympathetic tracts usually above T6

VSITE tip: similar self-limiting phenomena occur in vasovagal syncope and spinal anesthesia.

Treatment Principles

- Prevent secondary injury due to hypotension: first use volume to ensure preload
- Add vasopressors with inotropy and chronotropy
- First-line vasopressor is norepinephrine, second-line epinephrine. Phenylephrine will cause reflex bradycardia with worsening cardiac output (CO)
- Bradycardia can be treated with atropine or glycopyrrolate
- *Stop/remove epidural if iatrogenic*

Septic Shock

Life-threatening organ dysfunction caused by a dysregulated response to infection
- **Systemic inflammatory response syndrome (SIRS)** is an exaggerated defense response of the body to a noxious stressor (infection, trauma, surgery, acute inflammation, ischemia or reperfusion, or malignancy, to name a few) to localize and then eliminate the endogenous or exogenous source of the insult
- **SIRS criteria:** two or more of the following criteria
  - Temperature <36°C or >38°C
  - Heart rate (HR) >90 beats/min
  - Respiratory rate (RR) >20 breaths/min or $PaCO_2$ <32 mm Hg
  - White blood cell count >12,000. <4000. or >10% bands
  - Sepsis = SIRS + infection
  - *Septic shock* = sepsis + hypotension despite fluid resuscitation

Sequential organ failure assessment (SOFA) score: best for estimating mortality in sepsis

Organ System	SCORE				
	0	1	2	3	4
Respiratory: PaO_2/FIO_2 ratio	>400	≤400	≤300	≤200^c	≤100
Coagulation: platelets ($\times 10^3$ μ/L)	>150	≤150	≤100	≤50	≤20
Liver: bilirubin (mg/dL)	<1.2	1.2–1.9	2–5.9	6–11.9	>12
Cardiovascular: hypotension	No hypotension	MAP <70 mm Hg	Dop ≤5 or Dob any dose	Dop >5, Epi ≤0.1, or Nor ≤0.1	Dop ≥50, Epi >0.1, or Nor >0.1
Central nervous system: GCS	15	13–14	10–12	6–9	<6
Renal: creatinine (mg/dL) or daily urine output (mL)	<1.2	1.2–1.9	2–3.4	3.5–4.9 or <500	>5 or <200

Dob, Dobutamine; *Dop,* dopamine; *Epi,* epinephrine; *Fio₂,* fraction of inspired oxygen; *GCS,* Glasgow Coma Scale score; *MAP,* mean arterial blood pressure; *Nor,* norepinephrine; *Pao₂,* partial pressure of arterial oxygen.

Mean SOFA	% Mortality
2–3	20
3–4	36
4–5	73
>5	84

quick sequential organ failure assessment (qSOFA): Altered mental status, respiratory rate >22, SBP <100.

Pathophysiology

Dysregulated host response to infection.

- Early phase: activation of the inflammatory cascade, and alterations in hemostasis
  - Proinflammatory: tumor necrosis factor alpha (TNF-α), interleukin-1 beta (IL-1β), and nuclear factor-kappa B (NF-κB)
  - Antiinflammatory cytokines: IL-10
  - Anticoagulant factors: antithrombin III, activated protein C, protein S, and tissue factor pathway inhibitor are decreased → microthrombi → disseminated intravascular coagulation (DIC)
  - Early signs are mental status changes, hyperventilation (respiratory alkalosis), and hypotension
- Later stages: organ failure, immunosuppression, and apoptosis
  - Myocardial suppression can cause a mixed distributive and cardiogenic shock, especially with baseline CHF
  - Gram-negative sepsis
    - Most common organism is *Escherichia coli*
    - Endotoxin (lipopolysaccharide [LPS], lipid A portion) is a potent trigger of TNF-α. TNF activates inflammatory cascade
    - Early gram-negative sepsis: ↓ insulin, ↑ glucose (impaired utilization)
    - Late gram-negative sepsis: ↑ insulin, ↑ glucose (secondary to insulin resistance)

Treatment Principles

Early recognition, resuscitation, antibiotics, and source control are paramount!

- Early goal-directed therapy
  - 30 mL/kg bolus within 3 hours
  - Antibiotics within 1 h of recognition
  - Empiric broad-spectrum antibiotics initially with de-escalation according to culture results
  - Monitor for signs of adequate oxygen delivery: request
    - Serial lactate ± SVCO2 and CVP
    - MAP ≥65 mmHg
    - IVC size and respiratory cycle variation
    - Adequate urine output, mentation, and capillary refill
- Norepinephrine is the first-line vasopressor after volume expansion in shock
- Either epinephrine or vasopressin is second-line therapy
- If ↓ ejection fraction (EF) with euvolemia → consider epinephrine or dobutamine (dobutamine may ↓ SVR)
- Early source control reduces mortality

- Blood glucose goal <180 mg/dL is safer than 110 due to fewer hypoglycemia-induced cardiovascular events

Adrenal Insufficiency in Sepsis

- Inadequate physiologic response to stress of surgery or septic shock
- *VSITE tip: most common cause: withdrawal of exogenous steroid use*
- Common causative medications: propofol, etomidate
- Symptoms: fatigue, and GI complaints, including nausea, vomiting, and diarrhea. Hypotension unresponsive to fluids
- Free cortisol level >44 mcg/24 hours rules out diagnosis, <10 highly suggestive
- Adrenocorticotrophic hormone (ACTH) stimulation test no longer recommended by the Surviving Sepsis Campaign
- Common in liver failure and transplant community
- Indications for treatment: shock unresponsive to volume resuscitation and pressor support
- Treatment: hydrocortisone 200–300 mg/day (usually divided into 50 mg Q6) × 5 days prior to taper
- Fludrocortisone (mineralocorticoid) is not started until dose of hydrocortisone is under 100 mg/day
- Early stoppage may cause rebound shock

Anaphylaxis

Local response: two types of cellular responses to allergens result in mast cell and basophil degranulation that releases histamine, bradykinin, platelet-activating factor, tryptase, and leukotrienes.

1. Hypersensitivity reaction: IgE-mediated activation of mast cells and basophils
   - Causes: food, antimicrobials, neuromuscular blocking agents, blood products, latex, chlorhexidine, insect bites
   - Incidence of anaphylaxis with general anesthesia is 1–2:10,000
2. Anaphylactoid reaction: direct activation of mast cells and basophils
   - Causes: opiates, neuropeptides, intravenous (IV) contrast, compliment products

Disease course: onset is usually immediate but in rare cases can be delayed up to 72 hours.

Three patterns

1. Uniphasic: most common. Peaks at 30–60 minutes and resolves quickly without recurrence.
2. Biphasic: recurrence of the initial event up to 72 hours after, without a second exposure.
3. Protracted: rarely the inflammatory effects last for a number of days/weeks.

Systemic response: inflammatory cell activation results in an oxidative burst and diffuse capillary leak that affects every organ system.

- Skin and mucosa: 85%–90% of cases result in urticaria, flushing, angioedema

- Upper airway: 50%–60% result in oropharyngeal angio-edema, rhinitis, laryngeal edema
- Bronchopulmonary: 45%–50% result in bronchospasm, pulmonary edema, and respiratory failure
- Cardiovascular: 30%–50% result in myocardial depression, coronary vasoconstriction, and peripheral vasodilation resulting in decreased SVR. This can result in ischemia, arrhythmia, cardiac arrest, and a distributive shock
- GI: 25%–30% result in nausea, vomiting, and diarrhea
- Neurologic: confusion, lethargy, syncope
- Urologic: incontinence

Diagnosis
Clinical:
- Acute onset of mucocutaneous involvement with at least one other sign of end-organ dysfunction or
- Hypotension following exposure to a known allergen

Laboratory testing: used only for confirmation but should not preclude treatment
- Serum tryptase: peaks at 60–90 minutes. Detected in serum for <6 hours
- Plasma histamine: only lasts for 60 minutes after onset of symptoms
- Allergy testing: should be performed in all patients after the acute illness has subsided to identify the allergen

Treatment
First-line:
- Epinephrine:
  - Anaphylaxis: 0.3–0.5 mg imtramuscularly (IM) (0.15 mg in children weighing <30 kg). Repeat as needed (PRN) every 5–15 minutes for a maximum of three doses
  - Laryngeal edema: 2.5 mg (2 mL solution) via nebulizer
  - Anaphylactic shock: 5–15 mcg/min infusion
- Glucagon: used in patients receiving beta-blockers which may attenuate the effect of epinephrine. 1–5 mg IV over 5 minutes followed by 5–15 mg/min infusion titrated to response

Second-line:
- Antihistamines: diphenhydramine and ranitidine should be given together for cutaneous symptoms
- Bronchodilators: albuterol nebulizer
- Volume expansion: up to 35% of circulating volume can be lost within 10 minutes in severe reactions
- Corticosteroids: *not indicated* in anaphylaxis

PULMONARY

Tidal volume (VT): volume of gas the lung moves in one normal inspiration and expiration *at rest* total lung capacity (TLC) = Functional vital capacity (FVC) + residual volume (RV).

Vital capacity: volume moved between *maximal* expiration and maximal inspiration.

Functional residual capacity (FRC): total volume left in the lung after normal expiration (FRC = ERV + RV).

Residual volume: volume remaining after maximum expiration (increased in emphysema).

Dead space (VD): volume of air inhaled that does not take part in the gas exchange (airways, alveoli not being perfused) (Fig. 5.2).

Respiratory Failure

Risk factors for respiratory failure
- Emergency surgery, dependent functional status, sepsis, high American Society of Anesthesiologists (ASA) classification, large volume shifts (large blood loss or large

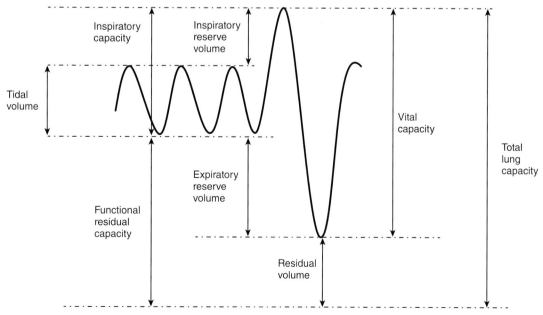

FIG. 5.2 **Lung Volumes**

area of dissection), thoracotomy, inspiratory weakness (phrenic nerve injury, myasthenia gravis, paralytics, ICU deconditioning, etc.)

Types of respiratory failure: hypoxic, hypercapnic, and mixed

1. Hypoxic respiratory failure:
   - Defined as Pao_2 <50–60
   - Extrapulmonary causes: atmospheric (altitude), hypoventilation (pneumothorax, neuromuscular, chest wall mechanical defect such as postburn eschar or flail segment)
   - Pulmonary: ventilation/perfusion mismatch or impaired gas diffusion (acute respiratory distress syndrome [ARDS], PE, restrictive lung disease, fibrosis, pulmonary edema, contusion)
   - Oxygen transport abnormalities: carboxyhemoglobin (carbon monoxide) and methemoglobinemia (nitroglycerin, nitroprusside)
2. Hypercapnic respiratory failure:
   - Defined as: $Paco_2$ >50 with pH <7.35
   - ↓ Minute ventilation (MV) causes hypercapnia
   - $MV = (VT - VD) \times RR$
   - Hypercapnia is caused by a decrease in RR, a decrease in VT, or an increase in VD
   - Causes of increased VD: hypovolemia, low CO, PE, high airway pressures
3. Mixed: most common

Acute Respiratory Distress Syndrome

Pathogenesis

- Most commonly precipitated by a systemic inflammatory response
- Sequestration of activated circulating neutrophils in the lung parenchyma leads to toxic degranulation and a respiratory burst. This causes obliteration of air spaces with inflammatory exudate that first damages pneumocytes and eventually causes pulmonary fibrosis due to progressive deposition of fibrin
- Damage to alveolar cells:
  - Type I pneumocytes: loss of barrier function causing edema and decreased clearance of exudate
  - Type II pneumocytes: loss of surfactant production causing alveolar collapse

Phases of ARDS

- Exudative (acute) phase: damage to pneumocytes with accumulation of interstitial and alveolar edema and inflammation (first 6 days)
- Proliferative (subacute) phase: infiltration of fibroblasts and reestablishment of type II pneumocytes (7–14 days)
- Fibrotic (chronic) phase: predominated by macrophages and mononuclear cells ongoing repair causes deposition of collagen and formation of fibrosis

Diagnosis

Berlin criteria:
- Onset within 1 week of clinical insult
- Pulmonary edema not fully explained by cardiac failure or fluid overload. Pulmonary arterial wedge pressure (PAWP) <18 is indicative of ARDS
- Diffuse bilateral pulmonary infiltrates

Kigali modification: ultrasonography can be used to detect bilateral diffuse edema, and that oxygenation criteria could be met with a pulse oximetric oxygen saturation $(Spo_2):F_{IO_2}$ ratio of ≤315 without the requirement for positive end-expiratory pressure (PEEP). Used in resource-limited settings.

Bronchoalveolar lavage: rarely used; high neutrophil counts and lavage fluid protein: plasma protein >0.7. Degree of ARDS is based on the degree of hypoxia while on a PEEP or continuous positive airway pressure (CPAP) of 5 cm/H_2O.

- Mild—$Pao_2:F_{IO_2}$ = 200–300   Mortality: 27%
- Moderate—$Pao_2:F_{IO_2}$ = 100–200   Mortality: 35%
- Severe—$Pao_2:F_{IO_2}$ = less than 100   Mortality: 45%

(F_{IO_2}, Fraction of inspired oxygen.)

This severity tool is predictive of mortality and duration of mechanical ventilation in survivors.

Prevention

Primary:
- Pneumococcal and influenza vaccination
- Aspiration precautions

Secondary:
- Restrictive resuscitation strategies both of blood products and crystalloid
- Early recognition and treatment of sepsis
- Lung protective ventilation: 6–8 mL/kg of predicted body weight (10 mL/kg during surgery)

Treatment

Noninvasive options:
- High-flow nasal cannula
- CPAP and bilevel positive airway pressure (BiPAP)

Ventilator management:
- Basic principles of mechanical ventilation:
  - ↑ PEEP increases FRC → ↑ oxygenation
  - PEEP ↓ venous return, ↑ pulmonary vascular resistance → decreases CO
  - PEEP ↓ renal perfusion and thus urine output
  - Excessive PEEP ↑ VD due to capillary compression
  - ↑ Rate or volume improves ventilation → ↓ CO_2
  - Wean F_{IO_2} <60% prior to weaning PEEP
  - Pressure support decreases work of breathing but may decrease MV
  - Volume control is the most protective form of ventilation

- Management of ARDS
  - Step 1:
    - Low VT: 6 mL/kg
    - PEEP of 5. Increase incrementally up to a maximum of 18–24
    - Lowest Fio_2 that achieves an SpO_2 of 88–95
    - High PEEP low Fio_2 strategy is generally preferred (refer to the ARDS Network protocol www.ardsnet.org)
  - Step 2:
    - Measure plateau pressure (Ppl)—if >30 cm H_2O, reduce VT by 1 mL/kg until either the Ppl <30 or VT = 4 mL/kg
  - Step 3:
    - Permissive hypercapnia: adjust MV to a goal pH >7.15
  - Step 4: consider alternative treatments
    - Prone position
    - Paralysis
    - ECMO

Physiologic Derangement

Intracranial hypertension:
- Caused by decreased cerebral venous outflow due to increased intrathoracic pressure. This is important to consider early in patients with intracranial hemorrhage as it decreases cerebral perfusion pressure (Monroe-Kellie doctrine)

Increased thoracic/intrapleural pressure:
- Decreased right heart compliance decreases CO, resulting in hypotension and decreased perfusion
- Increased afterload: further reduces CO

Pulmonary shunting can be caused by nitroprusside, nitroglycerine, or nifedipine and manifest as unresponsive hypoxia.

Increasing PEEP improves FRC and increases oxygenation. High PEEP can cause increase in intrathoracic pressure and decrease in RA filling with decrease in CO and decrease in urine output (*main cause of decrease in urine output with increase in PEEP*).

CARDIAC

Stroke volume (SV) = volume expelled by the ventricle in one contraction
$$CO = HR \times SV$$
$$Cardiac\ index\ (C) = CO/BSA$$
$$Mean\ arterial\ pressure: CO \times SVR$$
$$SVR = 80 \times [(MAP - CVP)/CO]$$

CO increases with HR up to 120–130 beats/min, then decreases because the ventricle does not have time to fill.

Preload: volume entering the ventricle creating pressure to stretch it open prior to contraction. This is linearly related to left ventricular end-diastolic pressure (LVEDP) and LV end-diastolic volume (LVEDV).

Atrial kick: increased CO by 20%.

Afterload: pressure the heart has to overcome to eject blood during systole. Is related to SVR. High afterload (high SVR) = ventricle has hard time ejecting blood. Low afterload (low SVR) = easier for ventricle to eject blood.

Starling law: the greater the preload (LVEDV). The greater the SV and with it the EF (right shift on the curve). *But too much right shift (too much preload) can lower EF due to overdistention of the ventricle. This is known as extreme right shift on the Starling curve.*

$$SV = LVEDV - LVESV$$
$$EF = SV/LVEDV$$

Oxygen delivery and consumption:

$$O_2\ delivery = CO \times arterial\ O_2\ content\ (Cao_2) \times 10$$
$$= CO \times [Hg \times 1.34 \times O_2\ arterial\ saturation] \times 10$$
$$O_2\ consumption\ (VO_2) = CO \times (CaO_2 - CvO_2)$$

Normally O_2 consumption is around 25% so the SvO_2 is 75%. CO will increase to keep this ratio constant.

Oxygen dissociation curve:
- Right shift: (oxygen unloading). $\uparrow CO_2$, $\uparrow$temperature, $\downarrow$pH, methemoglobin
- Left shift: (oxygen hoarding) $\downarrow CO_2$, $\downarrow$temperature, $\uparrow$pH, CO poisoning

Mixed venous saturation (SvO_2):
- Elevated SvO_2: shunting blood (septic shock, cirrhosis, arteriovenous [AV] shunt) or decrease extraction (hyperbaric, cyanide toxicity)
- Decrease SvO_2: increased O_2 extraction (malignant hyperthermia) of decreased O_2 delivery (hypoxia, cardiac shock)
- Renal veins have highest SvO_2 because of low O_2 use in kidney
- During hypoxia, and shock blood is shunted to heart and brain
- Drugs
  - Epinephrine: inotropy (beta-1 and beta-2 receptors) at lower doses (<5 mcg/min) and increased SVR (will increase afterload) via alpha-1 and alpha-2 (doses >5 mcg/min)
  - Dobutamine beta-1: inotropy and decreased SVR (will cause hypotension)
  - Milrinone: cAMP phosphodiesterase inhibitor with increased Ca influx into myocardium − Inotropy and pulmonary vasodilation + decreased SVR (will cause hypotension)
  - Vasopressin: (V1 receptors)
  - Nitroprusside: NO-mediated arterial dilation. Cyanide toxicity at high doses for >72 hours. Cyanide binds to cytochrome c in the mitochondria and disrupts electron transmission. Cell cannot use O_2 and therefore SvO_2 is high. Treat with amyl nitrite or sodium nitrite

- Nitroglycerine: Nitric oxide (NO)-mediated vasodilation. Used in MI to decrease wall tension by decreasing preload. High wall tension increases O_2 consumption more than HR
    - Hydralazine: vasodilator. Unknown mechanism
    - Labetalol: alpha-1 blocker (decrease BP) and beta-1 blocker (lower HR)

Cardiac Arrest in Trauma

- Penetrating: right ventricle most commonly injured
- Blunt:
    - Cardiac contusion
    - Cardiac herniation through a rent in the pericardium/diaphragm
- MI:
    - Injury to coronary arteries or
    - Ischemia due to hypovolemic shock
- Obstructive shock: cardiac tamponade, tension pneumothorax, massive hemothorax causes decreased venous return to the heart

Diagnosis

- Tamponade: Beck triad: JVD, muffled heart sounds and hypotension—FAST examination
- Tension pneumothorax: JVD, absent breath sounds unilaterally and hypotension—CXR
- Contusion: normal electrocardiogram (ECG) and troponins together approach 100% negative predictive value

Therapy

Resuscitative thoracotomy
- Indications:
    - Penetrating trauma with a witnessed arrest within 15 minutes of arrival
    - Blunt trauma with a witnessed arrest in the hospital

Postoperative Cardiac Arrest

- Continuation of rate control medications (beta-blockers) perioperatively reduces incidence
- Usually occurs within 48 hours of the operation
- Fluid shifts increase myocardial demand—most prominent when shifting back into the intravascular space around postoperative day 2 or 3
- Increased sympathetic tone increases myocardial oxygen demand.
- Sepsis—prolonged inflammatory response
- Electrolyte imbalances affect inotropy and may cause arrhythmias

Arrhythmias

Risk factors: age, electrolyte disturbances, QT-prolonging medications, PE, sepsis, pericarditis, mediastinitis, cardiac contusion, history of heart failure, coronary artery disease (CAD), or prior cardiac surgery.

Classification

- Tachyarrhythmias:
    - Sinus tachycardia: pain, anxiety, inflammation, hypovolemia, anemia, rebound from stopping medications. Treat underlying cause
    - Atrial fibrillation and flutter: pulmonary edema, hypoxia, hypercarbia, electrolyte disturbances, volume overload, pericarditis, mediastinitis
    - Premature ventricular contraction (PVC): anxiety, decongestants, and antihistamines, ethyl alcohol (ETOH), tobacco, cocaine, hypertension (HTN), CAD, CHF
    - Ventricular fibrillation/flutter: early postoperative MI
- Bradyarrhythmia/heart block:
    - First-degree: PR prolongation >0.2 second
        - Generally, no treatment is necessary
    - Second-degree
        - Mobitz I: functional AV suppression causing gradual PR prolongation with eventual AV block. (Drugs, reversible ischemia)—generally does not progress or need treatment unless hemodynamically unstable.
        - Mobitz II: structural conduction damage causing intermittent nonconducted P waves with the RR interval remaining constant. (Fibrosis, infarction/necrosis)—*requires pacing* as it has a high chance of progression to full block
    - Third-degree: complete AV dissociation (MI or drugs). PP and RR intervals are stable
        - Can cause severe bradycardia or sudden cardiac death.
        - Requires pacing

Treatment Principles

- Tachyarrhythmias:
    - If hemodynamically unstable → defibrillate ventricular tachycardia/fibrillation/and use synchronized cardioversion for narrow complex (supraventricular tachycardia [SVT], atrial fibrillation//flutter)
    - Avoid beta-blockers in heart failure and chronic obstructive pulmonary disease
    - Adenosine is for paroxysmal SVT, but amiodarone works as well
    - Atrial fibrillation >48 hours—consider anticoagulation depending on the patient's CHADS score
- Bradyarrhythmias:
    - Atropine, glycopyrrolate
    - Beta-agonists: epinephrine or dopamine
    - Transcutaneous pacing for hemodynamic instability

Pulseless electrical activity:
- Feel for pulse. If no pulse but electrical activity, start CPR. Give Epi. Give volume
- Figure out the cause
  - 6 H's (hypoxia, hypovolemia, hyper-or hypokalemia, hypothermia, hypoglycemia)
  - 5 T's (tamponade, tension pneumothorax, thrombosis, PE, toxins, and tables)

ECG findings:
ST elevation: acute MI
ST depression: active ischemia
Q waves: old MI

Heart Failure

Left-sided:
- Two types—reduced EF versus diastolic dysfunction (SV is low)
- Pulmonary edema in acute exacerbation
- Elevated LA = left atrial pressure (PCWP)

Right-sided:
- Elevated CVP
- Hepatic, renal dysfunction due to venous outflow obstruction
- LE edema
- In acute exacerbation, often left-sided failure causes right-sided dysfunction and subsequent systemic venous congestion

Treatment Principles

- Beta-blockers:
  - Improve long-term outcomes
  - Avoid in acute CHF exacerbation
  - Use with care perioperatively in case of hypotension
- Angiotensin-converting enzyme inhibitors:
  - Improve long-term mortality and are first-line therapy
  - Avoid in acute renal dysfunction and perioperatively until fluid shifts resolve
- Diuretics:
  - Symptoms of fluid overload
  - Avoid in the immediate perioperative period though may be helpful to resolve postoperative fluid overload

RENAL

Acute Renal Failure: abrupt dysfunction of previously normal or stable kidney function

Pathophysiology

- **Prenal:** decreased renal perfusion (hypovolemia, reduced effective circulating volume, abdominal compartment

syndrome, calcineurin, and renin-angiotensin-aldosterone system [RAAS] inhibitors potentiate it)
- **Intrinsic:** parenchymal injury (glomerular disease, vascular disease, tubulointerstitial nephritis [TIN], acute tubular necrosis [ATN], acute cortical necrosis)
- **Postrenal:** obstruction of urine outflow (ureteric or urethral obstruction/injury, nephrolithiasis, pyelonephritis, retroperitoneal fibrosis, neoplasia)
- 25% of the body's CO per minute
- Low O_2 extraction—renal vein O_2 saturation <90%
- Acute kidney injury (AKI) after cardiac surgery has been associated with increased mortality
- Sepsis and major abdominal surgery with hypotension are the most common causes
- Positive fluid balance is an independent risk factor for increased mortality in ATN
- Acute interstitial nephritis (AIN) is a hypersensitivity reaction: medications, infections, and autoimmune. Medications include antibiotics, anticonvulsants, nonsteroidal antiinflammatory drugs (NSAIDs), and proton pump inhibitors. AIN causes sterile pyuria, hematuria, eosinophilia, and fever
- Unilateral obstruction often does not result in oliguria

Classification

KDIGO Definition of Acute Kidney Injury

Stage	Creatinine Criteria	Urine Output Criteria
1	Cr 1.5–1.9 times baseline, or Cr increase >0.3 mg/dL	<0.5 mL/kg/h × 6–12 h
2	Cr 2–2.9 × baseline	<0.5 mL/kg/h for >12 h
3	Cr >3 × baseline, or Cr >4 mg/dL, or initiation of dialysis	<0.3 mL/kg/h for >24 h, or anuria >2 h

Patients are staged based on the single most concerning feature.
KDIGO, Kidney Disease Improving Global Outcomes.

- The clinical utility of an early AKI diagnosis is to optimize hemodynamics, promptly treat the underlying cause, and avoid potential nephrotoxins

Diagnosis and Treatment Principles

Optimize hemodynamics, avoid nephrotoxins, and treat the underlying cause.

$$FENa(\%) = \frac{U_{Na} \times S_{Cr}}{S_{Na} \times UCr} \times 100,$$

(U_{Na}, urine sodium; S_{Cr}, serum creatinine)
FENa <1% = prerenal   FENa >3% = parenchymal

	Prerenal	Intrinsic	Postrenal
Urine osmolality (mOsm/kg)	>500	<350	<350
Urine sodium (mEq/L)	<20	>40	Variable
FENa	<1%	>2%	>3%
FEUrea	<35%	50%–65%	
BUN:Cr ratio	>20	<15	Variable

FENa, Fractional excretion of sodium; *FEUrea*, fractional excretion of urea; *BUN/Cr*, blood urea nitrogen:creatinine

Postoperative Oliguria

First: rule out postrenal—flush Foley, renal ultrasound (US) looking for hydronephrosis, KUB looking for stone

Second: make sure the patient is euvolemic

Third: calculate FENa and resolve electrolyte disturbances—treat underlying cause

Fourth: dialysis if indicated

Indications for dialysis: *AEIOU*

Acidosis: pH <7.1 or if contributing to shock refractory to vasopressors

Electrolytes: K >6.5 or rapidly rising

Intoxicants: clearance of methanol, ethylene glycol, lithium

Overload: volume overload

Uremia: only when causing pericarditis or encephalopathy

Drugs toxic to kidneys:

- NSAIDs: inhibit prostaglandins and cause renal arterial vasoconstriction
- Aminoglycosides: directly injure renal tubules
- Contrast dye: the intravascular injection of a contrast drug causes rapid renal vasodilatation followed by long vasoconstriction, with a decrease in renal blood flow (RBF)
- Myoglobin: has a direct toxic effect on proximal renal tubules. Excessive myoglobin can interact with Tamm-Horsfall protein in the distal tubules and result in cast formation and tubular obstruction

Indication for dialysis:

- Fluid overload
- Increased K, Mg, PO$_4$, or BUN
- Metabolic acidosis
- Uremic encephalopathy

DERANGEMENTS OF ELECTROLYTES

Anatomy and Physiology

Total body water (TBW) (50%–60% body weight in kg)

- Extracellular fluids (1/3 of TBW) = plasma (5% TBW) + interstitial fluids (15% TBW)
- Intracellular fluids (2/3 TBW)
- Free water deficit = ([sodium]/140) − 1 × TBW

Sodium being the principal cation in extracellular fluids and potassium being the principal cation of the intracellular fluids.

Electrolyte Imbalances: Sign/Symptoms, Evaluation, and Treatment

- Sodium (136–145 mEq/L)
  - Hypernatremia (>145 mEq/L)
    - Signs/symptoms: thirst, dryness, skin turgor, reduced blood volume, and pressure
    - Cause: electrolytes are ingested or retained without corresponding amounts of water *or* water is lost faster than electrolytes. For example, diabetes
    - Treatment: ingestion of water or infusion of hypotonic solution
      - Rapid correction may lead to cerebral edema
      - Correction of acute and chronic: less than 8 mEq/L in 24 hours
  - Hyponatremia (<136 mEq/L): severe <120
    - Signs/symptoms: disturbed central nervous system (CNS) function, confusion, hallucinations, convulsions, coma, headaches, seizures, death in severe cases
    - Causes: excess extracellular free water relative to sodium concentration; for example, syndrome of inappropriate antidiuretic hormone secretion (SIADH)
    - Treatment: diuretic or infusion of salt solution
      - Rapid correction may lead to central pontine myelinolysis
        - Acute: 6–12 mEq/L/24 hours
        - Chronic: less than 8 mEq/L in 24 hours
- Potassium (3.5–5.5 mEq/L)
  - Hyperkalemia (>5.5 mEq/L)
    - Signs/symptoms: severe cardiac arrhythmias; muscle spasms
    - ECG, most commonly manifesting as peaked T waves and bradycardia
    - Causes: renal failure, use of diuretics, chronic acidosis
    - Treatment:
      - Temporary: intravenous calcium gluconate. IV insulin with glucose or beta-2 agonist by nebulizer
      - Total body potassium can be lowered with sodium polystyrene sulfonate (Kayexalate) and dietary restrictions
  - Hypokalemia (<5.5 mEq/L)
    - ECG: demonstrates prolonged QT interval (649 ms), ST-segment depression, prominent U waves
- Calcium (8.5–10.5 mg/dL)
  - Hypercalcemia (>10.5 mg/dL)
    - ECG shortening of the QT interval
  - Hypocalcemia (<8.5 mg<dL))

- Symptoms of hypocalcemia most commonly include paresthesia, muscle spasms, cramps, tetany, circumoral numbness, and seizures
- Hypocalcemia after large blood transfusion is caused by the anticoagulant citrate in the bag that donated blood
- ECG hypocalcemia causes QTc prolongation primarily by prolonging the ST segment. T wave is typically left unchanged. Torsades de pointes may occur, but is much less common than with hypokalemia or hypomagnesemia
- Magnesium (1.4–2.1 mEq/L)
  - Hypomagnesemia is associated with QT interval prolongation and an increased risk of ventricular arrhythmias including torsades de pointes
    - Correction of serum magnesium to >1.0 mmol/L, with concurrent correction of serum potassium to >4.0 mmol/L, is often effective in suppressing ectopy and supraventricular tachyarrhythmias
    - A rapid IV bols of magnesium 2 g is a standard emergency treatment for torsade's de pointes
- Phosphate (1.8–2.9 mEq/L)
  - Hypophosphatemia (<1.8 mEq/L)
    - Muscle weakness including diaphragm. May make weaning from ventilator difficult
    - Phosphate should be checked when initiating nutrition in patients at risk for refeeding syndrome. Patients with diabetic ketoacidosis or hyperosmolar hyperglycemic nonketotic syndrome (HHNS). Patients on continuous renal replacement therapy (CRRT)

HEPATIC FAILURE AND HEPATORENAL SYNDROME

Acute liver failure (ALF) is massive hepatocyte necrosis resulting in international normalized ratio (INR) >1.5, transaminitis, hyperbilirubinemia, encephalopathy, no history of cirrhosis/liver disease, and <26 weeks since symptoms onset.

Etiology of Acute Liver Failure

- Acetaminophen (most common in the United States)—transaminitis often >3500 IU/L
- Idiosyncratic drug-induced liver injury—common culprits include antibiotics, NSAIDs, and anticonvulsants
- Viral hepatitis (most common in developing countries)—hepatitis A, B, D, and E uncommonly B, herpes simplex virus, varicella zoster, Epstein-Barr virus, and cytomegalovirus
- Autoimmune hepatitis: confirmed by testing for antinuclear antibody (ANA), anti-smooth muscle antibody (SMA), and anti-liver microsomal antibody

- Hypoperfusion (1%–2.5%) leading to ischemia (1%–2.5%): CHF/sepsis, Budd-Chiari syndrome, and arterial constriction (cocaine, methamphetamines)
- Acute fatty liver of pregnancy/HELLP: hemolysis, elevated transaminitis, and thrombocytopenia
- Toxins: *Aminita phalloides* mushroom and carbon tetrachloride

Hepatorenal Syndrome

- Defined as splanchnic vasodilation in the presence of cirrhosis and portal HTN, which decreases renal artery perfusion. Consequently, renal dysfunction is propagated by the renin-angiotensin system and sympathetic nervous systems, which further reduces glomerular filtration rate (GFR)
- Hepatorenal syndrome—diagnosis of exclusion: increasing serum creatinine, oliguria, sodium excretion in urine <10 mEq/L, no improvement in GFR with administration of fluids and withholding of diuretic, urine RBC <50 cells/high-power field, and protein excretion <500 mg/day
  - Type 1 hepatorenal syndrome: Cr doubles within 2 weeks and reaches at least 2.5 mg/dL
  - Type 2 hepatorenal syndrome: ascites and kidney impairment that does respond to diuresis
- Treatment for hepatorenal syndrome: improvement with octreotide or terlipressin: causing splanchnic vasoconstriction and midodrine: causing systemic vasoconstriction. Otherwise CRRT/hemodialysis (HD)

Outcomes

- 45% of patients with ALF will recover without need for transplant with acetaminophen overdose the most likely to recover spontaneously
- 25% of patients with ALF will require transplantation; of those undergoing transplantation, 20% mortality at 1 year
- Patient with hepatorenal syndrome often die within weeks of onset, many of those who receive liver transplant will achieve complete recovery

ABDOMINAL COMPARTMENT SYNDROME

Normal intraabdominal pressure (IAP): 5–7 (corresponds to CVP and RA pressure)
Intraabdominal hypertension (IAH):
- Grade I: 12–15
- Grade II: 16–20
- Grade III: 21–25
- Grade IV: >25
Abdominal compartment syndrome: *IAP > 20 mm Hg with new-onset organ dysfunction*

Risk Factors

- Trauma (especially with large-volume resuscitation), open AAA repair, peritonitis, pancreatitis, ascites, intraabdominal or retroperitoneal hemorrhage, mesenteric ischemia (especially after reperfusion), bowel obstruction or ileus, pregnancy

Physiologic Derangement

Increased intraabdominal pressures:
- Compression of the IVC: decreases preload, resulting in decreased CO and increased venous pressures that further reduces end-organ perfusion.
- Compression of the renal veins: results in decreased renal perfusion, decreased urine output, and a prerenal AKI.
- Compression of visceral venous outflow can cause hepatic dysfunction and intestinal ischemia.

Diagnosis

A high suspicion is necessary in patients who are at risk.

Bladder pressure: measured at end-expiration in supine position, preferably with the patient paralyzed

Apart from the measurement (IAP > 20 mm Hg) there must be concurrent signs of *new* end-organ dysfunction

Management

Nonoperative

- Reduce intraabdominal volume: gastric decompression, paracentesis, diuresis in volume overload
- Decrease abdominal tone: management of pain/agitation/delirium, paralysis

Operative

- Decompressive laparotomy: open the entire length of the linea alba using a temporary closure device such as a vacuum-assisted device, Bogota bag
- Delayed primary closure: when primary closure of the anterior fascia cannot be achieved without causing IAH. This can be tested by monitoring vent pressures while approximating facia using clamps. Bowel coverage is accomplished using skin flaps, skin grafts, absorbable mesh, or bioprosthetic

SPINAL CORD ISCHEMIA (SCI) AFTER ARTERIAL REPAIR

- SCI deficit is classified as paraplegia (defined as minimal function) and paraparesis (patient had motion against resistance or gravity across all joints)

- The location of the deficit is limited to the lower body musculature
- The deficit can be left-side predominant, right-side predominant, or symmetric
- The deficit is predominantly motor with proximal muscles affected more
- Sensory deficits, neuropathic pain, and bowel/bladder dysfunction have also been observed
- Neuroprotective therapy, pharmacologic elevation of the BP, and the institution of spinal drainage to increase the spinal cord perfusion pressure

BRAIN DEATH

Uniform Determination of Death Act (UDDA) in 1981: "irreversible cessation of all functions of the entire brain, including the brain stem."

Criteria:
1. Known cause and presence of coma
2. Absence of brainstem reflexes
3. Apnea

Each state has specific statutes for the determination of brain death, including algorithms to test for it. It is thus important to understand local hospital policies.

Brain Death Examination

- Unresponsive to painful stimuli to the extremity, trunk, and face
- No spontaneous respiration
- Absent brainstem reflexes (oculovestibular, corneal, pupillary, oculocephalic, cough, and gag)
- The patient may still have deep tendon reflexes with brain death

Apnea Test

- Step 1: the patient is oxygenated via a catheter placed at the carina with oxygen at 8 L/min. The patient's PCO_2 should be normal before the start of the test
- Step 2: disconnect the patient from ventilator for 10 minutes
  - A CO_2 >60 mm Hg or increase by 20 mm Hg without spontaneous respiration is considered a positive test for apnea (meets brain death criteria)
  - Criteria to abort testing:
    - Hypotension (SBP <90 mm Hg)
    - Hypoxia (SpO_2 <85%)

Conditions That Limit Appropriate Testing

- Cervical spinal cord injury
- Ocular injury

- Therapeutic hypothermia (must wait 72 h after return of spontaneous circulation [ROSC])
- Sedative drug administration

Confirmatory Tests if the Examination or Apnea Test Is Not Possible

- Nuclear perfusion scan, CTA, cerebral angiography, electroencephalography, transcranial Doppler ultrasonography

DELIRIUM

Postoperative delirium is associated with an increase in mortality, length of stay, cost of care.

Epidemiology

- Delirium: causes are multifactorial, prevention is best. Risk can be calculated
  - Mnemonic: I CAN STOP A DELIRIUM
    - **I**mpairment in activities
    - **C**NS pathology (cerebrovascular accident [CVA], dementia, depression)
    - **A**lcohol/drug withdrawal, age >70 years
    - **N**ew tethers (restraints, Foley, IV, telemetry)
    - **S**urgery
    - **T**rauma, toxins
    - **O**piate use
    - **P**ain (uncontrolled), polypharmacy
      - Benzodiazepines, anticholinergics, antihistamines, antipsychotics
    - **A**nesthesia (general)
    - **D**eficiencies (B_{12}, thiamine, folate, niacin) drugs
    - **E**ndocrine (hyper/hypo), environmental
    - **L**ow oxygen
    - **I**nfection
    - **R**etention urine
    - **I**CU admission
    - **U**ndernutrition, underhydration
    - **M**etabolic (renal/hepatic/electrolytes/glucose)

Risk Factors

- Delirium risk calculator: 0 pt.: 2%; 1–2 pt.: 11%; >3 pt.: 50%
  - Age >70 years (1 pt.)
  - Alcohol abuse (1 pt.)
  - Cognitive impairment (1 pt.)

- Abnormal electrolytes Na <130 or >150 mol/L, K <3.0 or >6 mol/L, or glucose <60 or >300 mg/dL (1 pt.)
- Poor function status (1 pt.)
- Type of surgery (noncardiac thoracic surgery or open AAA) (1 pt.)

Sign/Symptoms of Disease

- Delirium: *acute onset*: changes in sleep-wake cycle, hallucination, delusions, mood changes, autonomic dysregulation
  - Three types
    - Hyperactive: restless and agitated
    - Hypoactive: lethargic/apathetic: high mortality
    - Mixed
- Diagnostic evaluation: various scoring systems
  - Delirium
    - CAM score, Four A's Test (Arousal, Attention, Abbreviated mental test, and Acute changes)
- Treatment (best treatment is prevention)
  - Preventing delirium remember: A DELIRIUM
    - **A**cute stressors: treat infection, metabolic disorders, other acute illness
    - **D**eficits: provide hearing aids, glasses, dentures, O_2, nutrition, electrolytes, prevent constipation, urinary retention
    - **E**nvironmental factors: stimulation control, lighting, orientation, familiar surroundings, noise reduction, uninterrupted sleep
    - **L**ongevity: age >70 years
    - **I**mpaired function: early mobilization, physical therapy (PT)/occupational therapy (OT)
    - **R**estraints
    - **U**ncomfortable: pain control (multimodal: acetaminophen, gabapentin, low-dose opioid)
    - **M**edications: especially benzodiazepines
      - Benzodiazepines should only be used in sedative-hypnotic withdrawal
  - Antipsychotics are not indicated in hypoactive delirium
  - Hyperactive delirium
    - Use of antipsychotics should be smallest dose for shortest length of time
      - Sedative effects: haloperidol > risperidone > olanzapine > quetiapine
      - Extrapyramidal symptoms: haloperidol < risperidone < olanzapine < quetiapine

ETOH withdrawal:
- HTN, tachycardia, mental status changes, seizures
- Treatment: thiamine, B_{12}, Mg, K
- Lorazepam (Ativan) for agitation, clonidine for HTN

CHAPTER 6

Aortic Dissection

BRIAN M. SHEEHAN, MD and JORDAN R. STERN, MD

EPIDEMIOLOGY

- Acute aortic dissection occurs in 2.9–3.5 per 100,000 person-years[1,2]
- 2:1 male:female ratio[3]
- Type A dissections: 67%; type B dissections: 33%[4]
- 93% of dissections occur in individuals 40 years of age or older[3]
- Predicted mortality of acute type A dissection: 30% at 24 hours and 57% at 30 days; type B: 10% and 28%[5]

RISK FACTORS

Genetic/Congenital

- Connective tissue disorders (Marfan syndrome, Ehlers-Danlos syndrome, Loeys-Dietz syndrome), bicuspid aortic valve, congenital malformations (coarctation, tetralogy of Fallot, Turner syndrome)

Medical/Acquired

- Hypertension, atherosclerosis, inflammatory/infectious conditions (giant cell arteritis, syphilis), pregnancy, previous aortic surgery

Modifiable

- Smoking, use of cocaine/methamphetamine and other illicit drugs[6]

TEMPORAL CLASSIFICATION

- Hyperacute: <24 hours, acute: 1–14 days, subacute: 15–90 days, chronic: >90 days[7]

ANATOMY OF ARTERIAL WALL

- Tunica intima: endothelium, internal elastic lamina
- Tunica media: smooth muscle cells, external elastic lamina
- Tunica adventitia: vasa vasorum, connective tissue[8]

PATHOPHYSIOLOGY OF DISSECTION

- Intimal tear and degeneration of media layer of aorta[9]
- Initial tears tend to occur in areas with high shear stress[10]:
  - Type A—right lateral wall of ascending aorta
  - Type B—ligamentum arteriosum
  - Progressive separation of intima and media leads to propagation between layers,[10] development of true and false lumens, separated by a septum (Fig. 6.1)
- Direction of propagation depends on pressure gradients between true and false lumens but typically antegrade[8]

DEFINITIONS

- False lumen: blood-filled space between intima and adventitia

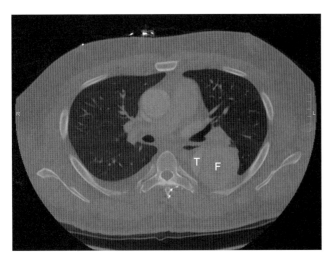

FIGURE 6.1 Progressive separation of intima and media leads to development of true *(T)* and false *(F)* lumens, separated by a septum.

- Fenestration: tear in intima allowing for flow of blood between true and false lumens. May also be referred to as "entry tear" for primary fenestration or "reentry tear" for secondary fenestration
- Septum: intimal flap which separates true and false lumens[8]

ACUTE PRESENTATION

- Abrupt onset of chest, back, or abdominal pain ("tearing" sensation); refractory hypertension; blood pressure discrepancy; neurologic deficits; diastolic murmur; pulse deficit[11,12]
- End-organ dysfunction—may include:
  - Type A: aortic valvular insufficiency, tamponade, neurologic deficits, myocardial ischemia
  - Type B: spinal cord ischemia, renal failure, mesenteric ischemia, limb ischemia[8,11]

ANATOMIC CLASSIFICATION SYSTEMS

- Generally described by the location of the primary entry tear/fenestration

DeBakey Classification

- Type I: dissection begins in the ascending aorta and continues into the descending and/or abdominal aorta for a varying distance
- Type II: dissection begins in, and is confined to, the descending aorta
- Type IIIa: dissection begins in the descending aorta (i.e., distal to left subclavian) and does not extend into abdominal aorta
- Type IIIb: dissection begins in the descending aorta and extends for a varying distance into the abdominal aorta[13]

Stanford Classification

- Type A: dissection begins proximal to left subclavian artery
- Type B: dissection begins distal to left subclavian artery[14]

CLASSIFICATION BY CLINICAL STATUS

- Traditionally divided into complicated (rupture, malperfusion) vs. uncomplicated
- Newer classification system proposed by both The Society for Vascular Surgery (SVS) and The Society of Thoracic Surgeons (STS) with an intermediate category of high-risk features (Table 6.1)

This system also includes an anatomic descriptor based on the location of the primary entry tear, as well as proximal/distal extent of dissection:
- Type A: dissection begins in the ascending aorta to include the brachiocephalic artery (zone 0)
- Type B: dissection begins distal to the brachiocephalic artery (zone $\geq$1)
- Type I: unidentified/indeterminate primary entry tear location

SVS nomenclature: type $(A,B,I)_{proximal\ extent\ (0-12),\ distal\ extent\ (0-12)}$

For example, type A_9, type B_{3-10}. If primary entry tear is in zone $\geq$1 but there is retrograde, ascending involvement, this would be classified as type B (e.g., type B_{0-9})[7]

TABLE 6.1   SVS/STS Reporting Standards for Type B Aortic Dissection

Uncomplicated	High-Risk Features	Complicated
No high-risk features	Refractory pain	Rupture
No malperfusion	Refractory hypertension	Malperfusion
No rupture	Bloody pleural effusion	
	Aortic diameter $\geq$40 mm	
	Radiographic only malperfusion	
	Readmission	
	Entry tear on lesser curve	
	False lumen diameter $\geq$22 mm	

Adapted from Lombardi JV, Hughes GC, Appoo JJ, et al. Society for Vascular Surgery (SVS) and Society of Thoracic Surgeons (STS) reporting standards for type B aortic dissections. *J Vasc Surg.* 2020;71(3):723-747.

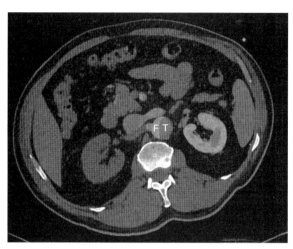

FIGURE 6.2 Propagation of dissection flap can result in malperfusion of branch arteries and their respective vascular territories. *F,* False; *T,* true.

MALPERFUSION

- Propagation of dissection flap can result in malperfusion of branch arteries and their respective vascular territories (renovisceral, extremity, spinal cord) (Fig. 6.2)
  - Dynamic obstruction: compressed aortic true lumen with movement of the dissection flap during cardiac cycle leads to intermittent obstruction of flow
  - Static obstruction: aortic true lumen cannot accommodate enough blood flow to vascular branch territory due to:
    - Flap results in a mechanical obstruction, blocking the ostium of the true lumen
    - Dissection propagates into branch vessel, resulting in narrowing of the true lumen; false lumen may thrombose[15]

INITIAL EVALUATION AND DIAGNOSIS

- Electrocardiogram (ECG): can help differentiate etiology of chest pain[11]
- Chest x-ray: findings (e.g., widened mediastinum) typically nonspecific and not diagnostic[8,11]
- Labs: may provide early indication of malperfusion (elevated creatinine, lactic acidosis, elevated troponin I)
- Computed tomography angiography (CTA): gold standard. CTA of chest, abdomen, and pelvis is sensitive and specific. ECG-gated CTA reduces motion artifacts, particularly of ascending aorta, arch, and proximal descending aorta
  - Provides anatomic detail necessary to aid in planning repair:
    Identification and measurement of true/false lumen (Fig. 6.1)
    - True lumen identification: may need to look at axial, coronal, sagittal views to establish path of

continuity with undissected aorta. Generally smaller and more rounded[16]
- False lumen identification: generally larger, beak sign within false lumen, intraluminal thrombus, absence of outer wall calcification[16]
  - Location of entry tear and other fenestrations
  - Identify rupture or radiologic malperfusion (diminished or absent contrast opacification)
  - Access planning including evaluation of extension into iliofemoral system[17]
- Magnetic resonance angiography (MRA): limited utility in acute dissection due to examination time, expense. High sensitivity and specificity. May be useful for evaluating chronic dissection patients with renal insufficiency[18]
- Echocardiography: transthoracic exam can be performed in emergency department but has low sensitivity and specificity. Transesophageal echocardiogram (TEE) is more sensitive and specific, but requires anesthesia; can be performed in the operating room during intervention, operator dependent
- Digital subtraction angiography: no longer performed as diagnostic tool, but useful during repair

INITIAL MANAGEMENT

Medical/pharmacologic:
- Pain control
- Heart rate/impulse control <60 beats/min: first line—intravenous beta-blocker; second line—nondihydropyridine calcium channel blocker
- Systolic blood pressure control/permissive hypotension <120 mmHg: if still elevated after rate control, nitroprusside and angiotensin-converting enzyme (ACE) inhibitor can be used[19]

INDICATIONS FOR INTERVENTION

Type A Dissection

- Repair is mandatory to protect coronaries from dissection (open surgery)
- Replacement of arch depends on several factors: location of tear, involvement of head vessels, prior surgery, additional pathology, connective tissue disorders, etc.
- Options for repair include ascending repair only, hemiarch replacement, total arch with elephant trunk (extension of graft into descending) or frozen elephant trunk (thoracic endovascular aortic repair [TEVAR] into descending aorta)[20,21]

Complicated Type B Dissection

- Absolute indications: rupture, spinal cord ischemia, visceral or limb malperfusion. Relative indications include SVS/STS "high-risk" features noted earlier

- Intervention generally not performed for uncomplicated type B dissection, though controversial
- If no urgent need to revascularize, outcomes are best if intervention delayed until subacute phase[22]
- Open repair of type B dissection now uncommon due to high morbidity/mortality
  - Open options include: open fenestration, resection/interposition, debranching

ENDOVASCULAR INTERVENTION FOR ACUTE TYPE B DISSECTION

- Managed primarily with TEVAR—placement of stent graft (Fig. 6.3)
- Short-term goals of intervention: occlude primary entry tear, preferentially pressurize true lumen, improve visceral/spinal/limb perfusion or seal rupture
- Long-term goals of intervention: promote positive remodeling, prevent late aneurysmal degeneration[23]
  - Access can be percutaneous or open
  - Need approximately 2 cm of proximal seal[8]
  - Hydrophilic wire will easily cross through fenestrations, curved catheter used without a wire more likely to stay in true lumen
  - Super stiff wire (double-curved Lunderquist) placed in ascending aorta
- Digital subtraction angiography—provides information on flow, end-organ perfusion. May be difficult to discern true vs. false lumen location
- Intravascular ultrasound (IVUS)—facilitates detailed examination of true lumen, false lumen, and branch vessels

Identification of major and minor fenestrations. Evaluate mobility of the dissection flap and dynamic obstruction. Ensure wire path is entirely in true lumen prior to deploying TEVAR. Accurate diameter measurements

ADJUNCTIVE PROCEDURES

- PETTICOAT: Provisional ExTension To Induce COmplete ATtachment. Uncovered, self-expanding stent deployed at the distal end of thoracic endograft to promote aortic remodeling. Can be deployed through visceral aorta due to open-cell design[24]
- STABILISE: Stent-Assisted Balloon-Induced intimal disruption of reLamination in aortic dISsection rEpair. Used in conjunction with PETTICOAT, balloon angioplasty of entire stented aorta to rupture the septum and occlude the false lumen.[25,26] May carry risk of aortic rupture, particularly in acute phase[27]
- Percutaneous fenestration: creates communication between true and false lumens at the level of malperfused branch, equalizes pressure between true and false lumens. Generally reserved for when TEVAR is not possible or there is inadequate expansion of true lumen[28]
- Visceral stenting: for static obstruction that does not resolve with TEVAR or other adjuncts. May require traversing fenestration from true lumen into target vessel. Self-expanding stent preferred[29]
- Cervical debranching: may be required if <2-cm landing zone and graft deployed proximal to zone 3
  - Left subclavian artery provides spinal cord collaterals via vertebral artery, other pathways

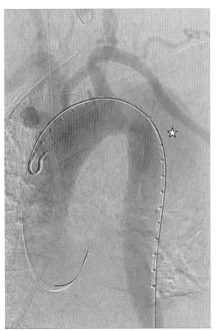
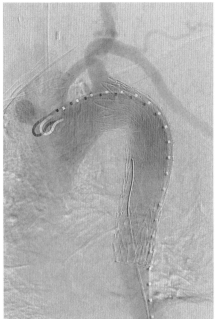

FIGURE 6.3   Thoracic endovascular aortic repair (TEVAR) placement of stent graft. (☆) Star represents the filling of the false lumen prior to placement of the endograft

- Indications for left subclavian artery revascularization: dominant left vertebral artery or vertebral that ends in terminal posterior inferior cerebellar artery, arm ischemia, previous left internal mammary coronary artery bypass[30]

MAJOR RISKS OF ENDOVASCULAR INTERVENTION

- Stroke: risk factors include proximal intervention, arch manipulation, severe arch atherosclerosis[31,32]
- Spinal cord ischemia: risk increases with >20 cm of aortic coverage
  - Highest-risk area is coverage within 5 cm proximal to celiac axis (T9–12)
    - Coverage of artery of Adamkiewicz
  - Other important collateral pathways include: hypogastric arteries, subclavian arteries[33]
- Retrograde type A dissection: risk factors include graft oversizing, bare-metal configuration, and balloon molding[34]
- Stent graft–induced new entry (SINE) tears: risk factors include stent-graft oversizing. Can repressurize false lumen[35]
- Entry flow into the false lumen following endovascular repair:
  - Type IA—proximal perigraft entry flow
  - Type IB—distal perigraft entry flow (including SINE)
  - Type II—retrograde flow through arch vessel branches, bronchial or intercostal arteries
  - Type R—antegrade entry flow from true to false lumen through distal fenestrations[7]

CHRONIC TYPE B DISSECTION

- Long-term sequelae primarily related to persistent false lumen perfusion, can lead to late aneurysmal degeneration

Indications for intervention:

- Recurrence of symptoms or malperfusion
- Aneurysmal dilation >55 mm
- Increase in diameter >4 mm/y[19]

Surgical Intervention for Chronic Dissection:

- Open repair
  - Replace aneurysmal segment, may require formal open thoracoabdominal repair
- Endovascular intervention
  - Septum becomes thick and fibrotic, making intervention difficult
  - Seal fenestrations and depressurization of false lumen
  - May require advanced maneuvers for management of septum

FOLLOW-UP

- Patients require long-term follow-up and medical optimization due to sequelae of chronic dissection
- Triple-phase CTA at 30 days, 3 months, 6 months, and then annually for at least 5 years[7]

REFERENCES

1. Clouse WD, Hallett JW Jr, Schaff HV, et al. Acute aortic dissection: population-based incidence compared with degenerative aortic aneurysm rupture. *Mayo Clin Proc.* 2004;79:176-180.
2. Mészáros I, Mórocz J, Szlávi J, et al. Epidemiology and clinicopathology of aortic dissection. *Chest.* 2000;117:1271-1278.
3. Januzzi JL, Isselbacher EM, Fattori R, et al. Characterizing the young patient with aortic dissection: results from the International Registry of Aortic Dissection (IRAD). *J Am Coll Cardiol.* 2004;43:665-669.
4. Pape LA, Awais M, Woznicki EM, et al. Presentation, diagnosis, and outcomes of acute aortic dissection: 17-year trends from the International Registry of Acute Aortic Dissection. *J Am Coll Cardiol.* 2015;66:350-358.
5. Melvinsdottir IH, Lund SH, Agnarsson BA, Sigvaldason K, Gudbjartsson T, Geirsson A. The incidence and mortality of acute thoracic aortic dissection: results from a whole nation study. *Eur J Cardiothorac Surg.* 2016;50:1111-1117.
6. Braverman AC. Acute aortic dissection: clinician update. *Circulation.* 2010;122:184-188.
7. Lombardi JV, Hughes GC, Appoo JJ, et al. Society for Vascular Surgery (SVS) and Society of Thoracic Surgeons (STS) reporting standards for type B aortic dissections. *J Vasc Surg.* 2020; 71:723-747.
8. Sidawy AN, Perler BA. *Rutherford's Vascular Surgery and Endovascular Therapy.* 9th ed. Elsevier; 2019.
9. Patel PD, Arora RR. Pathophysiology, diagnosis, and management of aortic dissection. *Ther Adv Cardiovasc Dis.* 2008;2: 439-468.
10. Gawinecka J, Schönrath F, von Eckardstein A. Acute aortic dissection: pathogenesis, risk factors and diagnosis. *Swiss Med Wkly.* 2017;147:w14489.
11. Levy D, Goyal A, Grigorova Y, Farci F, Le JK. Aortic dissection. In: *StatPearls.* StatPearls Publishing; 2021.
12. Hiratzka LF, Bakris GL, Beckman JA, et al. 2010 ACCF/AHA/ AATS/ACR/ASA/SCA/SCAI/SIR/STS/SVM guidelines for the diagnosis and management of patients with thoracic aortic disease: a report of the American College of Cardiology Foundation/American Heart Association Task Force on Practice

Guidelines, American Association for Thoracic Surgery, American College of Radiology, American Stroke Association, Society of Cardiovascular Anesthesiologists, Society for Cardiovascular Angiography and Interventions, Society of Interventional Radiology, Society of Thoracic Surgeons, and Society for Vascular Medicine. *Circulation.* 2010;121:e266-e369.

13. Debakey ME, Henly WS, Cooley DA, Morris GC Jr, Crawford ES, Beall AC Jr. Surgical management of dissecting aneurysms of the aorta. *J Thorac Cardiovasc Surg.* 1965;49:130-149.

14. Daily PO, Trueblood HW, Stinson EB, Wuerflein RD, Shumway NE. Management of acute aortic dissections. *Ann Thorac Surg.* 1970;10:237-247.

15. Williams DM, Lee DY, Hamilton BH, et al. The dissected aorta: percutaneous treatment of ischemic complications—principles and results. *J Vasc Interv Radiol.* 1997;8:605-625.

16. LePage MA, Quint LE, Sonnad SS, Deeb GM, Williams DM. Aortic dissection: CT features that distinguish true lumen from false lumen. *AJR Am J Roentgenol.* 2001;177:207-211.

17. Roos JE, Willmann JK, Weishaupt D, Lachat M, Marincek B, Hilfiker PR. Thoracic aorta: motion artifact reduction with retrospective and prospective electrocardiography-assisted multi-detector row CT. *Radiology.* 2002;222:271-277.

18. Sentz A. The role of CTA, MRA, and sonography in aortic dissection. *J Diagn Med Sonogr.* 2015;31:235-240.

19. Fattori R, Cao P, De Rango P, et al. Interdisciplinary expert consensus document on management of type B aortic dissection. *J Am Coll Cardiol.* 2013;61:1661-1678.

20. Hussain ST, Svensson LG. Surgical techniques in type A dissection. *Ann Cardiothorac Surg.* 2016;5:233-235.

21. Çekmecioğlu D, Köksoy C, Coselli J. The frozen elephant trunk technique in acute DeBakey type I aortic dissection. *Turk J Thorac Cardiovasc Surg.* 2020;28:411-418.

22. Torrent DJ, McFarland GE, Wang G, et al. Timing of thoracic endovascular aortic repair for uncomplicated acute type B aortic dissection and the association with complications. *J Vasc Surg.* 2021;73:826-835.

23. Nienaber CA, Rousseau H, Eggebrecht H, et al. Randomized comparison of strategies for type B aortic dissection: the INvestigation of STEnt Grafts in Aortic Dissection (INSTEAD) trial. *Circulation.* 2009;120:2519-2528.

24. Antonello M, Squizzato F, Colacchio C, Taglialavoro J, Grego F, Piazza M. The PETTICOAT technique for complicated acute Stanford type B aortic dissection using a tapered self-expanding nitinol device as distal uncovered stent. *Ann Vasc Surg.* 2017;42:308-316.

25. Hofferberth SC, Newcomb AE, Yii MY, et al. Combined proximal stent grafting plus distal bare metal stenting for management of aortic dissection: superior to standard endovascular repair? *J Thorac Cardiovasc Surg.* 2012;144:956-962.

26. Lopes A, Melo RG, Gomes ML, et al. Aortic dissection repair using the STABILISE technique associated with arch procedures: report of two cases. *EJVES Short Rep.* 2019;42:26-30.

27. Melissano G, Bertoglio L, Rinaldi E, et al. Satisfactory short-term outcomes of the STABILISE technique for type B aortic dissection. *J Vasc Surg.* 2018;68:966-975.

28. Iwakoshi S, Watkins CA, Ogawa Y, et al. "Cheese wire" fenestration of dissection intimal flap to facilitate thoracic endovascular aortic repair in chronic dissection. *J Vasc Interv Radiol.* 2020;31:150-154.e2.

29. Barnes DM, Williams DM, Dasika NL, et al. A single-center experience treating renal malperfusion after aortic dissection with central aortic fenestration and renal artery stenting. *J Vasc Surg.* 2008;47:903-910.e3.

30. Matsumura JS, Lee WA, Mitchell RS, et al. The Society for Vascular Surgery Practice Guidelines: management of the left subclavian artery with thoracic endovascular aortic repair. *J Vasc Surg.* 2009;50:1155-1158.

31. Gutsche JT, Cheung AT, McGarvey ML, et al. Risk factors for perioperative stroke after thoracic endovascular aortic repair. *Ann Thorac Surg.* 2007;84:1195-1200; discussion 1200.

32. Feezor RJ, Martin TD, Hess PJ, et al. Risk factors for perioperative stroke during thoracic endovascular aortic repairs (TEVAR). *J Endovasc Ther.* 2007;14:568-573.

33. Wortmann M, Böckler D, Geisbüsch P. Perioperative cerebrospinal fluid drainage for the prevention of spinal ischemia after endovascular aortic repair. *Gefasschirurgie.* 2017;22:35-40.

34. Chen Y, Zhang S, Liu L, Lu Q, Zhang T, Jing Z. Retrograde type A aortic dissection after thoracic endovascular aortic repair: a systematic review and meta-analysis. *J Am Heart Assoc.* 2017; 6:e004649.

35. Burdess A, Mani K, Tegler G, Wanhainen A. Stent-graft induced new entry tears after type B aortic dissection: how to treat and how to prevent? *J Cardiovasc Surg (Torino).* 2018;59:789-796.

CHAPTER 7

Thoracic Aorta Aneurysmal Disease— Open Repair

BRANDI MIZE, MD, MONSERRAT P. ESCOBAR, MD, and
GUILLERMO A. ESCOBAR, MD

CHAPTER OUTLINE

ANATOMY AND CLASSIFICATIONS

Crawford TAAA Classification

In 1991 Stanley Crawford[1] proposed *four* types of thoracoab-dominal aortic aneurysms (TAAAs) based on the differences in their open surgical approach and expected complications.

They remain a useful predictor for operative risk (even with modern repair).

Extent I, distal to the left subclavian artery (SCA) to above the renal arteries.

Extent II, distal to the left SCA to below the renal arteries.

Extent III, from the sixth intercostal (IC) space to the renal arteries.

Extent IV, visceral abdominal aorta from the diaphragm down *(only one that can be repaired without entering the chest via incision in the 10th IC space).*

Extent V (addition by Safi), beginning below the sixth inter-costal space to just above the renal arteries.[2]

- Incidence of TAAAs by Crawford classification type: extent I (9%), extent II (23%), extent III (15%), and *extent IV (52%)*[3]

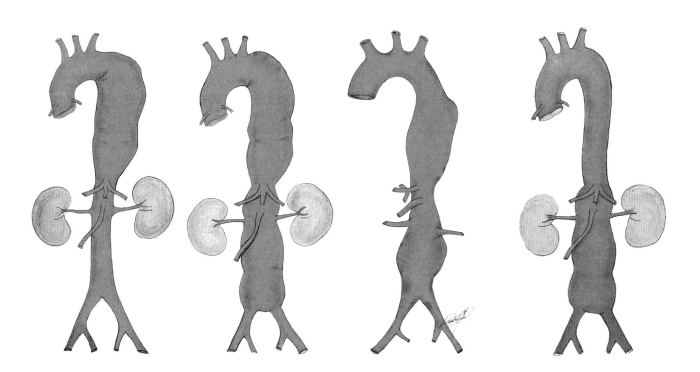

51

> **VSITE Tip:** Most common TAAA is Extent IV. Most common causes for Extent II are Dissection > Marfan. Highest risk for paraplegia and death is Extent II.

Aortic Zones

Use of zones, designed to standardize reporting in thoracic endovascular aortic repair (TEVAR) treatment to better evaluate outcomes and approaches according to coverage, but has become standard to describe thoracic aortic aneurysms (TAAs) and dissections as well. Important to know.[4]

> **VSITE Tip:** In the arch each zone (0–2) includes the next branch vessel, and again from the celiac to renals (Zone 6–8). Ensure you learn the regions commonly involved in trauma, dissection, and highest risk for spinal cord injury (SCI).

Zone 0: ascending aorta and innominate artery (IA)
Zone 1: distal to the IA and left common carotid artery (LCCA)
Zone 2: distal to the LCCA and left SCA
Zone 3: curve of the descending thoracic aorta (DTA) (<2 cm from left SCA) or until "straight"
Zone 4: ~2 cm distal to the SCA extending to proximal, "straight" top half of thoracic aorta (to ~T6)
Zone 5: distal half of DTA proximal to CA
Zone 6: CA until the superior mesenteric artery (SMA)
Zone 7: SMA until the renals
Zone 8: perirenal aorta (all aorta with renals)
Zone 9: infrarenal aorta (including inferior mesenteric artery [IMA])
Zone 10: common iliac arteries
Zone 11: external iliac arteries[2]

> **VSITE Tip:** Most common site for traumatic aortic injury is Zone II–III, highest risk for SCI is intervening in Zone 5, highest risk of stroke is working in zones 0–2, deep hypothermic arrest is needed for open repair of Zone 0–1.

Aortic Arch Types

Aortic arches were classified in 2008 to predict the risk/complexity of supraaortic procedures (originally transfemoral carotid stenting by S. Madhwal et al.[5]).
Type I: origin of the IA is almost even with the top of the arch

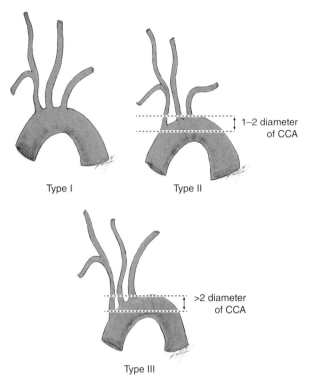

Type I   Type II

1–2 diameter of CCA

Type III

>2 diameter of CCA

CCA, common carotid artery

Type II: origin of the IA is lower off the arch by a distance <2 times the diameter of the CCA
Type III: origin of the IA is lower off the arch by a distance >2 times the diameter of the CCA

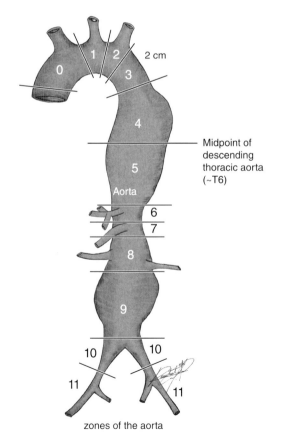

zones of the aorta

EPIDEMIOLOGY AND CLASSIFICATION OF TAAA

- TAAAs differ from TAAs because TAAAs involve the infradiaphragmatic aorta, and generally require entry into the chest and/or division of the diaphragm to repair open
  - Both start distal to the left SCA
- Specific epidemiology is hard to obtain because TAAs and TAAAs are often (erroneously) reported as one entity (possibly due to their lower incidence)
- TAAAs are less common than all other aortic aneurysmal diseases (root, ascending, arch, or abdominal)—less than 1000 TAAAs are repaired each year compared with nearly 100,000 AAA repairs[6,7]
- TAAAs account for approximately 10% of all thoracic aneurysms[8]
- Population-based studies have found between 5.9 and 10.4 new TAAs per 100,000 person-years[3,8-11]
- Familial clusters are common with 20% of patients with TAA having a first-degree relative with a TAA
- However, incidence of thoracic aortic disease among men and women increased to nearly 16.3 and 9.1 per 100,000 per year, respectively[12]
- Male:female ratio 1.7:1, with males diagnosed between 63 and 65 years of age compared with 75–77 years of age in women[8]
  - Rupture rate may appear falsely equivalent among genders when assessing patients who present alive upon rupture. However, when comparing all patients with TAAA rupture, including deceased patients, nearly 75% are female[10,12]
- Inheritable syndromes associated with TAA and TAAA include Marfan syndrome (*FBN1* mutation spontaneous in ~25% of cases), Turner syndrome, type IV Ehlers-Danlos syndrome (*CPL3A1* for type 1 collagen—autosomal dominant and usually spontaneous), and polycystic kidney disease
- Nearly one-quarter of TAA will have concomitant AAA → incidental findings of either warrant assessment of the entire aorta for aneurysmal disease[8]

RISK FACTORS FOR TAAA DEVELOPMENT, RUPTURE, AND DEATH

- Risk factors are similar to other aneurysms: hypertension, smoking, atherosclerosis leading to medial degeneration (~80%)
- Most common single risk factor is chronic aortic dissection (approximately 15%–20%)
- "Connective tissue" and inherited disorders: Marfan syndrome, Ehlers-Danlos syndrome, Loeys-Dietz syndrome (LDS), Turner syndrome, and others like familial thoracic and aortic aneurysm and dissection (TAAD)
  - Note: Marfan syndrome and LDS will almost always have an ascending aortic aneurysm, and LDS is less

common to be a primary TAAA, but rather follows aortic dissection
- Risk of TAAA rupture is based upon maximal aortic diameter:
  - <5 cm is <1% annually
  - >6-cm risk ranges from 37.5% to 62.5% per year[13]
  - Untreated 6.0-cm TAAs have a 5-year survival of 54% and a risk of dying of ~12% per year
  - TAA grows an average of 0.10 cm/y (0.07 cm for the ascending aorta and 0.19 cm for the DTA)
- Risk factors for rupture: chronic obstructive pulmonary disease (COPD) (odds ratio [OR] 3.6), increasing age per decade (OR 2.6), pain (OR 2.3), descending aortic and abdominal aortic diameter/per centimeter increase (OR 1.9 and OR 1.5, respectively)[14]
  - Hypertension (HTN)—specifically diastolic (usually >100 mm Hg)—is commonly associated with increased risk of growth and rupture

Open Repair[15]

Mortality in the largest series is <9% (all extents). The average is ~15%.

Most common complication is respiratory (>20%)

Risk Factors for Death

Combined two or more: age >79, emergency, congestive heart failure (CHF), diabetes mellitus (DM) = 50% mortality.

Postoperative acute renal failure (especially in dialysis) = up to 70% mortality and increases risk of neurological, gastrointestinal (GI), and respiratory complications (and sepsis syndrome). One-third of acute renal failure stay on dialysis. Highest risk is after emergencies and preoperative chronic kidney disease (CKD).

Spinal Cord Ischemia

Largest series' (over >100 cases reported) incidence average <5% for all extents. This is much higher in other series (likely average in experienced centers 10%–15%).

The lowest risk is in extent IV and the highest is in extent II. *The highest risk is in surgery excluding flow between T8 and T12 (especially extent II).*

Adjuncts to prevent/treat SCI include: mean arterial pressure (MAP) >90, spinal drain with goal intraspinal pressure (ISP) 10 ± 5 cm H$_2$O (range according to symptoms of ischemia), reattachment of large/poor flow intercostals (either in an island attached via fenestration of the main graft or a side branch), lowering core temperature to 32°C–34°C during clamp, left-heart bypass during clamp, spinal cooling, intravenous steroids (pre- or postoperative), deep hypothermic arrest, and naloxone infusions. Largest-volume centers routinely use left-heart bypass, core cooling, spinal drainage, and intercostal reimplantation.[16,17]

REPAIR TYPES/TECHNIQUES

- "Clamp and sew": oldest method and largely replaced by other approaches. Aorta is clamped proximally and distally and depends on speedy anastomosis. Preferred for type I. Visceral branches are reimplanted in groups using island (Corell) patches of aneurysmal tissue. Downside: highest overall risk of organ ischemia and SCI. Islands become aneurysmal over time (especially in patients with genetic syndromes). Long ischemia time to the last organ/patch reperfused
- "Pick off": left heart bypass (or other adjunct—see next column) continuously perfuses the viscera as the clamp is moved down. Each visceral vessel is individually connected end-to-end to a branch of a thoracoabdominal aortic graft. Best to avoid late patch aneurysm. Ischemia to organs is the shortest and similar
- Ballard: only for extent III or IV TAAA. A bifurcated end-to-side aortic graft has two additional grafts added. An end-to-side anastomosis is done off the normal, proximal aorta. The pick-off technique to each visceral branch follows. Then end-to-end anastomosis of the aneurysmal aorta is done with a separate tube graft. Benefits: no need for an extracorporeal pump, but minimal visceral ischemia. Downside: only for extent III or IV TAAA, one extra anastomosis[18,19]
- Debranching: hybrid approach. four visceral vessels gain flow from the iliacs (or unaffected abdominal aorta/graft) via long grafts in a retrograde manner and a TEVAR is done to exclude the TAAA. Benefit: avoids entry to the chest and no aortic cross-clamp. Low mortality overall, especially in low-risk patients (as low as ~3%) and low SCI (~6%). Not very useful for extent II, still has pulmonary complications, TEVAR needed[20]

REFERENCES

1. Crawford ES, Coselli JS. Thoracoabdominal aneurysm surgery. *Semin Thorac Cardiovasc Surg*. 1991;3:300-322.
2. Juvonen T, Ergin MA, Galla JD, et al. Prospective study of the natural history of thoracic aortic aneurysms. *Ann Thorac Surg*. 1997;63:1533-1545.
3. Johansson G, Swedenborg J. Little impact of elective surgery on the incidence and mortality of ruptured aortic aneurysms. *Eur J Vasc Surg*. 1994;8:489-493.
4. Upchurch GR Jr, Escobar GA, Azizzadeh A, et al. Society for Vascular Surgery clinical practice guidelines of thoracic endovascular aortic repair for descending thoracic aortic aneurysms. *J Vasc Surg*. 2021;73(1S):55S-83S.
5. Madhwal S, Rajagopal V, Bhatt DL, Bajzer CT, Whitlow P, Kapadia SR. Predictors of difficult carotid stenting determined by aortic arch angiography. *J Invasive Cardiol*. 2008;20(5):200-204.
6. Escobar GA, Upchurch GR Jr. Management of thoracoabdominal aortic aneurysms. *Curr Probl Surg*. 2011;48(2):70-133.
7. Cowan JA Jr, Dimick JB, Henke PK, Huber TS, Stanley JC, Upchurch GR Jr. Surgical treatment of intact thoracoabdominal aortic aneurysm in the United States: hospital and surgeon volume-related outcomes. *J Vasc Surg*. 2003;37:1169-1174.
8. Cowan JA Jr, Dimick JB, Henke PK, Rectenwald J, Stanley JC, Upchurch GR Jr. Epidemiology of aortic aneurysm repair in the United States from 1993 to 2003. *Ann N Y Acad Sci*. 2006;1085:1-10.
9. Bickerstaff LK, Pairolero PC, Hollier LH, Melton LJ, Van Peenen HJ, Cherry KJ. Thoracic aortic aneurysms: a population-based study. *Surgery*. 1982;92(6):1103-1108.
10. Clouse WD, Hallett JW, Schaff HV, Gayari MM, Ilstrup DM, Melton LJ. Improved prognosis of thoracic aortic aneurysms: a population-based study. *JAMA*. 1998;280:1926-1929.
11. Johansson G, Markstrom U, Swedenborg J. Ruptured thoracic aortic aneurysms: a study of incidence and mortality rates. *J Vasc Surg*. 1995;21:985-988.
12. Hansen PA, Richards JM, Tambyraja AL, Khan LR, Chalmers RTA. Natural history of thoracoabdominal aneurysm in high-risk patients. *Eur J Vasc Endovasc Surg*. 2010;39:266-270.
13. Olsson C, Thelin S, Ståhle E, Ekbom A, Granath F. Thoracic aortic aneurysm and dissection increasing prevalence and improved outcomes reported in a nationwide population-based study of more than 14000 cases from 1987 to 2002. *Circulation*. 2006;114:2611-2618.
14. Kim JB, Kim K, Lindsay ME, et al. Risk of rupture or dissection in descending thoracic aortic aneurysm. *Circulation*. 2015;132:1620-1629.
15. Moulakakis KG, Karaolanis G, Antonopoulos CN, et al. Open repair of thoracoabdominal aortic aneurysms in experienced centers. *J Vasc Surg*. 2018;68(2):634-645.e12.
16. LeMaire SA, Price MD, Green SY, Zarda S, Coselli JS. Results of open thoracoabdominal aortic aneurysm repair. *Ann Cardiothorac Surg*. 2012;1(3):286-292.
17. Estrera AL, Sandhu HK, Charlton-Ouw KM, et al. A quarter century of organ protection in open thoracoabdominal repair. *Ann Surg*. 2015;262(4):660-668.
18. Ballard JL. Thoracoabdominal aortic aneurysm repair: historical review and description of a re-engineered technique. *Perspect Vasc Surg Endovasc Ther*. 2005;17(3):207-215.
19. Ballard JL. Thoracoabdominal aortic aneurysm repair with sequential visceral perfusion: a technical note. *Ann Vasc Surg*. 1999;13(2):216-221.
20. Escobar GA, Oderich GS, Farber MA, et al. Results of the North American Complex Abdominal Aortic Debranching (NACAAD) Registry. *Circulation*. 2022;146(15):1149-1158.

CHAPTER 8

Thoracic Aortic Aneurysmal Disease Endo

BENJAMIN JAY PEARCE, MD, FACS, and JACOB WEBER, MD

CHAPTER OUTLINE

INDICATIONS FOR THORACIC ENDOVASCULAR AORTIC REPAIR (TEVAR)

- Thoracic aortic aneurysms, aortic trauma, penetrating aortic ulcer/intramural hematoma, aortic dissection, congenital aortic anomalies
- No randomized trials, but several observational studies demonstrate benefits to endovascular approach over open[1]
  - Less surgical stress intraoperatively
  - Fewer cardiovascular complications postoperatively
  - Improved 30-day mortality
  - Decreased spinal cord injury
  - Decreased hospital length of stay

THORACIC AORTIC ANEURYSMS

- Multiple trials have demonstrated noninferiority of TEVAR versus open surgical repair
  - International controlled clinical trial of thoracic endovascular aneurysm repair with the Zenith TX2 endovascular graft (Cook Medical) 1-year results: 230 patients received Zenith endograft for thoracic aneurysms with 30-day survival rate of 98% versus 94% in open ($P <$ .01, noninferiority). Patients also had decreased postoperative cardiovascular and pulmonary adverse complications (no change in neurologic events). One-year follow-up identified aneurysm growth in 7.1%, endoleak in 3.9%, and migration in 2.8%[2]
- Results of endovascular treatment with the Gore TAG device (Gore & Associates) at 5 years compared with open repair of thoracic aortic aneurysms: 140 TAG patients versus 94 open controls. TAG patients at 5 years had decreased aneurysm-related mortality (2.8% vs. 11.7%) but no difference in all-cause mortality (68% vs. 67%). Major adverse events decreased in the endo group at 5 years (57.9% vs. 78.7%)[3]

BLUNT THORACIC AORTIC INJURY

- (See also, trauma chapter.)
- Common in high-speed deceleration injuries, most common at ligamentum arteriosum
- Aortic dissection/aortic intramural hematoma/penetrating ulcer
- Aortoesophageal fistula (malignancy, aneurysm, stent graft)
- TEVAR as a temporizing measure prior to open repair

CONGENITAL ANOMALIES

- Aberrant right subclavian with dysphagia lusoria or associated Kommerell diverticulum
- Right-sided aortic arch with Kommerell diverticulum at left subclavian origin
- Coarctation of aorta

ANATOMIC CONSIDERATIONS

- Size/health of access vessels (consider conduits)
- Iliac arteries should have minimal calcification (especially anterior) and tortuosity. Table 8.1 lists current US Food and Drug Administration (FDA)-approved devices

TABLE 8.1   Current Food and Drug Administration–Approved Devices for Access Requirements

Manufacturer	Device	Sheath Sizes	Minimum Iliac Diameters (mm)	Graft Diameters (mm)	Intended Treatment Diameters (mm)	Length of Seal IFU (mm)
Gore	cTAG	18–24 Fr (ID)	6.8–9.1	21–45	16–42	20
Terumo	Relay	22–26 Fr (OD)	NL	22–46	19–42	15–25 (proximal), 25–30 (distal)
Terumo	Relay Pro	19–23 Fr (OD)	NL	22–46	19–42	22–30 (proximal), 25–30 (distal)
Cook	Zenith Alpha	16–20 Fr (OD)	NL	18–46	15–42	20
Cook	Zenith TX2	20–22 Fr (OD)	NL	28–42	20–38	20
Medtronic	Valiant	22–25 Fr (OD)	NL	22–46	18–44	20

Fr, French; *ID*, inner diameter; *IFU*, instruction for use; *NL*, not listed in IFU; *OD*, outer diameter.

- Adequate seal zone for TEVAR on proximal and distal ends of endograft without sacrifice of critical branch vessels
  - Instruction for use (IFU) most approved devices require a 2-cm segment of normal diameter aorta to achieve a seal (proximal and distal)
  - Branch technology for arch vessels currently in trial only
  - Seal zone should be free of atheroma or severe calcification
  - Landing in healthy aorta is the single strongest predictor of freedom from retrograde type A dissection and need for reintervention
  - Appropriate to land in zone 2 to achieve adequate seal
  - Intentional coverage of celiac artery generally well tolerated to achieve distal seal (Fig. 8.1A–B)
  - Evaluation of patency of gastroduodenal artery (GDA) or prior foregut surgery before planned coverage
  - Increased incidence of spinal cord ischemia (SCI) in this cohort likely due to increased length of coverage and likely coverage of artery of Adamkiewicz

PREOPERATIVE EVALUATION

- Computed tomography angiography (CTA) chest, abdomen, and pelvis gold standard
- Abdomen/pelvis computed tomography (CT) critical for all patients considering TEVAR to evaluate access vessels for both size and quality
- Determine length and diameter of seal zones for proximal and distal
- Calculate total length of coverage necessary to seal adequately
- Calculate degree of obliquity and cranial/caudal tilt to remove parallax (Fig. 8.2), especially when landing close to internal carotid arteries (can be done automatically on most three-dimensional imaging software)

- Deployment of first graft distally if tapering is required with two pieces
- Majority of endografts can seal if native aorta in seal zone is between 18 and 42 mm
  - 9%–20% oversizing is recommended
  - 15%–20% oversizing in aneurysm cases
- Dissection/trauma/intramural hematoma cases should attempt to oversize no more than 10% to decrease risk of retrograde dissection
- Careful evaluation of zones of TEVAR deployment and aortic arch configuration (Fig. 8.3)[4]

VARIATIONS OF AORTIC ARCH BRANCHING

Variations in the origin of the aortic arch branches. (A) and (B) represent the majority of anomalies found in the general population (Fig. 8.4).

(A) Common origin of the left common carotid artery and brachiocephalic artery (bovine arch). Represents 73% of all branch variations.

(B) Origin of the left common carotid from the mid- to upper brachiocephalic artery. Represents 22% of all branch variations.

(C) Common carotid trunk giving origin to the left subclavian artery (LSCA).

(D) Common carotid trunk, independent from both subclavian arteries.

(E) Left and right brachiocephalic arteries.

(F) Single arch vessel (brachiocephalic artery) originates from the left common carotid and left subclavian arteries.

(G) Aberrant takeoff of the right subclavian artery from the left and passing behind the aortic arch vessels. With this anomaly, dilation of the proximal subclavian can occur and is termed a Kommerell diverticulum.[5,6]

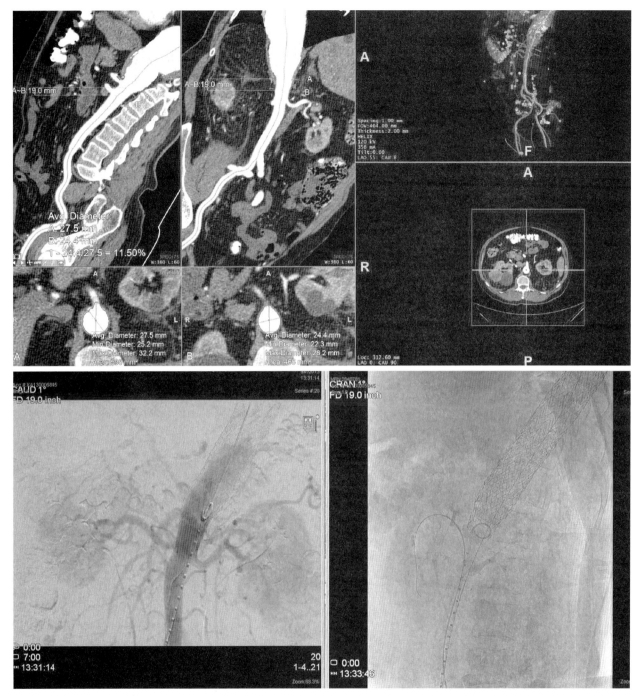

FIG. 8.1   (A) Three-dimensional rendering demonstrating additional 2-cm distal seal with coverage of celiac artery. (B) Intraoperative images of the same patient demonstrate adequate seal with celiac coverage; note parallax on anteroposterior (AP) view but clear salvage of superior mesenteric artery with catheter in place on lateral view.

INTRAOPERATIVE TECHNICAL CONSIDERATIONS

- Femoral cutdown versus percutaneous access to bilateral groins
  - Percutaneous is acceptable if access vessel is free of anterior wall calcium, adequate length of common femoral artery accessible below inguinal ligament/above femoral bifurcation, and is greater than the outer diameter (OD) of the device sheath
- Intravascular ultrasound (IVUS) is not indicated in all TEVAR for aneurysm, but can yield critical information about the quality/size of access iliac vessels
- Gantry/image intensifier (II) should be adjusted to remove all parallax

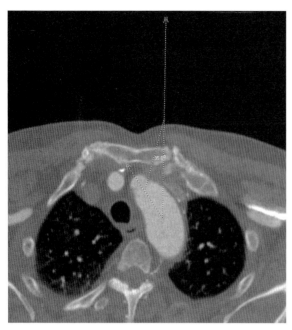

FIG. 8.2   Base of left common carotid artery is at a 35-degree angle from vertical axis, and thus left anterior oblique of 65 degrees will account for parallax.

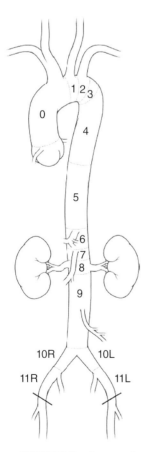

FIG. 8.3   **Zones of TEVAR Deployment and Aortic Arch Configuration**

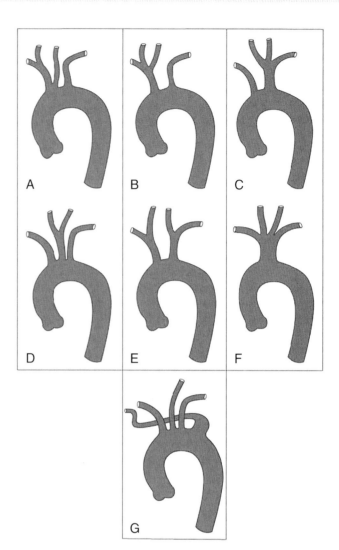

FIG. 8.4   **Variations of Aortic Arch Branching (Reproduced with permission from Uflacker R.** *Atlas of Vascular Anatomy: An Angiographic Approach.* 2nd ed. Lippincott Williams & Wilkins; 2007. Copyright © 2007, Lippincott Williams & Wilkins.)

- Consider placing patient in "surrender" position to allow for full 90 degrees of C-arm rotation to image steep arch angles or origin of abdominal visceral branches
- Consider permissive hypotension/atropine dosing/intentional overpacing to decrease mean arterial pressure (MAP) prior to proximal device deployment to increase accuracy of proximal deployment
- Use of *compliant* balloon in seal and overlap zones after deployment in *aneurysm* cases
- Controversy exists with balloon molding of endograft in nonaneurysm pathology but most recommend against this to decrease incidence of retrograde type A aortic dissection (RTAD)
- Completion angiography to ensure branch vessel patency, presence of endoleak, patency of access vessels

COMPLICATIONS/OUTCOMES

- Mortality 2%–3% electively
- Emergent TEVAR (dissection, rupture) has higher mortality at 30 days at 23% versus 6.2% elective in National Surgical Quality Improvement Program (NSQIP) study[7]
  - Mortality was 5.7% at 30 days and 15.6% at 1 year (endo) versus 8.3% at 30 days and 15.8% at 1 year (open) with *P* = .2/.9. *4.3% of endo and 7.5% of open patients had SCI* (*P* = .08). Strongest risk factor remained extent of disease
- Retrograde dissection after TEVAR most lethal complication
  - Metaanalysis of 8969 patients. RTAD seen in 2.5% of patients, 37.1% mortality percentage in those in which it occurred. Risk associated with hypertension (HTN), previous vascular surgery. Risk was higher in patients with acute dissection
- Aortobronchial or aortopulmonary fistulas—usually related to compression of aerodigestive structure secondary to endoleak causing sac expansion or continued pressurization of aneurysm

Access Site Complications

- 12% complication rate
- Risk factors: female gender, arterial-brachial indices (ABIs), average/minimal iliac diameters, iliac morphology[8]

Spinal Cord Ischemia

- Risk between 3% and 11%
- Spinal blood flow predominately from anterior and posterior spinal arteries, which are branches of vertebral arteries
- Largest radicular artery supplying collateral flow to spinal cord is the artery of Adamkiewicz, which has a variable origin from intercostal vessels between T9 and T12 in 75% of patients
- TEVAR has "lower rate" of SCI than open operation
- Risk factors for SCI are extent of coverage, perioperative hypotension, procedure duration, occluded hypogastric arteries, coverage of LSCA, intrabdominal aortic aneurysm, or prior infrarenal aortic repair

Cerebrovascular Accident (CVA)

- Patients are at risk of embolic strokes due to proximity of carotid arteries and vertebral arteries to the area of stent graft deployment, wire/catheter manipulation, and air/thrombus within endograft packaging
  - Stroke risk was 4.1% overall. Stroke risk was lower if LSA was not covered (3.2%) versus if it was covered

after revascularization (5.3%) or covered without revascularization (8%)[9]

Extremity Ischemia

- Ischemia is infrequent but Society for Vascular Surgery (SVS) guidelines recommend revascularization of LSCA in patients undergoing elective repairs requiring landing in zone 2

Postimplantation Syndrome

- Leukocytosis, fever, elevation of C-reactive protein (CRP)
- Due to endothelial activation by the prosthetic (worse with Dacron grafts)
- Development of uni-/bilateral pleural effusions is common

Endoleak

- Broad incidence between 3.9% and 15.3%
- Type II endoleak most common at the LSA

Graft Migration

- 1%–2.8% annual percentage
- Increased risk including device oversizing, tortuosity of seal zone

Acute Kidney Injury

- Independent predictors of acute kidney injury (AKI) included preoperative depressed estimated glomerular filtration rate, extent of thoracoabdominal repair, and postoperative transfusion
- <15% of TEVAR experience some degree of AKI
  - Any kidney injury associated with worse long-term survival

LUMBAR DRAINS (LDs)

Indication for Preoperatively Placed LDs

- Prior infrarenal repair (12.5% vs. 1.2% risk of spinal cord injury) (place reference here)
- Presence of abdominal aortic aneurysm (AAA)
- Hypogastric artery occlusion
- Planned LSCA coverage without revascularization
- Coverage of >20 cm of thoracic aorta[10]
- Staged repair in patients in whom extensive spinal cord coverage will be required helps to reduce the incidence of SCI

- Median time between operations was 5 months (minimum 1). SCI in the staged group was 11% versus 37.5% (P = .03). All neurologic injuries in the staged group were temporary[11]
- Spinal drainage decreases pressure in the subarachnoid space

  Spinal cord perfusion pressure = MAP − cerebrospinal fluid (CSF) pressure
- LD can rescue patients with delayed onset of neurologic deficits

LEFT SUBCLAVIAN REVASCULARIZATION

- Approximately 40% of TEVARs require coverage of left subclavian artery (LSCA) for appropriate seal
- Risk of stroke (CVA) and SCI are the two major neurologic complications observed with TEVAR
- Risk of both increased with zone 2 TEVAR
- Risk of both increased with zone 2 TEVAR if LSCA not revascularized
- The LSCA gives rise to the left vertebral artery which supplies the anterior spinal artery. It also gives rise to the left internal mammary artery which supplies intercostal branches
- Left subclavian coverage without revascularization leads to a fourfold increased risk of SCI[12]
- In elective TEVAR, coverage of the LSCA should be preceded by carotid subclavian revascularization to reduce risk of stroke, SCI, and upper extremity ischemia
- In patients without high-risk features for SCI (see earlier sections) elective revascularization did not significantly reduce neurologic complications or mortality
  - Five studies of 444 patients receiving TEVAR with revascularization versus 717 without. No difference in stroke (P = .15), SCI (P = .09), or mortality (P = .56)[13]
  - Retrospective review of 394 TAA treated with TEVAR and 180 were revascularized. Predictors of SCI included emergent operations, renal failure, HTN, and number of stents placed. Revascularization was not protective for SCI or CVA[14]

Absolute Indication for Revascularization With TEVAR

- Patients with dominant left vertebral artery (or hypoplastic right vertebral)
- Incomplete circle of Willis
- Left internal mammary to coronary bypass graft (CABG)
- Functioning left upper extremity (LUE) arteriovenous fistula (AVF)/arteriovenous graft (AVG)
- Systematic review from 99 studies and 4906 patients. Looked at incidence of left arm ischemia (0% vs. 9.2%,

P = .002) and stroke (4.7% vs. 7.2% P > .001) were significantly less following revascularization of LSCA[15]

SPECIAL CONSIDERATIONS

TEVAR for Mycotic Aneurysm

- 0.6%–2% of aortic aneurysms are mycotic in Western countries, with higher ratios in Eastern countries
  - Mycotic thoracic aortic aneurysms bear high morbidity and mortality
  - Conventional treatment consists of open repair with resection of the aneurysm with broad local debridement and revascularization
  - 30% intraoperative and postoperative mortality and >50% morbidity
  - Paucity of data comparing open repair and endovascular repair
    - 50 patients with mycotic thoracic aortic aneurysms received endovascular intervention and had good 30-day survival (92%), with 78% and 71% survival at 1 and 5 years
  - 17% had infectious complications of which 67% were fatal
- The most common pathogens identified in thoracic mycotic aneurysms have been
  1. *Staphylococcus*
  2. *Streptococcus*
  3. *Salmonella*
- Favorable endovascular treatment strategies of mycotic aneurysm include
  - Long-term antibiotic administration
  - Close follow-up with trends of inflammatory markers (erythrocyte sedimentation rate [ESR], CRP)
  - Routine interval imaging
- Recurrent infectious complications after TEVAR for mycotic abdominal aorta aneurysm (MAAA) have a high mortality (>50%)

SPECIAL CONSIDERATION: TEVAR FOR CONGENITAL ANOMALIES

Aberrant Right Subclavian Artery (ARSCA) (Fig. 8.5)

- 0.5%–2.5% reported incidence in CT reviews of large population (3:1 prevalence in women)
- Most aberrant SCA course behind the esophagus (80%) but can be between esophagus and trachea (15%) or anterior to trachea (5%)
- Concordant 0.4%–1.8% incidence of clinical syndrome of dysphagia lusoria
- In pediatric patients, symptoms often caused by direct compression from the diverticulum or restriction from

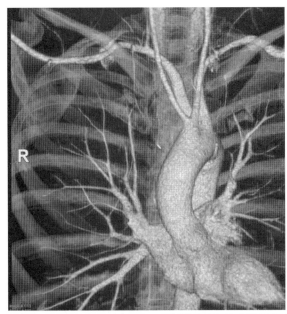

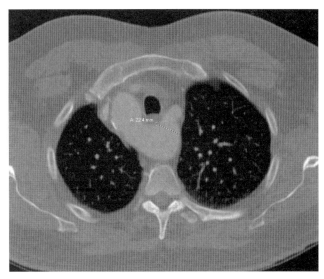

FIG. 8.6 Right-sided aortic arch with normal left subclavian order but retroesophageal course and 2.2-cm Kommerell diverticula.

- In addition to ARSCA, can be associated with right-sided aortic arch and normal branching pattern at LSCA ostium (Fig. 8.6)
- Kommerell diverticulum is often asymptomatic but carries a risk of rupture or dissection as high as 19%–53%

Surgical Indication for Kommerell Diverticulum

Severe esophageal or tracheal compressive symptoms are definitive indications. In asymptomatic patients criteria are not well-established. Some advocate for repair based on high rupture rate. Given the high rupture risk diverticulum >50 mm should be repaired or for orifice diameter of the SCA >30 mm

- Aberrant subclavian surgical indications: dysphagia, subclavian steal syndrome, subclavian aneurysm, arm claudication

Treatment

Open Repair
- Resection of the diverticulum (graft replacement of the descending aorta) and reconstruction/relocation of the ARSCA
  - Review of 47 cases of graft replacement from 2004 to 2014, early mortality was 11% (5.3% in elective cases). Postoperative complications seen in 11 cases (2 mediastinitis, 1 chylothorax, 2 respiratory failures, 2 bleeding, 2 nerve injuries, 1 pulmonary embolism [PE], 1 transient ischemic attack [TIA])[16]
- Reconstruction of the aberrant SCA:
  - Initially treated with ligation (may still be OK in pediatric patients); however, significant ischemic complications identified in 64% of adults

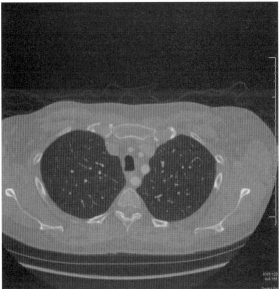

FIG. 8.5 Normal left-sided aortic arch with aberrant right subclavian artery (ARSCA) coursing retroesophageal without Kommerell diverticula.

vascular ring formation. Respiratory symptoms more common due to absence of tracheal rigidity
- Adult patients only 5% present with symptoms
  - Dysphagia, chest pain, blood pressure (BP) discrepancy (aberrant side may be diminished due to punctate opening of the SCA, caliber change between diverticulum and SCA)
- Associated with Kommerell diverticula (>50% of all Kommerell diverticula in ARSCA)

Kommerell diverticulum is a congenital aortic diverticulum that arises due to a persistent remnant of the fourth dorsal aortic arch due to failed regression.

- Thoracotomy with in situ reconstruction
- Supraclavicular versus cervical incision with carotid to SCA bypass
- Translocation of the aberrant artery to the carotid

Treatment: TEVAR

- Surgical debranching of aberrant subclavian
  - Subclavian to carotid transposition with proximal ligation of ARSCA preferred but bypass acceptable
  - Bypass will require endovascular obliteration of origin of ARSCA
  - Majority of cases require concomitant LSCA transposition or bypass as well due to proximity of origin of subclavian vessels
- TEVAR as described earlier
  - Higher risk than aneurysm disease for intraoperative dissection
- Overall mortality 2%–10%
- Late complications
  - Usual for TEVAR as discussed earlier
  - Migration of plug/coils from origin resulting in expansion of Kommerell diverticula
  - Aortoesophageal fistula

- Either due to endoleak with persistent pressurization or of foreign body occluders in origins of subclavian vessels
- Total endovascular repair likely in future as advent of branch technology improves
- Coarctation of aorta
- Most commonly found in infancy
  - Occurs at insertion of ductus arteriosum in most patients
  - TEVAR emerging modality for treatment of late restenosis of prior open repair
- Diagnosed in adults with early-onset HTN associated with headaches and claudication
- Discrepant pulses between upper and lower extremities
- Markedly enlarged internal mammaries/epigastric arteries on CT
- Indications to repair
  - 20-mm Hg resting gradient in catheterization
  - Evidence of left heart failure
- Initial studies of endovascular therapy used serial dilation of balloon expandable uncovered stents
- TEVAR decreases risk of perforation and intraoperative dissection

REFERENCES

1. Walsh SR, Tang TY, Sadat U. Endovascular stenting versus open surgery for thoracic aortic disease: systematic review and meta-analysis of perioperative results. *J Vasc Surg.* 2008;47(5):1094-1098.
2. Matsumura JS, Cambria RP, Dake MD, et al. International controlled clinical trial of thoracic endovascular aneurysm repair with the Zenith TX2 endovascular graft: 1-year results. *J Vasc Surg.* 2008;47(2):247-257.
3. Makaroun MS, Dillavou ED, Wheatley GH, Cambria RP, Gore TAG Investigators. Five-year results of endovascular treatment with the Gore TAG device compared with open repair of thoracic aortic aneurysms. *J Vasc Surg.* 2008;47(5):912-918.
4. Charlton-Ouw KM, Estrera AL. Thoracic endovascular aortic repair for aneurysm: how I teach it. *Ann Thorac Surg.* 2018;106(3):646-650.
5. Gafoor S, Stelter W, Bertog S, Sievert H. Fully percutaneous treatment of an aberrant right subclavian artery and thoracic aortic aneurysm. *Vasc Med.* 2013;18(3):139-144.
6. Erben Y, Brownstein AJ, Velasquez CA, et al. Natural history and management of Kommerell's diverticulum in a single tertiary referral center. *J Vasc Surg.* 2020;71(6):2004-2011.
7. Greenberg RK, Lu Q, Roselli EE, et al. Contemporary analysis of descending thoracic and thoracoabdominal aneurysm repair: a comparison of endovascular and open techniques. *Circulation.* 2008;118(8):808-817.
8. Vandy FC, Girotti M, Williams DM, et al. Iliofemoral complications associated with thoracic endovascular aortic repair: frequency, risk factors, and early and late outcomes. *J Thorac Cardiovasc Surg.* 2014;147(3):960-965.
9. von Allmen RS, Gahl B, Powell JT. Editor's choice - incidence of stroke following thoracic endovascular aortic repair for

descending aortic aneurysm: a systematic review of the literature with meta-analysis. *Eur J Vasc Endovasc Surg.* 2017;53(2):176-184.
10. Felix JV, Schlösser FJV, Hence JM, et al. TEVAR following prior abdominal aortic aneurysm surgery: increased risk of neurological deficit. *J Vasc Surg.* 2009;49(2):308-314.
11. O'Callaghan A, Mastracci TM, Eagleton MJ. Staged endovascular repair of thoracoabdominal aortic aneurysms limits incidence and severity of spinal cord ischemia. *J Vasc Surg.* 2015;61(2):347-354.e1.
12. Buth J, Harris PL, Hobo R, et al. Neurologic complications associated with endovascular repair of thoracic aortic pathology: incidence and risk factors. a study from the European Collaborators on Stent/Graft Techniques for Aortic Aneurysm Repair (EUROSTAR) registry. *J Vasc Surg.* 2007;46(6):1103-1111.
13. Hajibandeh S, Hajibandeh S, Antoniou SA, Torella F, Antoniou GA. Meta-analysis of left subclavian artery coverage with and without revascularization in thoracic endovascular aortic repair. *J Endovasc Ther.* 2016;23(4):634-641.
14. Maldonado TS, Dexter D, Rockman CB, et al. Left subclavian artery coverage during thoracic endovascular aortic aneurysm repair does not mandate revascularization. *J Vasc Surg.* 2013;57(1):116-124.
15. Rehman SM, Vecht JA, Perera R, et al. How to manage the left subclavian artery during endovascular stenting for thoracic aortic dissection? An assessment of the evidence. *Ann Vasc Surg.* 2010;24(7):956-965.
16. Kimyaghalam A, Gabay A, Singh K. Aberrant right subclavian artery: a case of vertebrobasilar insufficiency. *J Surg Case Rep.* 2023;2023(4):rjad199.

CHAPTER 9

Abdominal Aortic Aneurysmal Disease—Open

WILLIAM JORDAN, MD and AMANDA FOBARE, MD

TRIALS (OPEN VS. ENDO)

EVAR 1

- 1082 patients, 34 hospitals in the United Kingdom, enrolled from 1999 to 2004
- Selection: age >60 years, infrarenal abdominal aortic aneurysm (AAA) >5.5 cm, suitable for either endovascular aneurysm repair (EVAR) or open repair
- Mean age 74 years, 91% men, median aneurysm diameter was 6.2 cm
- Median follow-up was 2.9 years
- Short-term outcomes
  - Improved survival in the EVAR group at 30 days
  - All-cause mortality was similar between groups
  - Persistent reduction in aneurysm-related death in the EVAR group (4% vs. 7%, $P = .04$)
  - Proportion of patients with postoperative complications within 4 years of randomization: ($P < .0001$)
    - 41% EVAR group
    - 9% open group
  - Health-related quality of life (HRQL)
    - Open group had a diminished HRQL at 0–3 months
    - This recovered by 3–12 months and 12–24 months after randomization

- Mean hospital cost per patient up to 4 years
  - EVAR £13257, £9946 open
  - Mean difference £3311
- Long-term outcomes
  - In the first 6 months: total and aneurysm-related mortality was lower in the EVAR group
  - In the late follow-up: patients who had an EVAR showed greater aneurysm-related mortality and total mortality
    - The increase in aneurysm-related deaths was predominantly from secondary sac rupture
    - The rate of reintervention was higher in the EVAR group at all timepoints
    - Conclusion: survival was the same in both groups but reinterventions were higher for EVAR, thought to be related to the pursuit of endoleaks, which is done less frequently today

DREAM

- 345 patients, 28 centers (24 in the Netherlands, 4 in Belgium), enrolled from November 2000 to December 2003
- Selection: AAA >5 cm, suitable for either EVAR or open repair
- Median follow-up was 10.2 years
- Surveillance with computed tomography (CT) dropped off after 5 years in both groups (greater drop in the open group)
- Results: at 12 years
  - Survival rate of 42.2% (open) vs. 38.5% (EVAR), $P = .48$
  - No difference in the aneurysm mortality between groups
  - No difference in all-cause mortality, mortality due to cardiovascular (CV) or malignant disease
  - Freedom from intervention: 78.9% (open) vs. 62.2% (EVAR), $P = .01$
  - While more patients who underwent EVAR required reintervention, survival was the same between both groups

OVER

- 881 veterans, 42 centers, enrolled from October 2002 to October 2008
- Selection
  - AAA >5 cm OR AAA >4.5 cm with rapid enlargement (0.7 cm in 6 months or 1 cm in 12 months) OR saccular morphology
  - Mean aneurysm diameter was 5.7 cm
  - Candidates for either open repair or EVAR
  - CT scans for all visits following EVAR, CT scan at 1 year following open repair
- Short-term outcomes
  - Perioperative mortality was higher for open repair at 30 days (0.2% vs. 2.3%, P =.006)
  - No significant difference in all-cause mortality at 2 years
  - No differences between the groups with regard to procedure failures, secondary therapeutic procedures, aneurysm-related hospitalizations, or 1-year major mortality
  - No differences between the two groups in HRQL at 2 years
- Long-term outcomes
  - Reduction in perioperative mortality with EVAR was sustained at 2 years, but not thereafter
  - In patients younger than 70 years old, EVAR led to improved long-term survival
    - But, tended to reduce survival in older patients
  - Number of rehospitalizations was similar between groups
  - Aneurysm rupture following repair was uncommon, but only occurred in the EVAR group
  - Number of reinterventions was similar between groups
  - Hernia repair was the most common intervention in the open group
  - Endovascular procedures were the most common intervention in the EVAR group

INDICATIONS FOR SURGERY

- Risk factors for AAA development: male gender, increasing age, family history of aneurysmal disease, hyperlipidemia, smoking, hypertension
  - Smoking is the strongest risk factor
- Aneurysm defined:
  - Enlargement of the aorta to 1.5 times the normal diameter, which is approximately 2 cm (men: 1.9–2.3 cm, women: 1.7–1.9 cm)
  - Repair is indicated for aortic diameter >5.5 cm in men, >5 cm in women

- Rapid growth
  - Rate of expansion is ≥10 mm in a 12-month period
- Risk of rupture
  - Risk factors: female gender, hypertension, current smoking, chronic obstructive pulmonary disease (COPD), and family history of AAA

AAA Diameter (cm)	Rupture Risk (%) in 12 months
3.0–3.9	0.3
4.0–4.9	0.5–1.5
5.0–5.9	1–11
6.0–6.9	11–22
>7	>30

OPEN REPAIR FOR RUPTURED AAA

Approach

- Transperitoneal
  - Indications: most common approach. May be used when there is a need for full abdominal assessment (ex: intestinal examination). Reconstruction requiring aortoiliac configuration
  - Positioning: supine, arms extended
- Retroperitoneal
  - Indications: prior intraperitoneal surgeries, intraperitoneal infections, bowel resections with the creation of stomas, and in the setting of an inflammatory aneurysm
  - Positioning: right lateral decubitus position, on a beanbag. The torso is rotated approximately 45 degrees, with the pelvis flat in the supine position. Typically, an axillary roll is used under the right upper extremity, and an arm sling is used for the left upper extremity. The bed is maximally flexed to open the space between the left costal margin and the anterior superior iliac spine (ASIS). Pillows are placed between the legs, the knees are slightly bent, and the ankles are padded
  - Incision
    - Thoracoabdominal: used for aneurysms that require supraceliac clamping, or access to the descending thoracic aorta
      - In the eighth intercostal space, an incision is made from the posterior midaxillary line, through the intercostal space, to the border of the left rectus, at the level between the umbilicus and the pubic bone
    - Abdominal: used for aneurysms that do not require clamping superior to the renal arteries
      - In the 10th intercostal space a curvilinear incision is made at the costal margin, to the border of the left rectus, at the level between the umbilicus and the pubic bone

Technical Considerations

- Proximal clamp
  - Placed superior to the target anastomosis site, at the level of renal arteries in most patients. Be aware of the diseased aorta that can lead to "retrograde embolization" into renals or superior mesenteric artery (SMA)
  - Aim to clamp as low as possible in relation to the mesenteric vessels or renal arteries if able, to avoid mesenteric and renal ischemia time
- Distal clamp
  - Placed distal to the target anastomosis site (common iliac arteries, external iliac arteries, or common femoral arteries)
  - In patients with significant iliac calcifications and plaque, occlusive balloon catheters may be used as a substitution for clamps
- Conduit
  - Appropriately sized bifurcated polyester or polytetrafluoroethylene (PTFE) graft
  - Cryopreserved aorta (requires rapid access to the product, which may not be available)
- Reimplantation of the inferior mesenteric artery (IMA): should be considered if the IMA has poor back bleeding, large-caliber IMA with a diseased celiac/SMA/internal iliac arteries, prior history of colonic surgery, or a poorly perfused colon based on intraoperative examination
- Retroaortic left renal vein—requires caution during mobilization of the aorta as it can be injured during dissection and clamping
  - If injured, transect the aorta at the location of the injury for exposure and repair

Complications

- Intestinal ischemia
- Ileus
- Prolonged ventilatory support
- Renal failure

Postoperative Management

- If stable from a cardiopulmonary standpoint, these patients are extubated in the operating room (OR)
- Admitted to the intensive care unit (ICU) following surgery
- Frequent laboratory monitoring and correction of coagulopathy and anemia are imperative
  - Bowel function is monitored, and enteral nutrition is resumed with the passage of flatus and/or bowel movements (must monitor for blood in the stool)

Follow-up

- Aortoiliac ultrasound at, 6 months, and yearly thereafter; CT scan (axial imaging) is suggested at 5 years
- Patients with aortobifemoral reconstruction should be monitored for aneurysmal degeneration at their femoral anastomosis sites

INFLAMMATORY AAA

Epidemiology

- Accounts for 5%–10% of aortic aneurysms

Etiology

- Local inflammation surrounds the affected vessel, with deposition of fibrous tissue
- Numerous underlying etiologies have been postulated including: chronic subacute rupture, retroperitoneal fibrosis variant, and an exaggerated variation of the normal inflammatory response

Sign/Symptoms of Disease

- Weight loss, malaise, abdominal pain

Diagnostic Evaluation

- Labs: white blood cell (WBC), erythrocyte sedimentation rate (ESR), C-reactive protein (CRP)
- Computed tomography angiography (CTA)
  - Thick, inflammatory tissue surrounding the affected vessel
  - "Rind" may extend to encroach on adjacent structures
  - May be associated with ureteral obstruction, as the ureters and retroperitoneal space can also be involved (in up to 25% of cases)

Treatment

- Endovascular-stent grafting has been shown to promote the resolution of perianeurysmal inflammation
- Open approach—retroperitoneal approach should be considered to minimize the mobilization of adjacent structures during a transperitoneal approach
  - If there is concern for acute expansion or impending rupture, a classic transperitoneal approach may be used

Complications

- Local inflammation around the aorta increases the technical difficulty of dissection
- Ureteral injury
- Duodenal injury

INFECTED AAA

Epidemiology

- Can occur in any vessel
  Incidence is increased in patients with a history of illicit drug use/injection, and in populations that are immunosuppressed (e.g., cancer patients, transplant recipients, and those with HIV and AIDS)
- Accounts for 0.65%–1.5% of all aortic aneurysms
- Between 47% and 73% of patients have a contained or free rupture
- Mortality ranges from 5% to 36%, though mortality is higher for patients who present with free rupture

Etiology

- Can be caused by numerous organisms, including bacteria, fungi, tuberculosis, and syphilis
- The most frequently identified organisms are *Staphylococcus*, *Streptococcus*, *Salmonella*, and *Escherichia coli*

Sign/Symptoms of Disease

- Abdominal pain, fevers, weight loss

Diagnostic Evaluation

- Labs: blood cultures, WBC, ESR, CRP
- CTA abdomen and pelvis—periaortic fat stranding and inflammation, lymphadenopathy, occasionally fluid
  - There may be local destruction of periaortic tissues and adjacent structures (kidney, vertebral column)
  - Morphology of the aneurysm tends to be saccular or lobulated, with irregular borders

Treatment: Repair and Resection

- General principles
  - Open repair may be more difficult than expected, given the level of inflammation of the periaortic tissues

- Resection of infected tissue and debridement of the retroperitoneum is the mainstay of treatment
- Rifampin-soaked Dacron
  - Aneurysms infected with low-virulence organisms, such as *Staphylococcus epidermidis*, may be the ideal population for this reconstruction
  - Rifampin soaking in 1200 mg/20 mL of normal saline for 15 minutes prior to graft implantation
- Endovascular stenting (long-term success is not well defined)
  - Can be used as a bridge to definitive therapy or palliation
- Neoaortoiliac system (NAIS)
  - Resistant to reinfection
  - Helpful to image the deep femoral veins for patency of the vein and adequate size (6.0 mm at least)
  - Good size match for reconstruction
  - Does require additional operative time for harvest
  - Can be staged with exposure of the vein during one operation and reconstruction during the second operation
- Cryopreserved aorta
  - Prone to aneurysmal degeneration with graft disruption
  - Higher cost
  - Requires advanced planning
- Extraanatomic bypass
  - The aortic stump is closed with a two-layer suture technique (horizontal mattress, followed by a simple suture)
  - The stump is covered with a pedicled omental flap
  - Risk of stump blowout (20%)
  - Axillobifemoral bypass

AAA WITH IVC FISTULA

Epidemiology

- Occurs in 1% of asymptomatic, and 3%–4% of symptomatic aneurysms

Etiology

- Can occur after an aneurysm ruptures into the neighboring vein, causing a persistent fistula

Sign/Symptoms of Disease

- Abdominal or back pain
- Pulsatile abdominal mass with a continuous bruit
- Unilateral or bilateral lower extremity venous congestion
- High-output heart failure
- Hematuria

Diagnostic Evaluation

- Echocardiogram (ECHO)
- CTA A/P
  - Contrast will be enhanced in both the aorta and inferior vena cava (IVC)

Treatment

- Endovascular
- Open repair
  - Foley balloon catheters or other types of occlusive balloons may aid in control of venous bleeding; qualified assistant can hold manual pressure to aid with hemostasis
  - The fistula is repaired from within the aortic sac
  - Care must be taken not to embolize thrombus through the venous system, as these pulmonary embolisms can be devastating

Complications

- Intraoperative hemodynamic compromise, as venous return to the heart may be temporarily interrupted during closure of the fistula

AAA WITH AORTOENTERIC FISTULA

Epidemiology

- Typically occurs >6 months following aortic surgery
- Incidence in patients with AAA is 0.69%–2.46%
- Male:female prevalence 3:1

Etiology

- Primary
  - Communication between the gastrointestinal (GI) tract and the native aorta
  - In the majority of cases, the aneurysmal component of the aorta is associated with the fistula (83%)
  - More rare causes of primary aortoenteric fistulas: foreign bodies, mycotic aneurysms, prior radiation therapy
- Secondary
  - Communication between the GI tract and the reconstructed aorta
  - The proximal suture line of the graft erodes into the duodenum (third and fourth portions), most commonly

Sign/Symptoms of Disease

- Abdominal pain, fever, and GI bleeding (hematemesis)
- May have a "herald bleed" followed by massive bleeding (though the time interval between the two may be hours, up to months)

Diagnostic Evaluation

- Labs: blood cultures, WBC, ESR, CRP
- CTA A/P: will typically demonstrate periaortic gas/air, stranding, loss of the fat plane between the duodenum and the aorta
- Esophagogastroduodenoscopy (EGD): pulsatility of the duodenum, clot (should not be disturbed)

Treatment

- General principles
  - Nasogastric tube should be placed at the beginning of the case
  - The bowel should be repaired in two layers
    - If primary repair is not feasible, resection with a Roux-en-Y reconstruction may be required
  - The aorta must be debrided back to healthy tissue
  - An omental flap should be placed between the aorta and the bowel
- Extraanatomic bypass
  - Can be done in a single operation, or staged over 1–3 days
  - Traditionally an axillobifemoral configuration is used
  - The aortic stump is oversewn in two layers of nonabsorbable, monofilament suture
  - Pledgets should be avoided as they may be a source of persistent infection
  - An omental flap is created and placed in between the duodenum and the aortic stump
- NAIS
  - Resistant to reinfection
  - Requires duplex that demonstrates patency of the vein, and adequate size (6.0 mm at least)
  - Good size match for reconstruction
  - Does require additional operative time for harvest
  - Can be staged with exposure of the vein during one operation, and reconstruction during the second operation
- Endovascular stenting
  - May be used as a temporizing measure to exclude the fistula, with the plan to resuscitate, nutritionally optimize, and plan for definitive resection and reconstruction

- May be used in patients who are moribund or palliative
- The stent graft will likely be seeded with enteric contents
- Rifampin-impregnated Dacron graft
  - The graft should be soaked for at least 30 minutes in a 600-mg rifampin solution prior to implantation
- Cryopreserved aorta
  - Costly
  - Requires time to obtain preoperatively
  - Availability may be limited
  - Size mismatch
  - Prone to aneurysmal degeneration over time

Follow-up

- These patients should be imaged with CTA to evaluate for recurrence of the aortoenteric fistula or anastomotic aneurysms

INTESTINAL ISCHEMIA AFTER OPEN AAA

Epidemiology

- Prevalence (2.1%–3.6%) after open aortic repair
- Up to 15% of patients undergoing open aortic repair in the setting of rupture
- Increases the morbidity, length of hospital stay, and healthcare costs for patients undergoing open AAA repair
- Mortality >50%
- Risk factors: advanced age, female gender, diabetes, end-stage renal disease (ESRD), ruptured aneurysm, need for blood product transfusion, respiratory insufficiency, prolonged operative time, proximal clamp location during repair

Etiology

- Preoperative and sustained hypotension
- Prolonged use of vasopressor support in the pre- and postoperative setting
- Prolonged supraceliac clamping
- Loss of adequate flow to the mesenteric vessels
- In the setting of celiac and/or SMA stenosis/occlusion, the IMA may be the dominant vessel for intestinal perfusion
- If the IMA is sacrificed, there is a theoretical increased risk for intestinal ischemia (data have been conflicting)
- Prior colonic surgery may be an indication to reimplant the IMA, given the altered collateral flow
- Hypogastric artery ligation leads to increased risk of intestinal ischemia as it provides the middle and inferior rectal arteries

Sign/Symptoms of Disease

- Hypotension, tachycardia
- Abdominal pain, abdominal distension, blood per rectum (only in 30% of cases)
- Decreased urine output

Diagnostic Evaluation

- Labs: elevated WBC, elevated lactic acid
- Flexible sigmoidoscopy (can be done in the ICU or the operating room [OR])
  - Mild: ischemia limited to the colonic mucosa and submucosa
    - On endoscopy: patchy mucosal erythema, ecchymosis, or pallor
- Most common form of colonic ischemia
  - Moderate: ischemia involving the muscularis
    - On endoscopy: extensive changes of the mucosa with large areas of involved colonic wall
  - Severe: ischemia involving the full thickness of the colonic wall
    - On endoscopy: mucosal friability, ulcerations, patches of necrotic wall, fissures
    - Least common form of colonic ischemia
- CT scan with intravenous (IV) contrast
  - Patients are usually severely ill by the time a CT scan shows the changes (pneumatosis intestinalis)

Treatment

- Nonoperative management
  - Reserved for patients who demonstrate mild or moderate ischemia
  - IV hydration, IV antibiotics, bowel reset
  - Continued monitoring of WBC, lactic acid, and urine output
  - Serial abdominal exams to monitor for improvement in abdominal pain and distention
- Resection of nonviable bowel
  - IV hydration, IV antibiotics
  - Take back to the OR for an exploratory laparotomy and resection of nonviable bowel
  - This typically results in fecal diversion and creation of an ostomy

Complications

- Short gut syndrome in the setting of small bowel ischemia
- Permanent ostomy
- Death

INFECTED AORTIC ENDOGRAFT EXPLANATION

Epidemiology

- Mortality of 12.5% (in infected aortic graft)
- Amputation rate 7% (in infected aortic graft)

Etiology

- *S. aureus*, *S. epidermidis*, and *E. coli* are the causative organisms in approximately 80% of aortic graft infections
- *Klebsiella*, *Proteus*, *Enterobacter*, and *Pseudomonas* are less likely
- *Pseudomonas* is most likely to cause hemorrhage due to graft disruption

Sign/Symptoms of Disease

- Abdominal pain, fevers, malaise

Diagnostic Evaluation

- Labs: blood cultures, WBC, ESR, CRP
- CTA A/P—periaortic fat stranding and inflammation, lymphadenopathy, fluid, loss of tissue planes, adjacent thickened bowel wall
- Leukocyte scintigraphy vs. fluorodeoxyglucose-positron emission tomography (fused with CT scan)

Treatment—Resection and Reconstruction

- Antibiotic-impregnated graft
- Extraanatomic bypass
- NAIS
- Cryopreserved aorta

POSTOPERATIVE MANAGEMENT

- Frequent lab checks and neurovascular assessment are necessary
- Foley catheters typically remain until the patient has demonstrated adequate resuscitation, normalization of creatinine and volume of urine
- Early mobilization out of bed improves pulmonary recovery and prevents deep vein thrombosis
- Monitoring for return of bowel function, with special attention to the presence of blood in the stool or tarry stool is important
- Appropriate prophylaxis for venous thromboembolism should be initiated as soon as safe after repair

SUGGESTED READINGS

DREAM Trial update: van Schaik TG, Yeung KK, Verhagen HJ, et al. Long-term survival and secondary procedures after open or endovascular repair of abdominal aortic aneurysms. *J Vasc Surg.* 2017;66(5):1379-1389. Erratum in: *J Vasc Surg.* 2018;67(2):683.

DREAM Trial: Prinssen M, Verhoeven EL, Buth J, et al. A randomized trial comparing conventional and endovascular repair of abdominal aortic aneurysms. *N Engl J Med.* 2004;351(16):1607-1618.

Erbel R, Aboyans V, Boileau C, et al. ESC guidelines on the diagnosis and treatment of aortic diseases: document covering acute and chronic aortic diseases of the thoracic and abdominal aorta of the adult. The Task Force for the Diagnosis and Treatment of Aortic Diseases of the European Society of Cardiology (ESC). *Eur Heart J.* 2014;35:2873-2926.

EVAR 1 Trial update: Patel R, Sweeting MJ, Powell JT, Greenhalgh RM; EVAR trial investigators. Endovascular versus open repair of abdominal aortic aneurysm in 15-years' follow-up of the UK endovascular aneurysm repair trial 1 (EVAR trial 1): a randomised controlled trial. *Lancet.* 2016;388(10058):2366-2374.

EVAR 1 Trial: EVAR trial participants. Endovascular aneurysm repair versus open repair in patients with abdominal aortic aneurysm (EVAR trial 1): randomized controlled trial. *Lancet.* 2005;365(9478):2179-2186.

EY Woo, SM Damrauer. Abdominal aortic aneurysms: open surgical treatment. In: Sidawy A, Perler BA, eds. *Rutherford's Vascular Surgery and Endovascular Therapy.* Philadelphia, PA: Elsevier; 2019:894-909 [chapter 71].

Gurakar M, Locham S, Alshaikh HN, Malas MB. Risk factors and outcomes for bowel ischemia after open and endovascular abdominal aortic aneurysm repair. *J Vasc Surg.* 2019;70(3):869-881.

Lawrence P, Rigbert DA. Arterial aneurysms: etiology, epidemiology, and natural history. In: Sidawy A, Perler BA, eds. *Rutherford's Vascular Surgery and Endovascular Therapy.* Philadelphia, PA: Elsevier; 2019:875-883 [chapter 69].

Milner R, Minc S. Local complications: aortoenteric fistula. In: Sidawy A, Perler BA, eds. *Rutherford's Vascular and Endovascular Therapy.* Philadelphia, PA: Elsevier; 2019:615-623 [chapter 49].

OVER Trial Update: Lederle FA, Freischlag JA, Kyriakides TC, et al. Long-term comparison of endovascular and open repair of abdominal aortic aneurysm. *N Engl J Med.* 2012;367(21):1988-1997.

OVER Trial: Lederle FA, Freischlag JA, Kyriakides TC, et al. Outcomes following endovascular vs. open repair of abdominal aortic aneurysm: a randomized trial. *JAMA.* 2009;302(14):1535-1342.

Tracci MC, Roy RA, Upchurch GR. Aortoiliac aneurysms: evaluation, decision making, and medical management. In: Sidawy A, Perler BA, eds. *Rutherford's Vascular Surgery and Endovascular Therapy.* Philadelphia, PA: Elsevier; 2019:884-893 [chapter 70].

CHAPTER 10

Endovascular Repair of Abdominal Aortic Aneurysms

STEVEN TOHMASI, MD and NII-KABU KABUTEY, MD

INTRODUCTION

- Endovascular aneurysm repair (EVAR) is a commonly available treatment option for patients requiring abdominal aortic aneurysm (AAA) repair who meet appropriate anatomic criteria
  - It has been estimated that nearly 80% of intact AAAs are repaired using EVAR in the United States[1]
- EVAR is a minimally invasive technique performed by inserting compressed graft components within a delivery sheath through the lumen of the common femoral artery (CFA) or iliac conduit and into the aorta. The endograft is properly positioned using fluoroscopic guidance. The components are deployed and adhere to the aortic wall proximally and iliac vessels distally to exclude the aneurysm from systemic blood flow and pressure
- In correlation with the widespread adoption of EVAR, the annual number of AAA ruptures and AAA-related mortality has significantly declined in the United States, likely due to the ability to offer EVAR to patients who would be considered poor candidates for open surgical repair (OSR)[2]

RANDOMIZED TRIALS COMPARING ENDOVASCULAR AND OPEN REPAIR

- The *Dutch Randomized Endovascular Aneurysm Management (DREAM)* trial, *Endovascular Aneurysm Repair Versus Open Repair in Patients with AAA (EVAR-1)* trial, *U.S. Veterans Affairs Open Versus Endovascular Repair (OVER)* trial, and *French Anevrysme de l'aorte abdominale: Chirurgie versus Endoprothese (ACE)* trial are four high-quality multicenter, prospective trials that collectively randomized 2790 patients to either EVAR or OSR[3]
  - A pooled analysis of all four trials revealed short-term mortality (including 30-day or in-hospital mortality) to be significantly lower with EVAR than with OSR (1.4% vs. 4.2%; odds ratio [OR]: 0.33; $P < .0001$)[3]
  - Mortality benefit did not persist as the authors reported no significant difference in intermediate (up to 4 years from randomization) and long-term mortality (beyond 4 years) between the EVAR and OSR cohorts[3]
  - Long-term reintervention rate was significantly higher with EVAR than OSR (OR: 1.98; $P = .02$)[3]
    - Recently published long-term data from the OVER trial also reaffirmed this finding as significantly more patients in the EVAR group underwent secondary procedures (26.7% vs. 19.8%)[4]
  - Operative complications (including the incidence of cardiac deaths and fatal strokes), health-related quality of life, and sexual dysfunction are generally comparable between EVAR and OSR[3]
  - In the OVER trial, patients randomized to the EVAR group had reduced median procedure time (2.9 vs. 3.7 hours), blood loss (200 vs. 1000 mL), transfusion requirement (0 vs. 1.0 units), duration of mechanical ventilation (3.6 vs. 5.0 hours), hospital stay (3 vs. 7 days), and intensive care unit stay (1 vs. 4 days) but required increased exposure to fluoroscopy and contrast[5]

INDICATIONS FOR EVAR

- The normal abdominal aorta measures 2.0–2.5 cm in diameter

- An AAA is defined as a dilated aortic segment measuring >50% in diameter relative to the normal aorta (i.e., >3.0 cm)
- AAA diameter predicts the risk of rupture and guides the decision for operative repair
  - The 1-year risk of rupture rises with increasing AAA diameter: 0.5%–5% per year for 4 to 5 cm, 3%–15% per year for 5 to 6 cm, 10%–20% per year for 6 to 7 cm, and 30%–50% per year for aneurysms >8 cm in size[6]
- Elective AAA repair is recommended for:
  - All individuals with an AAA >5.5 cm in diameter
  - Women with an AAA >5.0 cm in maximum diameter
  - Patients with a rapidly expanding AAA (>0.5 cm/6 ms or >1 cm/y) on serial imaging examinations
  - Patients with abdominal, back, or flank pain that is attributed to the AAA

Anatomic Considerations for EVAR

Aneurysm Involvement

- Infrarenal AAA: occurs below the level of the renal arteries
  - Approximately 80% of all AAAs
- Juxtarenal AAA: aneurysm's proximal extent abuts the origin of the renal arteries but does not involve them
  - Requires suprarenal aortic clamping during OSR
- Pararenal AAA: aneurysm involves at least one of the renal artery orifices and extends up to the superior mesenteric artery
- Although the majority of EVAR procedures are performed for infrarenal AAAs, there has been increasing utility of advanced endovascular techniques with specialized endografts for juxtarenal and Pararenal AAAs[7]

Preoperative Planning

- Successful EVAR relies upon adequate fixation and seal of the endograft to the arterial wall proximally at the aortic neck and distally in each of the iliac arteries
  - The proximal and distal attachment sites are referred to as the "landing zones"
- The technical success and durability of the repair are contingent on the radial forces generated by the graft at the landing zones
- Certain aortic anatomic considerations require evaluation via imaging, such as computed tomography angiography (CTA), fluoroscopy, or intravascular ultrasound (IVUS), to determine a patient's candidacy for EVAR (Fig. 10.1, Table 10.1)[8]

- The aortoiliac anatomy of some patients may not be suitable for deployment of an infrarenal EVAR device[9] The presence of the following may preclude EVAR:
  - Short or angulated landing zone
  - Excessive aortoiliac thrombus
  - Multiple large accessory renal arteries
  - Small, tortuous access vessels with concomitant occlusive disease

- EVAR ideally should be performed in a dedicated hybrid endovascular operating suite in which conversion to OSR can be performed efficiently, if needed
- General anesthesia, regional anesthesia, or local anesthesia with conscious sedation may be used
- The patient should be positioned supine, and a Foley catheter and arterial line should be placed for monitoring
- The locations of the distal lower extremity pulses are marked and the patient's abdomen and both groins should be exposed and prepped
- The CFAs are accessed using ultrasound guidance and the Seldinger technique or bilateral femoral artery cutdowns
- The patient is then systemically heparinized and wires are passed into the thoracic aorta from the CFAs
- Sheaths and catheters are then introduced bilaterally and an aortogram and pelvic angiography are performed to examine the aortoiliac and renal artery anatomy as well as to verify the aortic dimensions prior to endograft implantation
- The main body of the endograft is then inserted over a stiff wire, oriented under fluoroscopy to the desired position, and deployed just below the renal arteries
- The deployed contralateral gate is then carefully cannulated
  - Confirmation of gate cannulation can be done with IVUS, spinning a pigtail catheter within the endograft or partially inflating a compliant balloon within the gate and main body to confirm positioning
- The contralateral limb of the endograft is then introduced over the wire, docked into the main body with adequate proximal overlap, and deployed to the level of distal fixation ensuring preservation of perfusion into the internal iliac artery
- To ensure adequate fixation, balloon angioplasty is performed at the proximal landing zone, the sealing zones of the iliac limbs, and the segment of overlap between the endograft's main body and contralateral iliac limb
- Completion angiography is performed to confirm exclusion of the AAA and absence of endoleaks (Fig. 10.2)
- The wires and sheaths are then removed, the arteriotomies are closed either percutaneously or with open

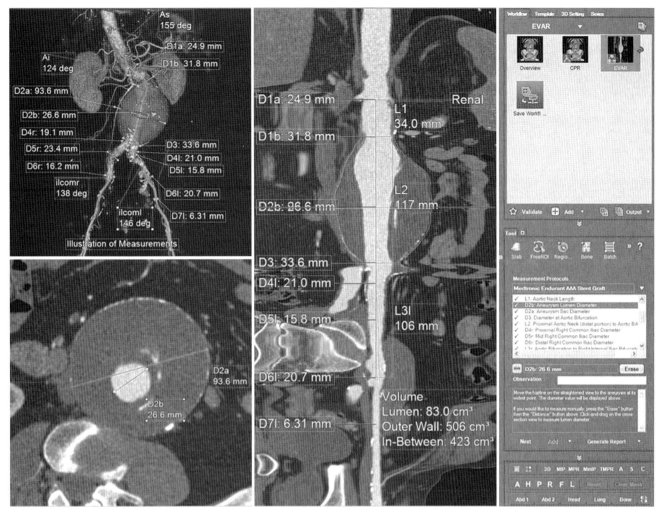

FIGURE 10.1 A series of walk-through steps on a vendor platform for preprocedure sizing of an abdominal aortic aneurysm endograft. (Reproduced from Greenberg RK. Computed tomography and computed tomographic arteriography in the evaluation of abdominal aortic aneurysms. In: Stanley JC, Veith FJ, Wakefield TW, eds. *Current Therapy in Vascular and Endovascular Surgery.* 5th ed. Elsevier; 2014.)

technique to ensure there is no narrowing of the access site, and the heparin can be reversed with protamine sulfate
- The groin incisions are closed in standard surgical fashion
- Distal extremity pulses should be checked prior to leaving the operating suite

EVAR FOR AAA RUPTURE

- A ruptured AAA is a true surgical emergency
  - Most patients with rupture die before hospitalization or ever undergoing an operation
- When a ruptured AAA is identified, emergent repair should be performed to give the patient the best chance of survival

- In a patient with hemodynamic instability of unclear etiology, a focused ultrasound examination can be quickly performed to evaluate for the presence of a ruptured AAA
- In a stable patient with a suspected AAA rupture, CTA can be performed to confirm the diagnosis and determine candidacy for EVAR
- Intravenous (IV) access should be established immediately with two large-bore peripheral IV lines
- Permissive hypotension, which refers to restricting aggressive fluid resuscitation as long as the patient maintains appropriate mental status and a systolic blood pressure between 70 and 90 mm Hg, should be implemented to limit excessive exsanguination
- In both stable and unstable patients with a ruptured AAA, transfemoral aortic balloon occlusion can be utilized for rapid proximal aortic control prior to proceeding with repair

TABLE 10.1 **Anatomic Considerations for Preoperative Planning Prior to Endovascular Abdominal Aortic Aneurysm Repair**

Anatomic Considerations	Definitions	Recommendations
Aortic neck diameter	Aortic diameter at the lowest renal artery	This diameter must be <32 mm. The required endograft diameter is determined by measuring the aortic neck diameter (e.g., 20 mm) and adding an additional 10%–20% (20 mm + 4 mm = 24 mm). Oversizing the endograft provides adequate radial force to provide sufficient seal and prevent device migration
Aortic neck length	Distance from the lowest renal artery to the origin of the aneurysm	This length should be >15 mm to provide an adequate proximal landing zone for endograft fixation
Aortic neck angulation	Angle formed between points connecting the lowest renal artery, the origin of the aneurysm, and the aortic bifurcation	The degree of angulation should be <60 degrees to facilitate implantation and prevent device migration, kinking, and endoleak
Accessory renal arteries	Present in 15%–20% of patients and occasionally may arise from the aneurysm[8]	Accessory renal arteries should be preserved at the time of EVAR if the artery is >3 mm in diameter or supplies more than one-third of the kidney
Iliac artery diameter and morphology	The iliac arteries must measure at least 6.5 mm in diameter and be without significant tortuosity, calcification/stenosis, or thrombus to allow delivery of the endoprosthesis	The common iliac arteries (CIAs) are the typical distal landing zones. Ectatic CIAs up to 2 cm in diameter are suitable landing zones for the endograft limbs. The length of normal diameter CIA into which the endograft limbs will be fixed should be >20 mm to achieve adequate distal seal. In certain cases, the external iliac artery may be used as the distal fixation site (e.g., CIA aneurysm). If the external iliac artery is used for fixation, the contralateral iliac artery should ideally be preserved to minimize gluteal claudication

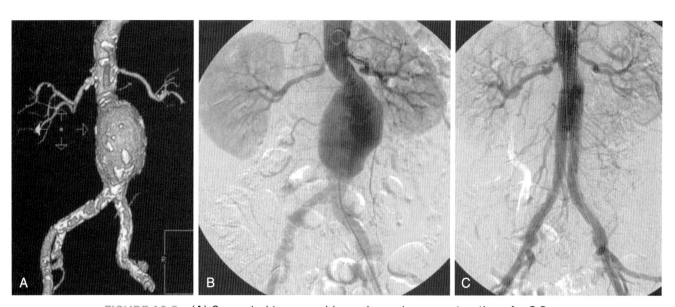

FIGURE 10.2 (A) Computed tomographic angiography reconstruction of a 6.3-cm abdominal aortic aneurysm (AAA). (B) Angiogram findings. (C) Completion angiography demonstrating AAA exclusion without endoleak. (Reprinted from Brinster CJ, Sternbergh WC 3rd. Endovascular aneurysm repair techniques. In: Sidawy AN, Perler BA, eds. *Rutherford's Vascular Surgery and Endovascular Therapy.* Vol. 1. 9th ed. Elsevier;2019.)

- A long sheath is required- to stabilize the compliant aortic balloon within a nonaneurysmal section of the descending thoracic aorta
- Once the balloon is inflated, anatomic feasibility for EVAR can be determined intraoperatively utilizing aortography or IVUS
- The Immediate Management of Patients with Rupture: Open Versus Endovascular Repair (IMPROVE) trial was a multicenter, pragmatic randomized trial that assigned 613 patients with suspected ruptured AAA to EVAR or OSR[10–12]
  - There was no significant difference in the 30-day mortality rate for patients with confirmed rupture between the EVAR and OSR groups (36.4% vs. 40.6%; $P = .31$), but more patients in the EVAR group were discharged directly to home (94% vs. 77%; $P < .001$)[10]
  - At 1-year follow-up, EVAR was more cost effective and offered significantly shorter length of hospital stay but did not offer a survival benefit in comparison to OSR[11]
  - At 3 years, mortality was significantly lower in the EVAR group (42% vs. 54%; OR: 0.62), but after 7 years there was no clear difference between the groups[12]
  - Reintervention rates up to 3 years were also not significantly different between the groups[12]
- The most recent published practice guidelines by the Society for Vascular Surgery recommend that EVAR be performed to treat a ruptured AAA when anatomically feasible[9]
- Abdominal compartment syndrome occurs after 8% of EVAR cases performed for a ruptured AAA and is typically due to large-volume retroperitoneal bleeding[13]
  - Characterized by high intraabdominal pressure leading to a bladder pressure >20 mm Hg and multiorgan dysfunction, including oliguria, increased peak airway pressures, hypoxemia, hypercapnia, hypotension, and decreased cardiac output due to inferior vena cava (IVC) compression
  - Early recognition and surgical decompression are recommended

ENDOLEAKS

- Endoleaks are caused by persistent blood flow into the aneurysm sac after endograft placement
- Overall incidence of 30.5% in the OVER trial[14]
- The presence of an endoleak indicates failure to completely exclude the aneurysm sac from arterial blood flow and pressure
- If left untreated, a clinically significant endoleak may lead to pressurization of the aneurysm sac with subsequent expansion and rupture
- Endoleak management depends on the type and presence of aneurysm sac enlargement

- Type I and type III endoleaks can occur as early or late complications but are usually identified on completion angiography
  - These should be treated as soon as they are recognized as they represent a direct communication between the systemic circulation and aneurysm sac
  - Type I and III endoleaks have been associated with an increased frequency of open conversions or risk of rupture of the aneurysm[15]
  - Commonly repaired using additional ballooning of the fixation sites or the placement of additional endograft components
- Type II endoleaks (T2Es) are the most commonly reported endoleak type, representing 76% of all endoleaks[14] (Fig. 10.3)
  - Often occur due to a patent inferior mesenteric artery or lumbar branches allowing retrograde flow into the aneurysm sac
  - Typically benign in nature and very rarely lead to aneurysm rupture
  - In a metaanalysis including 21,744 patients with 1515 T2Es following EVAR, the rupture rate of all T2Es was

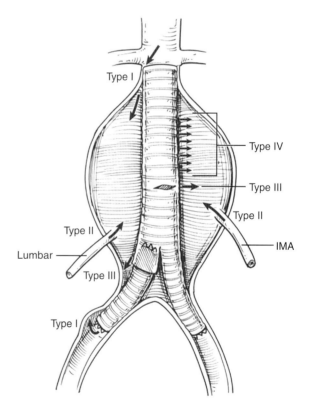

FIGURE 10.3 Endoleak classifications. *IMA,* Inferior mesenteric artery. (Reprinted from O'Brien GC, Qasabian RA, White GW. Endovascular treatment of nonruptured infrarenal aortic and aortoiliac aneurysms. In: Stanley JC, Veith FJ, Wakefield TW, eds. *Current Therapy in Vascular and Endovascular Surgery.* 5th ed. Elsevier Saunders; 2014.)

0.9%, with aneurysm sac expansion being absent in 43% of these cases[16]

- Silverberg et al. (data on 965 patients over an 8-year period at Mount Sinai Hospital) reported that 36% of T2Es sealed spontaneously, 8% experienced aneurysm sac enlargement >5 mm, and no patients with a T2E experienced rupture or required conversion to open repair during their follow-up (mean: 22.0 months)[17]
- *Close follow-up is a safe approach for most patients with a T2E and intervention is not recommended for endoleak persistence alone*
- Intervention may be considered for aneurysm sac expansion >5 mm during interval follow-up in the setting of a persistent T2E
- Transarterial embolization of the aortic branches feeding the aneurysm sac using coils, glues, thrombin, or Onyx (ethylene-vinyl alcohol copolymer) can be performed
- Translumbar and transcaval embolization techniques or an open or laparoscopic surgical approach can also be considered in cases of a persistent T2E with sac expansion refractory to embolization
- Type IV endoleaks result from the porosity of certain graft fabrics
  - More relevant with the earlier generations of endografts but are rare with the current generation of devices
  - Type IV endoleaks are self-limited, typically resolving without any intervention

TABLE 10.2   **Definitions for the Various Types of Endoleaks**

Type	Cause of Perigraft Flow
Ia	Inadequate seal at proximal end of endograft
Ib	Inadequate seal at distal end of endograft
Ic	Inadequate seal at iliac occluder plug
II	Flow from visceral vessel (lumbar, inferior mesenteric artery [IMA], accessory renal, hypogastric) without attachment site connection
IIIa	Flow from module disconnection
IIIb	Flow from fabric disruption
IV	Flow from porous fabric (30 days after graft placement)
Endoleak of undefined origin	Aneurysm enlargement but source of flow into the sac is unidentified

Reproduced from Chaikof EL, Blankensteijn JD, Harris PL, et al. Reporting standards for endovascular aortic aneurysm repair. *J Vasc Surg.* 2002;35(5):1048-1060.

POSTOPERATIVE IMAGING GUIDELINES

- Routine follow-up imaging is performed after EVAR to identify aneurysm sac growth, endoleak, device migration, or endograft failure (Fig. 10.4)
- Baseline imaging should be obtained 1 month after EVAR with CTA
  - If a T2E is observed 1 month after EVAR, CTA should be repeated at 6 months
- In the absence of an endoleak or aneurysm sac enlargement, imaging should be repeated in 12 months using CTA or duplex ultrasonography
- After 12 months, it is reasonable to use annual duplex ultrasound for routine surveillance in patients with no signs of an endoleak or aneurysm sac enlargement
- Any concerning interval findings should prompt CTA to rule out a type I or type III endoleak

LIMB ISCHEMIA AFTER EVAR

- Limb ischemia after EVAR is most often caused by endograft limb occlusion
  - Endograft limb occlusion occurs after 3%–7% of procedures, with most occurring within 6 months following the index operation[18-20]
- A distal landing zone in the external iliac artery (EIA), EIA of ≤10 mm, maximum AAA diameter of <59 mm, correction of endoleak after initial implant, and endograft kinking have been reported as predictors for limb occlusion[18]
  - First-generation endografts were at greatest risk for limb kinking compared with the newer generation of endografts[20]
- Prompt evaluation for possible graft limb occlusion is critical in patients who develop new-onset lower extremity claudication, ischemia, or reduction in ankle-brachial indices after EVAR
- Thrombolysis or mechanical thrombectomy, with or without adjunctive iliac stent placement, can be performed to recanalize graft limb occlusion
  - If unsuccessful, a femorofemoral bypass or axillofemoral bypass may be constructed to restore lower extremity perfusion

ILIAC BRANCH ENDOPROSTHESIS

- Concomitant iliac artery aneurysms occur in 15%–40% of patients with an AAA[21]
- The presence of an inadequate distal landing zone can complicate EVAR in patients with complex aortoiliac anatomy
- When the common iliac artery (CIA) diameter is larger than 2.5 cm or there is an aneurysmal proximal IIa per Table 10.2 present, extension of the endograft to the EIA can be performed to ensure adequate distal sealing

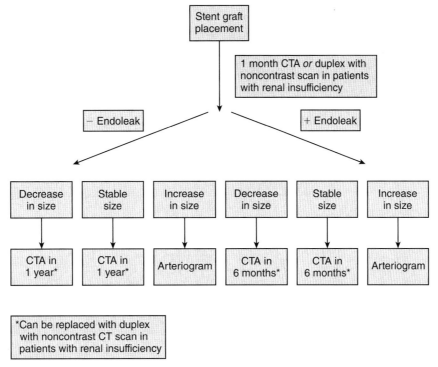

FIGURE 10.4 Recommended surveillance strategy following endovascular abdominal aortic aneurysm repair. *CTA,* Computed tomography angiography. (Reprinted from Fairman RM, Wang GJ. Abdominal aortic and iliac aneurysms. In: Sidawy AN, Perler BA, eds. *Rutherford's Vascular Surgery and Endovascular Therapy.* Vol. 1. 9th ed. Elsevier; 2019.)

- Coil embolization of the ipsilateral IIa is typically performed to prevent retrograde filling of the aneurysm
- IIa flow preservation can be performed in complex aortoiliac cases with construction of an EIA to IIa bypass or with the use of an iliac branch endoprosthesis (IBE)
- Current practice guidelines recommend preservation of flow to at least one IIa to reduce the risk for buttock claudication, erectile dysfunction, and spinal cord ischemia[9]
- In anatomically suitable patients, the use of an IBE is an effective and safe method to maintain flow into the IIa and exclude an aortoiliac aneurysm
  - These devices have a proximal limb that fits into the AAA endograft and distal limbs that extend down into the IIa and EIA (Fig. 10.5)
- The pErformance of iLiac branch deVIces for aneurysmS (pELVIS) multicenter registry studied 575 patients treated with an IBE[22]
  - The early (within 30 days) reintervention rate for occlusion or endoleak was low (1.6%)[22]
  - During a mean clinical follow-up period of ~33 months, 28 patients developed a type I endoleak and the overall postoperative reintervention rate was 9%[22]
  - A metaanalysis of 36 studies reporting on 1502 patients treated with an IBE found the technical success

of this procedure to be very high (97%).[23] The overall endoleak rate was 12.7% and the follow-up patency was around 94%.[23] The reintervention rate associated with IBEs was nearly 7%, and buttock claudication occurred in 2% of cases during the follow-up period[23]

INDICATIONS FOR ENDOANCHORS

- EndoAnchors (Aptus Endosystems) are small, helical "screws" that were designed to help prevent and treat type Ia endoleaks and endograft migration by providing greater radial fixation and sealing between the endograft and aortic wall (Fig. 10.6)
  - EndoAnchors have been shown to enhance endograft fixation to levels equivalent or superior to that of a hand-sewn anastomosis[24]
- May be implanted at the time of the initial EVAR or during a secondary procedure, such as repair of a type Ia endoleak or migrated graft
- Evidence for use of EndoAnchors comes from the *Aneurysm Treatment Using the Heli-FX* (Medtronic Vascular) *Aortic Securement System Global Registry* (ANCHOR) trial[25]
  - Prospective, multicenter trial that enrolled 319 patients who underwent EndoAnchor implantation

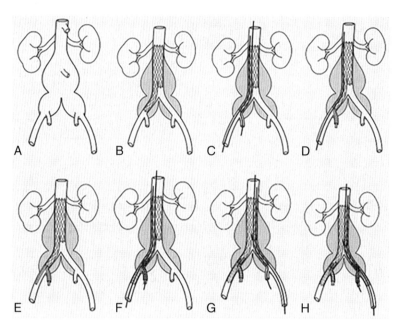

FIGURE 10.5 Key steps (A–H) of an endovascular repair of an aortoiliac aneurysm extending to the internal iliac arteries. (Reproduced from Lobato AC, Camacho-Lobato L. The sandwich technique to treat complex aortoiliac or isolated iliac aneurysms: results of midterm follow-up. *J Vasc Surg.* 2013;57(2):26S-34S.)

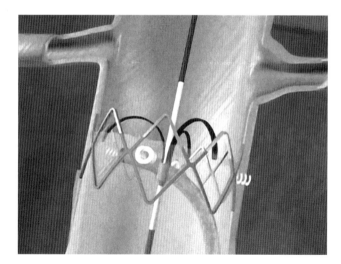

FIGURE 10.6 Deployment of Endo Anchors through the endograft and into the aortic wall. (Reprinted from Jordan Jr WD, Mehta M, Varnagy D, et al. Results of the ANCHOR prospective, multicenter registry of EndoAnchors for type Ia endoleaks and endograft migration in patients with challenging anatomy. *J Vasc Surg.* 2014; 60(4):885-892.)

at the time of initial EVAR (76%) or during revision for proximal neck complications after initial EVAR (24%)[25]

- The technical success rates of implantation were high and ~97% of the primary prophylactic patients were free from type Ia endoleak during follow-up.[25] Of the revision patients treated for type Ia

endoleak, 34% had evidence of type Ia endoleak during follow-up[25]

- In a separate propensity-matched cohort analysis including the subjects from the ANCHOR trial who received prophylactic EndoAnchors during EVAR, there was no significant difference in the rate of freedom from type Ia endoleak through two years between the ANCHOR and control cohorts (97% vs. 94%; $P =$ .34).[26] However, the rate of aneurysm sac regression through two years was significantly higher in subjects treated with EndoAnchors (81% vs. 49%; $P =$ .01)[26]

- While the use of EndoAnchors in EVAR and proximal aortic neck complications appears safe and technically feasible, additional studies with longer-term follow-up are necessary to determine which patients benefit the most from the use of these devices

OVERVIEW OF FENESTRATED EVAR

- Fenestrated endovascular aortic aneurysm repair (FEVAR) is intended to treat infrarenal AAAs with short proximal aortic necks (<10 mm) and juxtarenal AAAs
  - FEVAR utilizes openings within the graft fabric to incorporate the renal and/or mesenteric arteries into the proximal sealing zone
- The Zenith Fenestrated (Z-Fen) endograft (Cook Medical, Inc.) remains the only fenestrated device approved for use in the United States
  - Z-Fen endografts are manufactured specifically to fit each patient's aortic anatomy (Fig. 10.7)

- The safety and efficacy of the Z-Fen device was demonstrated in a prospective, multicenter study by Oderich et al., which included 67 patients treated for a juxtarenal AAA[27]
  - The 30-day mortality rate was only 1.5%.[27] At 5 years, freedom from all-cause mortality was 89% and freedom from aneurysm-related mortality was 97%.[27] Additionally, primary and secondary renal target patency was 83% and 96% at 5 years, respectively[27]
  - During the 5-year follow-up period, there was a relatively low rate of reported complications, including one type Ia endoleak (1.5%), one type Ib endoleak (1.5%), two device migrations (3%), and four aneurysm sac enlargements (6%)[27]
  - Overall, 81% of patients had sac shrinkage at 5 years and there were no aneurysm ruptures or conversions to open surgery[27]
  - Freedom from secondary intervention was approximately 64% at 5 years[27]
- An analysis of the American College of Surgeons National Surgical Quality Improvement Program Vascular Database comparing Z-Fen with OSR for complex AAAs found Z-Fen to be associated with lower rates of perioperative mortality (1.8% vs. 8.8%; $P =$ .001), postoperative

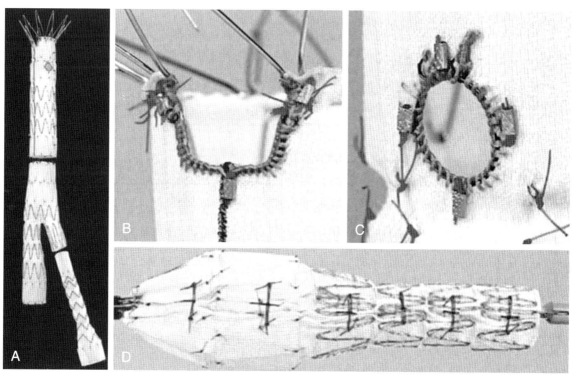

FIGURE 10.7   The Zenith Fenestrated abdominal aortic aneurysm endograft system (Cook Medical, Inc). (Reprinted from Robinson WP, Schanzer A, Simons JP, Upchurch GR Jr. Fenestrated and branched endograft treatment of juxtarenal, paravisceral, thoracoabdominal, and aortic arch aneurysms. In: Sidawy AN, Perler BA, eds. *Rutherford's Vascular Surgery and Endovascular Therapy*. Vol. 1. 9th ed. Elsevier; 2019.)

renal dysfunction (1.4% vs. 7.7%; $P = .002$), overall complications (11% vs. 33%; $P < .001$), blood transfusion requirement (22% vs. 73%; $P < .001$), and shorter length of stay (2 vs. 7 days; $P < .001$)[28]

INFECTED AORTIC ENDOGRAFTS

- Aortic endografts are at risk for infection by either direct contamination at the time of EVAR implantation or later via hematogenous seeding
- Endograft infection is rare and has been reported to occur in only 0.2%–0.7% of patients[29,30]
- The reported overall 30-day/in-hospital mortality rate is ~27% for cases of endograft infection following EVAR[30]
- Infection is most commonly attributed to *Staphylococcus aureus*[29]
- Patients presenting with an endograft infection typically have findings such as generalized sepsis, groin drainage, pseudoaneurysm formation, or ill-defined pain
- In the presence of extensive contamination and gross purulence, the preferred treatment approach is to explant all infected graft materials and perform extraanatomic vascular reconstruction and aortic debridement and resection
- In situ reconstruction using cryopreserved allografts, autologous vein grafts, or silver- or antibiotic-impregnated grafts may also be employed in certain cases
- Aortoenteric fistula formation is a potentially fatal complication of graft infection and may occur in 1%–2% of patients[9,31]
  - Any signs of gastrointestinal bleeding in a patient with an aortic graft should raise clinical suspicion for the presence of an aortoenteric fistula

- The diagnosis can be confirmed by endoscopy or computed tomography scan, and, if present, definitive surgical treatment is necessary

POTENTIAL COMPLICATIONS DURING EVAR AND TREATMENT

- Iliac on a stick
  - Iliac artery is torn and removed with the sheath
    - Keep wire access!
    - Place aortic occlusion balloon up contralateral side if still have access
    - Extend the limb to cover the defect
- Heavily calcified EIA and femorals
  - Unable to in large enough sheaths
    - Can sew an iliac conduit (retroperitoneal exposure)
    - Crack and pave
      - Angioplasty to the vessel followed by 10-mm self-expanding covered stent
- Loss of pulses post procedure from closure device
  - Femoral cutdown
  - Embolectomy if necessary
  - Primary repair of vessel
- Ruptured iliac after balloon molding the endograft
  - Careful inflation of balloon and distal aspect of limb
  - Can occur if balloon is outside the distal portion of the graft
    - Keep wire access
    - Aortic occlusion balloon if patient is hypotensive
    - Likely will need to embolize the hypogastric and extend the limb to cover the rupture site

REFERENCES

1. Beck AW, Sedrakyan A, Mao J, et al. Variations in abdominal aortic aneurysm care: a report from the International Consortium of Vascular Registries. *Circulation.* 2016;134(24):1948-1958.
2. Schermerhorn ML, Bensley RP, Giles KA, et al. Changes in abdominal aortic aneurysm rupture and short-term mortality, 1995-2008: a retrospective observational study. *Ann Surg.* 2012;256:651-658.
3. Paravastu SC, Jayarajasingam R, Cottam R, Palfreyman SJ, Michaels JA, Thomas SM. Endovascular repair of abdominal aortic aneurysm. *Cochrane Database Syst Rev.* 2014;(1):CD004178.
4. Lederle FA, Kyriakides TC, Stroupe KT, et al. Open versus endovascular repair of abdominal aortic aneurysm. *N Engl J Med.* 2019;380(22):2126-2135.
5. Lederle FA, Freischlag JA, Kyriakides TC, et al. Outcomes following endovascular vs open repair of abdominal aortic aneurysm: a randomized trial. *JAMA.* 2009;302(14):1535-1542.
6. Brewster DC, Cronenwett JL, Hallett JW Jr, et al. Guidelines for the treatment of abdominal aortic aneurysms: report of a

subcommittee of the Joint Council of the American Association for Vascular Surgery and Society for Vascular Surgery. *J Vasc Surg.* 2003;37(5):1106-1117.
7. Duong WQ, Fujitani RM, Grigorian A, et al. Evolving utility of endovascular treatment of juxtarenal, pararenal, and suprarenal abdominal aortic aneurysms associated with increased risk of mortality over time. *Ann Vasc Surg.* 2021;71:428-436.
8. Brewster DC, Retana A, Waltman AC, Darling RC. Angiography in the management of aneurysms of the abdominal aorta: its value and safety. *N Engl J Med.* 1975;292(16):822-825.
9. Chaikof EL, Dalman RL, Eskandari MK, et al. The Society for Vascular Surgery practice guidelines on the care of patients with an abdominal aortic aneurysm. *J Vasc Surg.* 2018;67(1):2-77.e2.
10. IMPROVE Trial Investigators, Powell JT, Sweeting MJ, et al. Endovascular or open repair strategy for ruptured abdominal aortic aneurysm: 30 day outcomes from IMPROVE randomised trial. *BMJ.* 2014;348:f7661.

11. IMPROVE Trial Investigators. Endovascular strategy or open repair for ruptured abdominal aortic aneurysm: one-year outcomes from the IMPROVE randomized trial. *Eur Heart J.* 2015;36(31):2061-2069.

12. IMPROVE Trial Investigators. Comparative clinical effectiveness and cost effectiveness of endovascular strategy *v* open repair for ruptured abdominal aortic aneurysm: three year results of the IMPROVE randomised trial. *BMJ.* 2017;359:j4859.

13. Karkos CD, Menexes GC, Patelis N, Kalogirou TE, Giagtzidis IT, Harkin DW. A systematic review and meta-analysis of abdominal compartment syndrome after endovascular repair of ruptured abdominal aortic aneurysms. *J Vasc Surg.* 2014;59(3):829-842.

14. Lal BK, Zhou W, Li Z, et al. Predictors and outcomes of endoleaks in the Veterans Affairs Open Versus Endovascular Repair (OVER) trial of abdominal aortic aneurysms. *J Vasc Surg.* 2015; 62(6):1394-1404.

15. Buth J, Harris PL, van Marrewijk C, Fransen G. The significance and management of different types of endoleaks. *Semin Vasc Surg.* 2003;16(2):95-102.

16. Sidloff DA, Stather PW, Choke E, Bown MJ, Sayers RD. Type II endoleak after endovascular aneurysm repair. *Br J Surg.* 2013; 100(10):1262-1270.

17. Silverberg D, Baril DT, Ellozy SH, et al. An 8-year experience with type II endoleaks: natural history suggests selective intervention is a safe approach. *J Vasc Surg.* 2006;44(3):453-459.

18. Faure EM, Becquemin JP, Cochennec F; ENGAGE collaborators. Predictive factors for limb occlusions after endovascular aneurysm repair. *J Vasc Surg.* 2015;61(5):1138-1145.e2.

19. Maldonado TS, Rockman CB, Riles E, et al. Ischemic complications after endovascular abdominal aortic aneurysm repair. *J Vasc Surg.* 2004;40(4):703-709; discussion 709-710.

20. Cochennec F, Becquemin JP, Desgranges P, Allaire E, Kobeiter H, Roudot-Thoraval F. Limb graft occlusion following EVAR: clinical pattern, outcomes and predictive factors of occurrence. *Eur J Vasc Endovasc Surg.* 2007;34(1):59-65.

21. Kirkwood ML, Saunders A, Jackson BM, Wang GJ, Fairman RM, Woo EY. Aneurysmal iliac arteries do not portend future iliac aneurysmal enlargement after endovascular aneurysm repair for abdominal aortic aneurysm. *J Vasc Surg.* 2011;53(2):269-273.

22. Donas KP, Inchingolo M, Cao P, et al. Secondary procedures following iliac branch device treatment of aneurysms involving the iliac bifurcation: the pELVIS registry. *J Endovasc Ther.* 2017;24(3):405-410.

23. Giosdekos A, Antonopoulos CN, Sfyroeras GS, et al. The use of iliac branch devices for preservation of flow in internal iliac artery during endovascular aortic aneurysm repair. *J Vasc Surg.* 2020;71(6):2133-2144.

24. Melas N, Perdikides T, Saratzis A, Saratzis N, Kiskinis D, Deaton DH. Helical EndoStaples enhance endograft fixation in an experimental model using human cadaveric aortas. *J Vasc Surg.* 2012;55(6):1726-1733.

25. de Vries JP, Ouriel K, Mehta M, et al. Analysis of EndoAnchors for endovascular aneurysm repair by indications for use. *J Vasc Surg.* 2014;60(6):1460-1467.

26. Muhs BE, Jordan W, Ouriel K, Rajaee S, de Vries JP. Matched cohort comparison of endovascular abdominal aortic aneurysm repair with and without EndoAnchors. *J Vasc Surg.* 2018;67(6):1699-1707.

27. Oderich GS, Farber MA, Schneider D, et al. Final 5-year results of the United States Zenith Fenestrated prospective multicenter study for juxtarenal abdominal aortic aneurysms. *J Vasc Surg.* 2021;73(4):1128-1138.

28. Varkevisser RR, O'Donnell TF, Swerdlow NJ, et al. Fenestrated endovascular aneurysm repair is associated with lower perioperative morbidity and mortality compared with open repair for complex abdominal aortic aneurysms. *J Vasc Surg.* 2019; 69(6):1670-1678.

29. Hobbs SD, Kumar S, Gilling-Smith GL. Epidemiology and diagnosis of endograft infection. *J Cardiovasc Surg (Torino).* 2010;51(1):5-14.

30. Argyriou C, Georgiadis GS, Lazarides MK, Georgakarakos E, Antoniou GA. Endograft infection after endovascular abdominal aortic aneurysm repair: a systematic review and meta-analysis. *J Endovasc Ther.* 2017;24(5):688-697.

31. Geroulakos G, Lumley JS, Wright JG. Factors influencing the long-term results of abdominal aortic aneurysm repair. *Eur J Vasc Endovasc Surg.* 1997;13(1):3-8.

CHAPTER 11

Aortoiliac Occlusive Disease

RICHARD A. MEENA, MD and OLAMIDE ALABI, MD

EPIDEMIOLOGY AND ETIOLOGY

- Aortoiliac occlusive disease (AIOD), a subtype of peripheral artery disease (PAD), includes a spectrum of partial to complete atherosclerotic obstruction of the aorta and/or iliac arteries
- Overall disease prevalence of 3%–10%
- As the population ages, so does the estimated prevalence of PAD, with more than 10% of patients aged 60–80 years diagnosed with PAD[1]
- Patients with PAD (including AIOD) present with a range of symptoms, from asymptomatic to claudication to rest pain and tissue loss. The ratio of asymptomatic to symptomatic patients has been estimated to be 3:1 based on several large cross-sectional studies[2]
- Risk factors associated with AIOD: non-White race, older age, cigarette smoking, diabetes mellitus, hypertension, dyslipidemia, elevated inflammatory markers, hyperviscosity/hypercoagulability, hyperhomocysteinemia, and chronic kidney disease[3,4]

SIGNS/SYMPTOMS OF DISEASE

- Based on anatomic distribution of disease, patients with AIOD may develop buttock or thigh claudication
- It is important to remember that patients with AIOD may first complain of generalized lower extremity claudication, not specifically of the thigh and buttocks
- Patients with chronic limb-threatening ischemia (CLTI) may present with pain at rest or with tissue loss
- Male patients with AIOD may develop impotence[5]

- The eponym Leriche syndrome refers to a triad of signs/symptoms often found at the time of AIOD diagnosis: claudication, impotence, and absent femoral pulses
- Cholesterol emboli embolizing in the dorsal digital arteries of the foot from the atherosclerotic aortoiliac disease may lead to blue-toe syndrome
- When the aortic atheromatous disease is nonconcentric and protruding into the vessel lumen, the aorta is often referred to as a "shaggy aorta," which is extremely friable and susceptible to embolization[6]

DIAGNOSTIC EVALUATION

- Evaluating bilateral femoral artery pulses can give great insight into the extent of AIOD, as can the evaluation of pedal pulses
- Arterial-brachial indices (ABIs) can provide detail of the degree of PAD and AIOD, with an ABI less than <0.9 indicating arterial insufficiency and an ABI greater than 1.3 indicating calcified vessels
- If ABIs at rest do not demonstrate findings consistent with PAD or AIOD, but clinical history and/or physical examination remains suggestive of the diagnosis, exercise ABIs can be performed
- If the ABI drops 30 mm Hg while exercising, or if there is a drop of greater than 20% in the ABI with exercise compared to baseline, this demonstrates significant disease
- Literature has shown greater than 90% sensitivity and specificity of duplex ultrasonography in preoperative diagnosis of AIOD[7]
- The most commonly used imaging modality is computed tomography angiography (CTA)[8]
- A systematic review of 10 studies demonstrated that CTA has a pooled sensitivity and specificity of 93% and 94%, respectively, when evaluating AIOD.[9] Given that resolution of CTA imaging may be negatively impacted by heavy calcific burden, magnetic resonance (MR) imaging can also be used. MR, specifically magnetic resonance angiography (MRA), is a useful imaging modality for those patients with chronic kidney disease or for those unable to tolerate iodine-based contrast.[10] Contrast-enhanced MRA has a sensitivity and specificity of 94% and 73%, respectively, for significant atherosclerotic lesions of the aortoiliac system[11]

Arteriography can also be used to assess disease burden. While CTA remains first-line for the diagnosis of AIOD, given its noninvasive nature, arteriography allows for a more robust evaluation of dynamic flow. Additionally, if endovascular means of revascularization are to be attempted, arteriography can be both diagnostic and therapeutic. When performing arteriography for AIOD, it may be necessary to obtain arterial access from an alternative source (such as the upper extremity), given the iliacs may be occluded.

TREATMENT

Nonoperative Intervention

All patients with AIOD do not need an operation. Determining whether a patient needs an operation is largely based on severity of symptoms. Patients with intermittent claudication from AIOD that is not lifestyle limiting, for example, may not require operative intervention, while those with rest pain or tissue loss may require more urgent intervention.

To modify risk factors, patients with AIOD and intermittent claudication should first be treated with optimal nonoperative medical management, including adherence to an antiplatelet agent and statin, blood pressure control, blood glucose control, smoking cessation, and structured exercise.

Open Reconstruction

When symptoms warrant an operation, the management of AIOD can be both endovascular and open. The gold standard of open repair is an aortofemoral bypass (AFB). To perform an AFB, bilateral groin incisions are made, and either a transperitoneal or retroperitoneal approach is utilized. The anterior surface of the aorta is carefully dissected, avoiding lateral injury to the inferior vena cava. The level of the proximal aortic clamp depends on the extent of calcific disease; if a suprarenal or supramesenteric clamp is required, the clamp can be placed more distally after the proximal anastomosis is created to perfuse the mesenteric and/or renal arteries. While the proximal anastomosis can be performed in an end-to-end or end-to-side fashion, if there are bilateral external iliac artery occlusions, the proximal anastomosis must be end-to-side (to preserve the hypogastric arteries). Typically, distal anastomoses are end-to-side. Providers should circumferentially control the common femoral, superficial femoral, and profunda arteries prior to clamping and suturing their distal anastomoses. AFB has been documented to have a 5-year primary patency rate of 88.5%, with a 5-year secondary patency rate of 96.5%.[12]

While AFB is the gold standard for open operative intervention, extraanatomical bypasses can be considered, particularly for patients who are unfit for the stress of aortic cross-clamping and in general for those who are poor surgical candidates. Axillofemoral bypasses avoid the need for cross-clamping of the aorta. To perform an axillofemoral bypass, an infraclavicular incision (typically on the patient's right side) is made, along with two groin incisions. The axillary artery and bilateral common femoral arteries are dissected and controlled. The graft is tunneled superficially to the chest wall.

While axillofemoral bypasses are a viable surgical option, their 5-year primary patency rate (67.7%) is inferior to that of AFBs. Studies suggest that axillofemoral grafts are associated with lower 1-year overall survival rates (67.0%), although this statistic may be due to the fact that these operations are often reserved for patients who are not good surgical candidates.[10,12] While primary patency rates and overall survival rates are clearly inferior in axillofemoral bypasses compared with AFB, 5-year limb salvage rates are comparable (92.9% axillofemoral versus 96.4% AFB), suggesting that axillofemoral bypasses remain a viable option for high-risk patients with symptomatic AIOD.[10]

Endovascular Repair

Endovascular approaches to AIOD have become more frequently utilized, with improving technology and increasing provider experience. These minimally invasive procedures are less morbid and are associated with decreased hospital length of stay.[13] For AIOD, stent angioplasty is more effective than percutaneous transluminal angioplasty (PTA). One study evaluating 1300 patients who underwent PTA and 816 patients who underwent stent angioplasty for AIOD demonstrated higher 4-year primary patency rates for those treated with stents, both for claudication (stenoses: 65% PTA versus 77% stents; occlusions: 54% PTA versus 61% stents) and CLTI (stenoses: 53% PTA versus 67% stents; occlusions: 44% polytetrafluoroethylene [PTFE] versus 53% stents).[14]

Both covered stents and bare-metal stents have been evaluated in the endovascular repair of AIOD depending on the extent of disease.[15] The COBEST (Covered versus Balloon Expandable Stent Trial) compared covered and bare-metal stents. For TransAtlantic Inter-Society Consensus (TASC) B lesions, no difference between freedom from binary restenosis was appreciated at 18 months. However, for TASC C and D lesions, covered stents were significantly more likely to be free from binary restenosis than bare-metal stents at 18 months.[16] When results were reassessed at 5 years, it was determined that covered stents had statistically significantly higher patency rates than bare-metal stents at 18 months (95.1% versus 73.9%), 24 months (82.1% versus 70.9%), 48 months (79.9% versus 63%), and 60 months (74.7% versus 62.5%).[17]

A metaanalysis including 14 studies, 8 of which were prospective clinical trials, found that covered balloon-expandable stents had a 1-year primary patency rate between 83.6% and 96.9% for AIOD.[18]

Several studies have aimed to determine whether endovascular or open operative techniques are superior in the treatment of AIOD. One study reviewed 75 consecutive patients undergoing repair of complex, TASC D aortoiliac occlusive lesions. In this study, endovascular therapy was associated with fewer in-hospital systemic complications than open repair, with high initial technical success rates. However, at a mean follow-up of 21.3 months, patients undergoing endovascular therapy had higher reintervention rates than those undergoing open repair. Importantly, at 2 years of follow-up, graft patency was higher in the open group (96.7% versus 80%).[19] Another study found that patients undergoing endovascular repair for AIOD had shorter hospitalizations (2.6 days versus 8.5 days) and shorter intensive care unit stays (0.1 days versus 0.9 days) than did those undergoing open repair, while their 5-year primary patency (81.4% endovascular versus 87.3% open) and limb salvage (98.4% endovascular versus 98.9% open) rates were comparable.[20] Ultimately, patient-specific factors must be considered and a detailed conversation with the patient must be had before determining the optimal operative approach for AIOD.

When treating AIOD, altering the aortic bifurcation is less ideal than reconstructing it, as can be appreciated when comparing AFB to axillofemoral bypasses (Table 11.1). CERAB (*Covered Endovascular Reconstruction of the Aortic Bifurcation*) is an endovascular technique that re-creates blood flow through a more normal anatomical configuration. This method was first introduced in 2013 in the Netherlands, when Goverde et al. published their data on using three covered balloon-expandable stents to recreate a neobifurcation.[21] The first results of this technique were published 2 years later, when CERAB was reported to have a 1-year primary patency rate of 87.3%, 1-year secondary patency rate of 95.0%, 2-year primary patency rate of 82.3%, and 2-year secondary patency rate of 95.0%.[22] A 3-year study from two centers reviewed 130 patients undergoing CERAB

and demonstrated primary patency rates of 86%, 84%, and 82% at 1, 2, and 3 years, respectively.[23]

AIOD and Aneurysmal Disease

In the setting of both AIOD and aneurysmal disease, endovascular repair of abdominal aortic aneurysms (EVAR) may require additional preoperative planning and operative steps. Small, stenotic or occluded, and tortuous vessels all provide additional challenges for surgeons. Further, calcified iliac vessels may limit sheath, catheter, or even wire advancement into the aorta.

Open retroperitoneal iliofemoral conduits can be created to improve access for EVAR in AIOD. Traditionally, to create an iliofemoral conduit, the distal common iliac artery is dissected and controlled via a retroperitoneal approach, and a 10-mm graft is anastomosed to the iliac. After completion of the EVAR, the conduit can be ligated, or its distal end can be anastomosed to the common femoral artery.[24]

Rather than performing a hybrid procedure, solely endovascular conduits (or "endoconduits") have also been described. Endoconduits can be created using the "pave and crack" technique, which involves placing covered stents along the diseased iliofemoral system. These covered stents are then dilated to create a controlled rupture of the vessel with an adequate diameter for sheath advancement.[25]

If bilateral hypogastric artery exclusion is deemed necessary, it is encouraged to stage exclusion. Concurrent bilateral hypogastric artery exclusion increases the risk of impotence, colorectal ischemia, and hip/buttock claudication. Staging these procedures, on the other hand, has been associated with decreased morbidity.[26]

POSTOPERATIVE COMPLICATIONS

Thrombosis

In the postoperative setting, complications from AIOD can vary based on type of intervention. After AFB graft creation, providers should have high suspicion for graft limb occlusion when patients present with acute changes in lower extremity symptoms. Smoking has been associated with increased risk of graft thrombosis. While thrombolysis can be attempted in the management of acute graft thrombosis, distal anastomotic reconstructions (i.e., graft interposition or patch angioplasty) have been associated with the highest patency rates and are more clinically appropriate in the setting of chronic limb occlusions. Graft thrombosis is a feared complication, with one study documenting a 5.6% operative mortality rate and a 14% amputation rate.[27] After endovascular interventions, in-stent thromboses can result in poor outflow and subsequent worsening of lower extremity ischemia. Taking antiplatelet agents poststent angioplasty for AIOD can help decrease the risk and severity of in-stent thromboses.

TABLE 11.1   Primary Patency Rates of Open and Endovascular Techniques in the Operative Management of Aortoiliac Occlusive Disease

Technique	Primary Patency Rate
Aortofemoral bypass	88.5% at 5 years
Axillofemoral bypass	67.7% at 5 years
Covered stent	74.7% at 5 years
Balloon-expandable Stent	62.5% at 5 years
Percutaneous transluminal angioplasty	65% at 4 years
Covered endovascular reconstruction of aortic bifurcation (CERAB)	82% at 3 years

Intestinal Ischemia

In addition to graft and in-stent thrombosis, a potential complication of AIOD repair is intestinal ischemia. Based on the proximal extent of the repair and atherosclerotic disease burden of the celiac, superior mesenteric, and inferior mesenteric arteries, poor perfusion of at least two of these vessels can result in mesenteric ischemia. Acute changes in bowel function, serum lactate levels, and abdominal pain can help raise concern for mesenteric ischemia.

Access Complications

Particularly in the presence of prosthetic bypasses, anastomotic pseudoaneurysmal degeneration can occur. The risk factors for this degeneration are varied, including hypertension, healing complications after surgery, infectious processes, excessive physical activity, forces from adjacent joints, defects in the structure of the graft material, and trauma. In vitro studies have found decreased bacterial adherence to expanded PTFE (ePTFE) compared with Dacron.[28] If an isolated femoral pseudoaneurysm is present without obvious involvement of the remainder of the graft, the surgeon can replace the infected graft segment with rifampin-soaked prosthesis, with or without a muscle flap, if there is concern for groin infection. Extraanatomic bypasses can also be performed to exclude the site of infection, including axillary artery to distal femoral or popliteal artery bypasses, as well as obturator bypasses. If reconstruction of the entire bypass is necessary, autologous conduits are preferred in the setting of infection.

In endovascular repair, hematomas can also occur at the site of access. Closure devices and manual pressure can be performed at the completion of the case to decrease the risk of groin bleeding, as can postoperative bedrest. Access sites should be monitored closely for prompt recognition and management.

FOLLOW-UP

Per Society for Vascular Surgery Guidelines published in 2018, follow-up after AFB for the indication of AIOD should include clinical examination and ankle-brachial indices, with or without duplex ultrasonography, in the early postoperative period to provide a new baseline after surgery. This evaluation should be repeated at 6 months, 12 months, and annually thereafter, pending any changes in clinical history prompting further evaluation (such as additional imaging).[29]

While similar follow-up can be implemented after endovascular treatment of AIOD, duplex ultrasonography becomes increasingly important, allowing for in-stent velocity measurements to be taken. Some suggest the same surveillance protocol, with clinical examination, ankle-brachial indices, and ultrasound versus contrast-enhanced CT at 1 month, 6 months, 12 months, and annually thereafter (pending any changes in clinical history or radiographic findings). Surveillance should be lifelong.

REFERENCES

1. Criqui MH, AboyansV. Epidemiology of peripheral artery disease. *Circ Res.* 2015;116(9):1509-1526.
2. Society for Vascular Surgery Lower Extremity Guidelines Writing Group, Conte MS, Pomposelli FB, et al. Society for Vascular Surgery practice guidelines for atherosclerotic occlusive disease of the lower extremities: management of asymptomatic disease and claudication. *J Vasc Surg.* 2015;61:2S-41S.
3. Neisen M. Endovascular management of aortoiliac occlusive disease. *Semin Intervent Radiol.* 2009;26(4):296-302.
4. Norgren L, Hiatt WR, Dormandy JA, et al. Inter-Society Consensus for the management of peripheral arterial disease (TASC II). *J Vasc Surg.* 2007;45:S5-S67.
5. Gür S, Oguzkurt L, Kaya B, Tekbas G, Ozkan U. Impotence due to external iliac steal syndrome: treatment with percutaneous transluminal angioplasty and stent placement. *Korean J Radiol.* 2013;14(1):81-85.
6. Serra R, Bracale U, Jiritano F, et al. The shaggy aorta syndrome: an updated review. *Am J Surg.* 2021;148(6):836-839.
7. Muela Méndez M, Morata Barrado PC, Blanco Cañibano E, García Fresnillo B, Guerra Requena M. Preoperative mapping of the aortoiliac territory with duplex ultrasound in patients with peripheral arterial occlusive disease. *J Vasc Surg.* 2018; 68(2):503-509.
8. Ahmed S, Raman S, Fishman EK. CT angiography and 3D imaging in aortoiliac occlusive disease: collateral pathways in Leriche syndrome. *Abdom Radiol (NY).* 2017;42(9): 2346-2357.
9. Sun Z. Diagnostic accuracy of multislice CT angiography in peripheral artery disease. *J Vasc Interv Radiol.* 2006;17: 1915-1921.
10. Igari K, Kudo T, Katsui S, Nishizawa M, Uetake H. The comparison of long-term results between aortofemoral and axillofemoral bypass for patients with aortoiliac occlusive disease. *Ann Thorac Cardiovasc Surg.* 2020;26(6):352-358.
11. Lundin P, Svensson A, Henriksen E, et al. Imaging of aortoiliac arterial disease. Duplex ultrasound and MR angiography versus digital subtraction angiography. *Acta Radiol.* 2000;41(2): 125-132.
12. Onohara T, Komori K, Kume M, et al. Multivariate analysis of long-term results after an axillobifemoral and aortobifemoral bypass in patients with aortoiliac occlusive disease. *J Cardiovasc Surg (Torino).* 2000;41(6):905-910.
13. Indes JE, Pfaff M, Farrokhyar F, et al. Clinical outcomes of 5358 patients undergoing direct open bypass or endovascular treatment for aortoiliac occlusive disease: a systematic review and meta-analysis. *J Endovasc Ther.* 2013;20(4):443-455.

14. Bosch JL, Hunink M. Meta-analysis of the results of percutaneous transluminal angioplasty and stent placement for aortoiliac occlusive disease. *Radiology.* 1997;204(1):87-96.

15. Grimme FA, Goverde P, Van Oostayen JA, Zeebregts CJ, Reijnen MM. Covered stents for aortoiliac reconstruction of chronic occlusive lesions. *J Cardiovasc Surg (Torino).* 2012;53(3):279-289.

16. Mwipatayi BP, Thomas S, Wong J, et al. A comparison of covered vs bare expandable stents for the treatment of aortoiliac occlusive disease. *J Vasc Surg.* 2011;54(6):1561-1570.

17. Mwipatayi BP, Sharma S, Daneshmand A, et al. Durability of the balloon-expandable covered versus bare-metal stents in the Covered versus Balloon Expandable Stent Trial (COBEST) for the treatment of aortoiliac occlusive disease. *J Vasc Surg.* 2016;64(1):83-94.

18. Mwipatayi BP, Ouriel K, Anwari T, et al. A systematic review of covered balloon-expandable stents for treating aortoiliac occlusive disease. *J Vasc Surg.* 2020;72(4):1473-1486.

19. Mayor J, Branco B, Chung J, et al. Outcome comparison between open and endovascular management of TASC II D aortoiliac occlusive disease. *Ann Vasc Surg.* 2019;61:65-71.e63.

20. Antonello M, Squizzato F, Bassini S, Porcellato L, Grego F, Piazza M. Open repair versus endovascular treatment of complex aortoiliac lesions in low risk patients. *J Vasc Surg.* 2019;70(4):1155-1165.e1.

21. Goverde PC, Grimme F, Verbruggen PJ, Reijnen MM. Covered endovascular reconstruction of aortic bifurcation (CERAB) technique: a new approach in treating extensive aortoiliac occlusive disease. *J Cardiovasc Surg (Torino).* 2013;54(3):383-387.

22. Grimme FAB, Goverde P, Verbruggen PJEM, Zeebregts CJ, Reijnen MMPJ. First results of the covered endovascular reconstruction of the aortic bifurcation (CERAB) technique for aortoiliac occlusive disease. *Eur J Vasc Endovasc Surg.* 2015;62(5):1371-1372.

23. Taeymans K, Jebbink EG, Holewijn S, et al. Three-year outcome of the covered endovascular reconstruction of the aortic bifurcation technique for aortoiliac occlusive disease. *J Vasc Surg.* 2018;67(5):1438-1447.

24. Hershberger R, Milner R. Conduit use during endovascular repair of AAAs. *Endovascular Today.* October, 2010:39-43.

25. Asciutto G, Aronici M, Resch T, Sonesson B, Kristmundsson T, Dias NV. Endoconduits with "pave and crack" technique avoid open ilio-femoral conduits with sustainable mid-term results. *Eur J Vasc Endovasc Surg.* 2017;54(4):472-479.

26. Wolpert LM, Dittrich K, Hallisey MJ, et al. Hypogastric artery embolization in endovascular abdominal aortic aneurysm repair. *J Vasc Surg.* 2001;33(6):1193-1198.

27. Pedrini L, Pisano E, Donato Di Paola M, Ballester A, Magnoni F. Late occlusion of aortofemoral bypass graft: surgical treatment. *Cardiovasc Surg.* 1994;2(6):763-766.

28. Seabrook GR, Schmitt D, Bandyk DF, Edmiston CE, Krepel CJ, Towne JB. Anastomotic femoral pseudoaneurysm: an investigation of occult infection as an etiologic factor. *J Vasc Surg.* 1990;11(5):629-634.

29. Zierler RE, Jordan W, Lal BK, et al. The Society for Vascular Surgery practice guidelines on follow-up after vascular surgery arterial procedures. *J Vasc Surg.* 2018;68(1):256-284.

CHAPTER 12

Cerebrovascular Disease

SHERNAZ S. DOSSABHOY, MD, MBA, and SHIPRA ARYA, MD, SM

EPIDEMIOLOGY AND PATHOPHYSIOLOGY OF ATHEROSCLEROTIC CAROTID ARTERY DISEASE

- Stroke is one of the leading causes of disability and death globally, with more than 795,000 new strokes in the United States every year[1]
- Atherosclerotic disease of the carotid artery is responsible for 15%–20% of all strokes[2]; the risk of stroke increases with increasing degree of stenosis from <1% stroke risk per year for <80% stenosis to 4.8% per year for >90% stenosis[3]
- Carotid artery disease begins as increased carotid intima-media thickness (defined as >1 mm) and develops into carotid plaque (1.5 mm–<50% luminal diameter), and ultimately to carotid stenosis (≥50% luminal diameter)[4]

- Plaque instability and mechanism of stroke
  - Atherosclerosis begins as the accumulation of lipids and immune cells in the intimal layer of the vessel wall, known as "fatty streaks," which are asymptomatic and do not cause stenosis themselves
  - Over time, inflammation, mediated by macrophages and other immune cells, causes the development of atherosclerotic plaque
  - Next, smooth muscle cells migrate from the adventitia to the media, leading to the formation of the fibrous cap, which surrounds the plaque
  - As atherosclerosis, now thought of as a systemic inflammatory state, progresses, apoptosis of smooth muscle cells and macrophages ensues, forming a lipid-rich necrotic core with plaque instability
  - Unstable plaque progresses until plaque rupture, during which the lipid core is exposed and serves as a nidus for thrombus formation
  - Cerebrovascular disease symptoms occur due to (1) *thrombotic event* leading to vessel occlusion at the location of the carotid plaque or (2) *embolic event* due to thrombi breaking off and traveling to the brain where they impede cerebral blood flow
  - Embolic events are more common causes of stroke compared to a low flow state
- Risk factors for carotid disease include older age, male sex, hypertension (HTN), diabetes, hyperlipidemia, genetics, poor diet, lack of exercise, and smoking[5]

IMAGING FOR CAROTID ARTERY DISEASE

- Duplex ultrasound (US)
  - Reports peak systolic velocity (PSV), end-diastolic velocity (EDV), and ratio of PSV of internal carotid artery (ICA) to common carotid artery (CCA)
  - 50%–69% ICA stenosis
    - PSV 125–229 cm/s
    - EDV 40–100
    - ICA/CCA PSV ratio 2–4
  - 70%–99% ICA stenosis
    - PSV ≥ 230
    - EDV >100 (EDV >140 most sensitive for stenosis >80%)
    - ICA/CCA PSV ratio >4

- Limitations—higher velocities may be seen in women and in the presence of contralateral ICA occlusion. US accuracy may be reduced if high carotid bifurcation, severe vessel tortuosity, increased calcifications, and in obese patients
- Computed tomography angiography (CTA)—fast, excellent resolution but requires contrast administration that carries risk of nephrotoxicity and allergic reaction as well as radiation exposure
- Magnetic resonance angiography (MRA)—no contrast, can analyze plaque morphology, but overestimates degree of stenosis
- Catheter-based angiography—still considered gold standard but reserved for patients with conflicting US/CTA/MRA imaging or patients considered for stenting; increased risk of stroke compared with noninvasive imaging (~1% risk)

SEMINAL CLINICAL TRIALS IN CAROTID ARTERY DISEASE MANAGEMENT

- Carotid endarterectomy (CEA) versus medical management for symptomatic disease
  - *North American Symptomatic Carotid Endarterectomy Trial (NASCET)*[6]
    - Symptomatic patients with moderate (50%–69%) and severe (>70%) stenosis, compared CEA versus medical management, multicenter randomized controlled trial (RCT) United States and Canada
      - Medical management was aspirin alone (this was before the era of statins and clopidogrel [Plavix])
    - For patients with <50% stenosis, no benefit demonstrated; for 50%–69% stenosis, only moderate benefit of CEA (5-year stroke—15.7% CEA vs. 22.2% medical)
    - *For >70% stenosis, 2-year stroke rate—9% CEA versus 26% medical = 17% absolute risk reduction (ARR) and benefit of CEA persisted through 8-year follow-up*
      - Given clear benefit to CEA, trial was stopped early for the >70% subset of patients and all received CEA
  - *European Carotid Surgery Trial (ECST)*[7]—demonstrated similar results to NASCET with benefit of CEA for >80% stenosis with 3-year stroke/death rate 14.9% CEA versus 26.5% medical = 11.6% ARR
    - ECST's 80%–99% stenosis was equivalent to 60%–99% for NASCET given different methods of determining stenosis
- CEA versus medical management for asymptomatic disease
  - *Asymptomatic Carotid Atherosclerosis Study (ACAS)*[8]
    - Asymptomatic patients with ≥60% stenosis, compared CEA versus medical management in low-risk patients, multicenter RCT United States and Canada (N = 1662)

- Medical management was aspirin 81 mg daily and "medical risk factor management" (prestatin and Plavix)
- 5-year stroke or death rate—5.1% CEA versus 11% medical
- Recommended CEA for patients (aged <80 years) as long as the expected combined stroke and mortality rate for the individual surgeon was not >3%
- ACAS subgroup analysis showed that CEA was less effective in women with 5-year stroke/death—7.3% CEA versus 8.7% medical—with higher rate of perioperative complications
- *Asymptomatic Carotid Surgery Trial (ACST)*[9]
  - European trial, similar to ACAS, with 5-year stroke/death for >70% stenosis in asymptomatic patients—6% CEA versus 12% medical
  - Medical management = aspirin and antihypertensives initially; statins were added later during the trial
- CEA versus carotid stenting trials—see Evidence summary of CEA versus CAS

BEST MEDICAL THERAPY (BMT) FOR ASYMPTOMATIC AND SYMPTOMATIC DISEASE

- HTN—target blood pressure (BP) <140/90 mm Hg by lifestyle interventions (diet, weight loss, exercise, etc.) or antihypertensives recommended for both asymptomatic carotid disease and those with transient ischemic attack (TIA) or stroke after acute phase
- Diabetes—target A1C <7% in diabetic patients to reduce microvascular (and possibly macrovascular) complications (see ACCORD and ADVANCE trials[10])
- Dyslipidemia—target low-density lipoprotein (LDL) is <70 mg/dL for anyone with ischemic stroke with atherosclerotic disease of cerebral vasculature.[11] The 2018 AHA/ACC guidelines on lipid management recommend high-intensity statins (atorvastatin 40/80 mg or rosuvastatin 20/40 mg) for all patients with atherosclerotic cardiovascular disease (ASCVD) irrespective of LDL levels[12]
  - Very high-risk patients: include a history of multiple major ASCVD events or one major ASCVD event and multiple high-risk conditions (age ≥ 65, heterozygous familial hypercholesterolemia, history of coronary artery bypass surgery or percutaneous coronary intervention, type 2 diabetes, HTN, chronic kidney disease, current smoking, persistently elevated LDL-C, or history of heart failure. In these patients, if LDL ≥70 despite highest-dose statin, it is reasonable to add ezetimibe followed by a PCSK9 inhibitor (e.g., alirocumab or evolocumab)
  - Not very high-risk patients: goal LDL reduction is 50% and if LDL>70 mg/dL, OK to add ezetimibe

- *Stroke Prevention by Aggressive Reduction in Cholesterol Levels (SPARCL)* trial showed intensive lipid lowering with atorvastatin (80 mg/day vs. placebo) reduces the risk of both cerebrovascular and cardiovascular events in patients with and without carotid stenosis with greater benefit in carotid patients: 33% risk reduction of any stroke (heart rate [HR] 0.67; 95% confidence interval [CI], 0.47–0.94; *P* =.02) and 56% reduction in need for later carotid revascularization (HR 0.44; 95% CI, 0.24–0.79; *P* =.006)[13]
- Smoking—increases risk of ischemic stroke 25%–50%. Tobacco cessation should be counseled by each physician, shown to be effective and reduces smoking in 10%–20% patients. Pharmacotherapies include varenicline (Chantix), bupropion, and nicotine replacement therapy (gum, lozenge, patch)
- Antiplatelet therapy—Most patients are placed on aspirin (81 or 325 mg daily) alone, clopidogrel (75 mg daily), or a combination of these drugs
  - Low-dose aspirin (75–150 mg) is thought to be protective in all patients at increased risk of occlusive vascular events[14]
  - Clopidogrel was compared with aspirin in the Clopidogrel versus Aspirin in Patients at Risk of Ischemic Events (CAPRIE) trial, which demonstrated an overall cardiovascular event rate of 5.32% in the clopidogrel group versus 5.83% in the aspirin group (*P* =.043).[15] However, this trial was not specific to stroke patients and does not consider the higher cost of clopidogrel versus aspirin
  - Symptomatic patients with recent TIA or cerebrovascular accident (CVA) could be placed on dual antiplatelet therapy (DAPT) with aspirin and clopidogrel (or other comparable agent like dipyridamole). In patients with recently symptomatic carotid stenosis, combination therapy with clopidogrel and aspirin is more effective than aspirin alone in reducing transcranial detected asymptomatic embolization (CARESS trial),[16] but no trial has shown a reduction in clinical events in symptomatic patients with DAPT

SURGICAL MANAGEMENT FOR ASYMPTOMATIC AND SYMPTOMATIC DISEASE

- 2021 Society for Vascular Surgery (SVS) Clinical Practice Guidelines for Management of Extracranial Cerebrovascular Disease[17]
  - CEA recommended as first-line treatment for symptomatic, low-risk patients with 50–99% stenosis and asymptomatic patients 70%–99% stenosis and perioperative stroke/death risk <3% to ensure benefit
  - If recent stable stroke, carotid revascularization appropriate in symptomatic patients with >50% stenosis

performed as soon as neurologically stable after 48 hours but before 14 days
- Screening the general population for clinically asymptomatic carotid stenosis in patients without CVA symptoms or risk factors is not recommended
  - In select asymptomatic patients at increased risk for carotid stenosis, screening is appropriate if patients are "fit for and willing to consider carotid intervention if significant stenosis is discovered"
- Patients with symptomatic stenosis 50%–99% requiring both CEA and coronary bypass graft (CABG) recommend CEA before or concomitant with CABG to reduce stroke and stroke/death risk but sequencing "depends on clinical presentation and institutional experience"

CAROTID ENDARTERECTOMY (CEA)

- First published in 1954 by Eastcott and long considered the gold-standard surgical treatment for carotid artery stenosis
- Indicated for asymptomatic high-grade (>70%) or symptomatic (>50%) carotid artery stenosis[17]
- For symptomatic patients with reported TIA or documented CVA, timing of CEA is important and should be performed in the following instances:
  - Acute stroke with neurologic deficit >6 hours and mild to moderate deficits may be considered for intervention after medical stabilization
  - When patients are neurologically and medically stable, intervention has maximal benefit >48 hours and ≤14 days from acute TIA/stroke. Natural history studies reported that the incidence of recurrent symptoms after the index TIA ranges from 5% to 8% at 48 hours, 4% to 17% at 72 hours, 8% to 22% at 7 days, and 11% to 25% at 14 days
  - Brain tissue with ischemic penumbra at risk for progression (urgent)
  - Unstable neurologic examination with evolving stroke or fluctuating/evolving neurologic deficit or crescendo TIAs (urgent)
  - CEA preferred to carotid artery stenting (CAS) in symptomatic patients due to potential increase for embolization from carotid lesions (see Evidence summary of CEA versus CAS)
  - Emergent CEA is reserved for crescendo TIAs or evolving stroke with an identifiable carotid lesion that can be corrected by surgery
  - Current guidelines recommend *against* revascularization regardless of the extent of stenosis in patients who have had a disabling stroke, have a modified Rankin score >3 (Table 12.1) whose area of infarction exceeds 30% territory, or who have altered consciousness to minimize the risk of postoperative parenchymal hemorrhage. These patients can be reevaluated

TABLE 12.1 The Modified Rankin Scale

Grade	Description
0	No symptoms
1	No significant disability despite symptoms; able to perform all usual duties and activities
2	Slight disability; unable to perform all previous activities but able to look after own affairs
3	Moderate disability; requires some help but able to walk without assistance
4	Moderately severe disability; unable to walk without assistance and unable to attend to own bodily needs without assistance
5	Severe disability; bedridden, incontinent, requiring constant nursing care and attention

Scale from Van Swieten JC, Koudstaal PJ, Visser MC, Schouten H, Van Gijn J. Interobserver agreement for the assessment of handicap in stroke patients. *Stroke*. 1988;19(5):604-607.

for revascularization later if neurologic recovery is satisfactory (Grade 1, Level of Evidence C)[18]

- Intraoperative techniques include CEA with patch angioplasty (Fig. 12.1) or eversion endarterectomy (Fig. 12.2), both of which are recommended over primary closure (Grade 1, Level of Evidence A)[19]
- Neuromonitoring and shunting is discussed in section on Use of shunts and neuromonitoring during CEA
- Potential nerve injuries and associated deficits: cranial nerve (CN) dysfunction is the most common complication of CEA (5%–20% incidence in case series, Carotid Revascularization Endarterectomy versus Stenting Trial [CREST] 4.7%). A vast majority are transient and subclinical. Risk of permanent nerve injury (<1%)[20]

- Hypoglossal (CN XII)—lies a few centimeters distal to the carotid bifurcation; injury results in ipsilateral tongue weakness and tongue deviation toward the side of the injury ("tongue licks the wound"). Most common CN injury (4%–17.5%). Higher exposure of ICA can be obtained by mobilizing the nerve medially and cephalad by dividing the ansa cervicalis and/or division of tethering branches of the external carotid artery (ECA) or internal jugular vein (IJV) (lower sternomastoid branch of the occipital artery)
- Vagus (CN X)—within the carotid sheath usually posterior and lateral to carotid (but can be anterior or medial as well) within the carotid sheath; injury occurs during clamping and results in voice hoarseness due to recurrent laryngeal nerve (RLN, which is a branch off the vagues in the mediastinum) dysfunction. Rarely RLN can arise from vagus near the carotid bifurcation (nonrecurrent). Injury of RLN leads to paralysis of ipsilateral vocal cord in paramedian position leading to hoarse voice and loss of effective cough reflex. In patients with prior neck surgery, vocal cord examination should be prior to surgery
- Marginal mandibular branch of facial nerve (CN VII)—injured due to retraction under the angle of the jaw during high dissections; results in ipsilateral lip corner droop and can sometimes be confused with a neurologic deficit postoperatively. The oblique incision for CEA should be angled posteriorly toward mastoid process below and a fingerbreadth away from angle of mandible to avoid this injury
- Glossopharyngeal (CN IX)—encountered with high dissections requiring division of the digastric muscle; injury results in difficulty swallowing, increased aspiration risk, and need for feeding tube in most severe cases
- Superior laryngeal nerve—arises from the vagus in the jugular foramen and lies posterior to ECA and ICA.

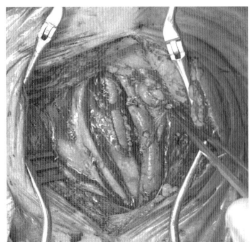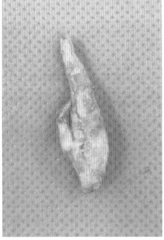

FIG. 12.1 Carotid endarterectomy with patch angioplasty.

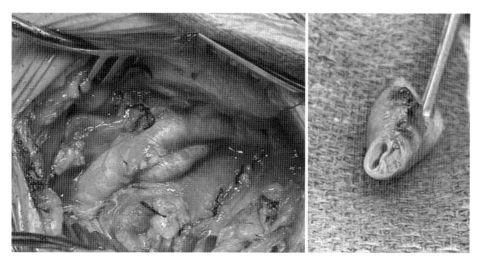

FIG. 12.2 **Eversion Endarterectomy.**

Usually not visualized in CEA. May be inadvertently injured if clamping is not done carefully and involves the posterior soft tissue planes. Results in easy fatigability and difficulty in high-pitched voice modulation (opera singers)

- Postoperative major complications after CEA including acute stroke (see Stroke after CEA), cerebral hyperperfusion (see Cerebral hyperperfusion after CEA) are discussed later

USE OF SHUNTS AND NEUROMONITORING DURING CEA

- Types of shunts (Fig. 12.3)
  - Two-way—Sundt, Javid, and Argyle
  - Three-way—Pruitt-Inahara, Brener, and Pruitt
- Practice patterns for shunting
  - Nonselective or routine shunting—shunt all CEA patients
  - Selective shunting—utilize adjunctive techniques to determine if shunting should be employed during CEA, including stump pressure, electroencephalogram (EEG), transcranial cerebral oximetry, awake neuromonitoring
- No shunting
- Indications for shunting—nonintact circle of Willis, recent neurologic ischemic event, carotid stump pressure <40 mm Hg, any neurologic or mental status change in awake patient, change in EEG suppression in intubated patient, contralateral ICA occlusion
  - NASCET identified increased perioperative stroke risk after CEA in patients with contralateral carotid occlusion from 5.8% to 14%[21]
- Assessing need for shunting
  - Stump pressure—used as a surrogate for cross-hemispheric (collateral) flow. The ICA, ECA, and CCA are clamped with placement of a butterfly needle attached to arterial-line pressure tubing into the bulb. The ICA is unclamped to record waveform and mean stump pressure. If stump pressure >40 mm Hg, with a pulsatile waveform on unclamping, proceed with CEA. If <40 mm Hg, place shunt
  - EEG monitoring—EEG leads are placed and monitored intraoperatively by technologist and neurologist (remotely). In general, the ICA is clamped and

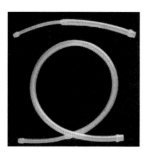 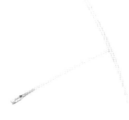 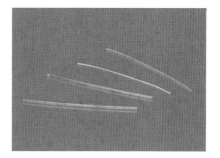 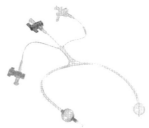

FIG. 12.3 **Types of Shunts for Carotid Endarterectomy (CEA).** (From *left* to *right*): Sundt, Javid, Argyle, and Pruitt.

EEG is monitored for any changes for 3 minutes before proceeding. If any neuro deficits, the ICA is unclamped, and normalization of EEG is awaited before proceeding

- Transcranial cerebral oximetry—noninvasive technique to monitor regional cerebral oxygen saturation using near-infrared spectroscopy to distinguish oxyhemoglobin from reduced hemoglobin
- Direct neuro monitoring (awake CEA) with local anesthesia—patient is awake and can move to command during the operation. Though increased cardiac stability with regional/local anesthesia has been demonstrated, no difference in primary outcome of stroke, death, myocardial infarction (MI) at 30 days (4.8% general vs. 4.5% local), or hospital length of stay[22]

STROKE AFTER CEA

- Differential diagnosis for acute ipsilateral stroke after CEA is broad, including:
  - Intracerebral hemorrhage due to heparinization or hyperperfusion
  - Watershed infarct
  - Hypoperfusion intraoperatively or postoperatively
  - Plaque or thrombus embolization intraoperatively
  - Embolization of plaque or thrombus that occurs postoperatively ± technical issue at endarterectomized site
  - Heparin-induced thrombocytopenia
  - ICA kinking or other abnormality resulting in obstructed low or no flow
  - Embolization from noncarotid site (e.g., cardiac)
- Workup and management
  - Diagnostic workup and management are dependent on timing of stroke relative to CEA (Fig. 12.4)

- Immediately postoperative—simultaneously prepare operating room for reexploration and perform duplex US to determine if there is thrombosis or intimal flap of the ICA
  - If CEA site thrombosed, redose with heparin and proceed to reexploration. Thrombosed CEA site usually due to fibrin and platelet adhesion or technical issue
    - On reexploration, first control the CCA, ICA, and ECA, but do not clamp! Risk of showering clot is too high. Remove the thrombus first, then clamp
  - If CEA site is open on duplex, reexploration is harmful as event may be due to intraoperative hypoperfusion or embolization. Proceed to head computed tomography (CT) and possible cerebral angiography
- Postoperative—if readily available, duplex US should be performed; if not available, then CT head without contrast to assess for hemorrhage followed by CTA head/neck to determine etiology
- Postoperative (hours–days)—CT head without contrast followed by CTA or MRA

CEREBRAL HYPERPERFUSION AFTER CEA

- Definition and risk factors
  - First described by Sundt in 1981 as the combination of increased arterial blood pressure with triad of ipsilateral migraine-like headache, seizure, and transient focal neurologic deficits in the absence of cerebral ischemia after CEA
  - Defined as ipsilateral headache, HTN, seizures, or focal neurological deficits, which can present 2–3 days after surgery

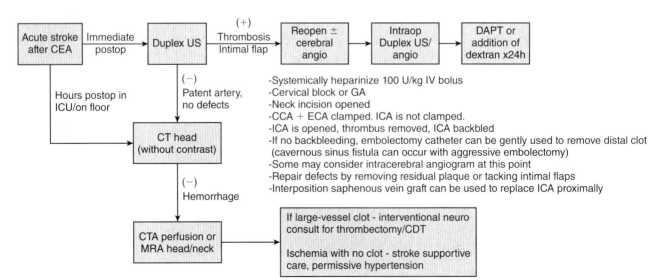

FIG. 12.4 **Diagnostic Workup and Management Flowchart.**

- Most important risk factor for hyperperfusion syndrome is *uncontrolled HTN* after CEA
- Additional risk factors: high-grade symptomatic ICA lesion, contralateral high-grade ICA stenosis or occlusion, urgent operation, and recent ipsilateral stroke
- Presents due to inability of intracerebral arterioles to autoregulate perfusion after sudden change from a chronic state of ischemia to high perfusion pressure with CEA
- Presentation
  - Often described as a throbbing, ipsilateral frontotemporal or periorbital headache
  - Patients may present with altered mental status, confusion, headache, cortical symptoms, seizure or signs/symptoms of intracranial hemorrhage
- Differential diagnosis
  - Migraine and cluster headaches
  - Postoperative stroke, especially if cortical symptoms are present
  - Seizure, which may be due to stroke, hemorrhage, trauma, or medication induced
  - Intracerebral hemorrhage, may occur due to stroke, trauma, malignancy, or uncontrolled HTN
- Workup
  - Patient should be referred to the emergency department for urgent workup of possible cerebral hyperperfusion with the following diagnostic studies considered
    - Duplex US scan—confirms ICA patency and rules out technical complication after CEA, including dissection, thrombosis, or occlusion
    - Transcranial Doppler (TCD)—if available, can measure cerebral blood flow in the middle cerebral artery (MCA); in cerebral hyperperfusion, TCD may show 150%–300% increase in velocity of ipsilateral MCA
    - CT head without contrast—initial screen for intracranial hemorrhage
    - MRI brain—distinguishes between cerebral edema and infarction
- Management
  - Continued close neurologic monitoring in intensive care unit (ICU) setting
  - For pain-related HTN, multimodal pain therapy including acetaminophen and narcotics can be used, but be careful to avoid oversedation, which may impair neurologic assessment
  - For HTN that is not pain-related:
    - Sodium nitroprusside or nitroglycerin—allow for rapid BP reduction with short half-life; patients should be monitored for reflex tachycardia
    - Beta-blockers—short-acting infusions such as labetalol are easily titratable and do not cause reflex tachycardia
  - In patients with early symptoms of cerebral hyperperfusion, holding antiplatelet and anticoagulation medications has been recommended as well to reduce

cerebral edema. Rarely, decompressive craniotomy may be needed
- Outcomes
  - Hyperperfusion syndrome is associated with a high mortality rate (38%)

EVIDENCE SUMMARY OF CEA VERSUS CAS

- *Stenting and Angioplasty with Protection in Patients at High Risk for Endarterectomy (SAPPHIRE)* study[23,24]
  - Evaluated CEA versus CAS with embolic-protection device in high-risk patients who were symptomatic with >50% stenosis or asymptomatic with >80% stenosis
  - CAS with embolic-protection device was noninferior to CAS with 3-year death/ipsilateral stroke 24.6% CAS versus 26.9% CEA (absolute difference for CAS −2.3%; 95% CI −11.8 to 7.0)
- *EVA-3S, SPACE,* and *ICST* in symptomatic patients
  - *EVA-3S* trial: the 30-day incidence of any stroke or death was 3.9% after CEA (95% CI, 2.0–7.2) and 9.6% after transfemoral carotid stenting (TF-CAS) (95% CI, 6.4–14.0); relative risk (RR) 2.5 (TF-CAS vs. CEA; 95% CI, 1.2–5.1)[25]
  - *Stent-Supported Percutaneous Angioplasty of the Carotid Artery versus Endarterectomy (SPACE)* trial: stopped after recruitment of 1200 patients due to futility of proving equivalence between the two treatments. The rate of death or ipsilateral stroke at 30 days was 6.84% for CAS and 6.34% for CEA in 1183 randomized patients.[26] However, this study was not powered appropriately and failed to show noninferiority of CAS compared with CEA (*P* <.09)
  - *International Carotid Stenting Study Trial (ICST)*: enrolled 1713 patients and demonstrated an increased periprocedural stroke risk for CAS (7.7%) compared with CEA (4.1%) in neurologically symptomatic patients (*P* <.002).[27] The rate of any stroke or death within 30 days of treatment in the stenting group was more than twice the rate recorded in the endarterectomy group (7.4% vs. 3.4%, *P* <.0004). In addition, the composite endpoint of stroke, death, and MI significantly favored CEA (5.2%) versus CAS (8.5%; *P* <.006)
- *Carotid Revascularization Endarterectomy versus Stenting Trial (CREST)*[28]
  - Compare CEA versus CAS in symptomatic and asymptomatic patients; multicenter RCT United States and Canada (*N* = 2502)
  - Composite endpoint of 30-day stroke, MI, or death or ipsilateral stroke within 4 years and was equivalent between CEA and CAS (6.8% vs. 7.2%, *P* = .51)
  - CEA had significantly higher incidence of MI (2.3% CEA vs. 1.1% CAS, *P* = .03), while CAS had significantly

higher incidence of stroke/death (6.4% CAS vs. 4.7% CEA, P = .03)

- Subgroup analysis identified higher stroke rate in older patients (>70 years) undergoing CAS, suggesting that older patients may benefit from CEA
- Predictors of increased stroke/death after CAS driven by anatomic characteristics—longer, sequential, or remote carotid lesions

- 2011 meta-analysis found CEA superior to CAS for perioperative and long-term results[29]
  - Included all prospective, controlled trials comparing CEA to CAS with outcomes of RR 30-day stroke, 30-day stroke/death, long-term stroke, restenosis
  - 30-day RR stroke for CAS was 1.6 times CEA, 30-day RR stroke/death was 1.5 times higher for CAS (both P <.01). CAS had higher risk of long-term stroke (RR 1.2) and restenosis (RR 1.8) than CEA (both P <.05)
- *Carotid Revascularization and Medical Management for Asymptomatic Carotid Stenosis Trial (CREST-2)*
  - Multicenter RCT that began in 2014 and currently ongoing to evaluate carotid revascularization (CEA or CAS) versus "intensive medical management" (includes statins and clopidogrel that were previously not included in NASCET or ACAS)
    - Medical management will address all stroke risk factors, including HTN, diabetes, hypercholesterolemia, cigarette smoking, physical activity, and diet

TRANSCAROTID ARTERIAL REVASCULARIZATION (TCAR) VERSUS TRANSFEMORAL STENTING (TF-CAS)

- TCAR—direct CCA access via supraclavicular incision with flow reversal, utilizes the best advantages of both CEA and CAS with direct CCA access and proximal CCA occlusion with flow reversal to allow for embolic protection during stenting
  - Flow reversal system—(1) placement of arterial sheath into CCA, (2) placement of venous sheath into common femoral vein (usually contralateral to CCA), and (3) arteriovenous (AV) shunt with flow reversal controller box[30]
- TF-CAS—percutaneous common femoral vein access to obtain wire access into the ICA, proximal balloon occlusion systems require 9-Fr sheath, which can increase risk of embolism in patients with tortuous or heavily calcified aortic arches
- *ROADSTER-1* trial[31]—single-arm feasibility study of transcarotid stenting with flow reversal for cerebral protection using the ENROUTE Transcarotid Neuroprotection System (NPS); Silk Road Medical). Results demonstrate safety and efficacy at preventing stroke during CAS with overall stroke rate 1.4%—lowest to date for any prospective, multicenter CAS trial

- *ROADSTER-2* trial[32]—prospective, open label, single-arm multicentral postapproval registry of TCAR. Primary endpoint procedural success, defined as technical success and the absence of stroke, MI, or death within 30 days (early outcomes have been published,[32] but the trial is ongoing)
- SVS VQI TCAR registry studies
  - Schermerhorn et al[33]—propensity-score matched n = 3286 pairs of patients who underwent TCAR or TF-CAS from 2016 to 2019 (from total 5 of 251 TCAR and 6640 TF-CAS). TCAR associated with significantly decreased in-hospital stroke or death (1.6% vs. 3.1%; P <.001), stroke (1.3% vs. 2.4%; P = .001), and death (0.4% vs. 1.0%; P =.008). On 1-year Kaplan-Meier (KM) analysis, TCAR had lower risk of stroke or death (5.1% vs. 9.6%; P <.001). TCAR had higher risk of access site complications requiring intervention (1.3% vs. 0.8%; P = .04), but TF-CAS had more radiation (median fluoroscopy time 5 min vs. 16 min; P <.001) and contrast use (30 mL vs. 80 mL; P <.001)
  - Malas et al[31]—compared TCAR March 2016–December 2017 (n = 638) with patients who underwent TF-CAS between 2005 and 2017 (n = 10,136). In-hospital TIA/stroke and TIA/stroke/death significantly higher in TF-CAS versus TCAR (3.3% vs. 1.9%; P = .04 and 3.8% vs. 2.2%; P = .04, respectively). Symptomatic patients had higher rates of TIA/stroke/death TCAR 3.7% versus 1.4% (P = .06) and TF-CAS 5.3% versus 2.7% (P <.001). TF-CAS associated with two times the odds of in-hospital neurologic event and TIA/stroke/death compared with TCAR (odds ratio [OR] 2.10; 95% CI, 1.08–4.08; P = .03)
- However, no head-to-head clinical trial comparison of TCAR versus TF-CAS exists currently

RESTENOSIS AFTER CEA

- Epidemiology and overview
  - Defined as intimal hyperplasia
  - Incidence of 4%–16% in patients followed with serial duplex after CEA[34]
  - Characteristic "homogenous neointimal lesion"
  - *Usually occurs within first 3 years after CEA*
  - Late occurrence (>3 years) is usually due to progressive atherosclerosis
- Presentation and risk factors
  - Most patients will be asymptomatic; if symptomatic, will present with ipsilateral stroke or TIA symptoms
  - Based on a secondary analysis of CREST data, risk factors for restenosis after CEA include female sex, HTN, diabetes, and dyslipidemia; smoking is an independent predictor for carotid restenosis[35]
  - Patch angioplasty closure during initial CEA operation decreases the risk of developing restenosis as compared with primary repair[36]

- Differential diagnosis
  - For symptomatic patients with stroke or TIA after CEA, in addition to carotid restenosis, consider
    - New-onset atrial fibrillation or cardioembolic disease
    - Vasculitis
    - Lacunar infarction
- Workup
  - Duplex US—most common way to diagnose restenosis after CEA as part of routine postoperative surveillance
    - SVS guidelines recommend all patients undergoing CEA have carotid duplex US within 30 days postoperatively. Most patients will have a repeat study at 6 months and annually thereafter
    - If duplex shows >50% stenosis, study should be repeated every 6 months or sooner if symptoms occur
    - New cervical bruit in asymptomatic patient after CEA should be evaluated with duplex
    - AbuRahma et al.[17] proposed duplex criteria for carotid restenosis: ICA PSV 274 cm/s correlated best with ≥70% restenosis with 99% sensitivity and 91% specificity[37]
  - Additional imaging with MRA or CTA can be used if duplex does not provide enough anatomic detail
- Management and treatment
  - Asymptomatic lesions that are low- or intermediate-grade can be managed with antiplatelet therapy and continued duplex surveillance
  - Symptomatic or high-grade (>80%) lesions or those with contralateral ICA occlusion should be considered for intervention
  - Preoperative assessment requires imaging to characterize the recurrent lesion and assessment of history and comorbidities to determine best treatment modality for individual patient
  - Redo CEA with patch angioplasty
    - Standard operation for both early and late carotid restenosis
    - Risk of CN injury increases to 7%–20%[38]
    - Data from regional database (VQI) suggest that redo CEA carries higher incidence of stroke/death/MI compared with index CEA with no difference in CN injury[39]
    - If redo CEA is not possible, CCA to ICA bypass using vein or graft conduit can be considered
  - Carotid artery stenting
    - More recently used as treatment option for restenosis after CEA
    - For early restenosis (<3 years), the lesion is secondary to myointimal hyperplasia, resulting in a smooth homogenous appearance, therefore less likely to result in embolization with wire passage[34]
    - Not recommended for late restenosis, which is due to progression of atherosclerosis, lesions with ulceration, thrombus, or tortuous carotid anatomy

- Benefits of CAS
  - Avoidance of dense scar tissue with redo open surgery
  - Use of local/regional anesthesia rather than general anesthesia
  - Not associated with CN injury
  - Consider in patients with prior nerve injury, history of neck radiation or extensive dissection, tracheostomy, limited neck/cervical spine mobility
- Stenting for restenosis is usually transfemoral via percutaneous groin access, though transcarotid (i.e., TCAR, see Transcarotid arterial revascularization [TCAR] versus transfemoral stenting [TF-CAS]) requiring open carotid cutdown may be considered
- Complications may include bradycardia during stent balloon inflation and access complications such as femoral pseudoaneurysm
- No RCT data comparing CEA to CAS for restenosis, but CAS should be considered for early restenosis and patients not suitable or too high risk for redo CEA or open surgical repair
- Postoperative management usually includes DAPT for 1 month, then single antiplatelet agent lifelong, with duplex imaging at 1 month, 6 months, and annually thereafter

STUMP SYNDROME

- Definition and presentation—TIA symptoms (e.g., amaurosis fugax, unilateral paresis or paralysis, slurred speech) or CVA in the setting of known ICA occlusion
- Due to emboli released from the ICA stump or ECA disease. Additional etiologies include cardioembolic and ascending aortic/arch disease
  - Asymptomatic occluded ICAs should not be treated
- Diagnosis
  - Carotid duplex US—demonstrates occluded ICA with stenosis of the ECA
  - CTA—performed in next step of workup to identify potential aortic arch pathology, confirm duplex findings of occluded ICA and stenotic ECA
  - Cardiac evaluation should include transesophageal echocardiogram (TEE) for preoperative risk assessment and evaluation of cardioembolic source
- Management
  - Open surgical management is the gold standard with ECA endarterectomy with patch angioplasty and ligation of the ICA to remove potential embolic source
    - ICA is suture ligated
    - Endarterectomy from CCA to ECA is completed
    - Patch closure with prosthetic, vein, or endarterectomized ICA
    - Superior laryngeal nerve injury should be avoided by dissection of ECA and its branches close to the vessel wall

CAROTID DISSECTION AND VERTEBRAL DISSECTION MANAGEMENT

- Presentation
  - Carotid artery dissection—acute-onset head and neck (or facial) pain, Horner syndrome (lid ptosis, miosis) due to injury of the ascending sympathetic chain, and stroke like symptoms in MCA, ACA territories
  - Vertebral artery dissection—typically presents as lower brain stem or cerebellar stroke
- Diagnosis
  - CTA head/neck or MRA—first-line imaging
  - Cervical/cerebral angiography
  - Radiographic findings
    - Intimal flap
    - Extracranial dissecting aneurysm
    - Smooth tapering or flame-shaped appearance may indicate expanding intramural hematoma
    - Luminal crescent or half-moon on axial CTA/MRA
    - Lesion location usually distal to carotid bifurcation
- Management
  - Initial treatment is antithrombotic with either antiplatelet or anticoagulation (Grade 1 recommendation, Level of Evidence C)[19]
  - If continued symptoms on medical therapy, consider intervention with surgical or endovascular treatment
  - Current comparative data are insufficient, but balloon angioplasty and stenting is preferred to open surgery if medical management fails for carotid artery dissection (Grade 2 recommendation, Level of Evidence C)[19]

CAROTID BODY TUMOR

- Presentation
  - Carotid body tumors (CBTs) are rare neoplasms developing within the adventitia of the medial carotid bifurcation
  - Carotid body is made of chemoreceptor cells surrounded by a vascular stroma
  - Can be sporadic (85%) or familial (10%–20%, younger patients)
    - Familial tumors commonly bilateral and multifocal; associated with *succinyl dehydrogenase (SDH) mutation*; obtain 24-hour urine metanephrine and catecholamine testing for these patients
    - Familial syndromes with CBTs include multiple endocrine neoplasia IIa and IIb as well as Carney complex
  - Most are slow-growing, presenting with asymptomatic palpable neck mass. Symptoms are usually related to local nerve compression. May have CN palsy (facial pain, hoarseness, dysphagia, Horner syndrome, shoulder drop) if involving hypoglossal (CN XII), glossopharyngeal (CN IX), recurrent laryngeal (CN X), or spinal accessory nerve (CN XI) or sympathetic chain
  - These tumors have a very rich vasculature and biopsy is contraindicated
  - Carotid body's prominent vascular supply comes from *ascending pharyngeal artery* branches, which are a branch of the ECA
  - Rarely can be malignant with lymph node involvement and distant metastases (5%). Radiotherapy has limited role in management of malignant CBTs
- Diagnosis
  - CTA or MRA head and neck is most useful for planning operative treatment
  - Shamblin classification—used to stage CBTs. Type I—small, can be easily dissected. Type II—medium, adherent to and partially encircling carotid vessels. Type III—large, encase carotid bifurcation
- Management
  - Most Shamblin type II and III CBTs require carotid resection and interposition graft placement
  - CBTs >4-cm diameter or 20-cm^3 volume should be considered for resection ± preoperative embolization
  - Preoperative embolization has mixed results in decreasing blood loss. May be beneficial for larger tumors. Commonly used embolic materials are particulate (glue), liquid embolic agents (Onyx; Micro Therapeutics), with super-selective catheterization of the feeding blood vessel to reduce the amount of tumor blush by >80%. Best done as close to surgery as possible (1–5 days) to maximize the benefits of embolization in decreasing tumor vascularity
  - For large tumors, located above C2 vertebral body level, nasotracheal intubation ± subluxation of the mandible may be necessary (20% of cases)
  - Large Shamblin type III CBTs have highest risk of CN injury, though most are temporary and resolve in 1 year unless transected
  - Radiation reserved for older patients or those with multiple medical comorbidities who are poor operative candidates, or patients with recurrent or malignant tumors

CAROTID TRAUMA

- Presentation
  - 90% of carotid injuries are penetrating (10% blunt)
  - Penetrating neck injury is defined by penetration of the platysma
  - Hard and soft signs of vascular injury
    - Hard signs
      - Active pulsatile bleeding
      - Large expanding or pulsatile hematoma
      - Absent or decreased distal pulse

- Bruit or thrill
- Refractory hypotension of unclear etiology
- Soft signs
  - Small or moderate stable hematoma
  - Minor bleeding
  - Mild hypotension, fluid responsive
  - Asymmetrical upper arm BP measurements
- Diagnosis
  - CTA—first-line diagnostic test in stable patients
  - Consider zones of the neck (Table 12.2) in defining the extent of the injury but realize the injuries can traverse multiple zones
- Management
  - Hard signs of vascular injury require emergent surgical exploration
  - Soft signs can be further investigated and selectively explored
  - Zone II injuries are most accessible for clinical examination and surgical exploration and should be treated this way
  - Surgical pearls
    - "Anticipate the unexpected"
    - Prep widely from chin to knees in the event median sternotomy is needed or greater saphenous vein harvested
    - Prepare multiple strategies for proximal and distal control of CCA, ICA, and ECA
  - Endovascular approach may be beneficial for stable patients with zone I or III injuries with pseudoaneurysm, incomplete transection, or AV fistula
    - Self-expanding covered stents
  - Airway and digesting tract must be evaluated for injury with endoscopy, contrast study, or direct inspection with consultation with ENT and thoracic surgery either at time of surgery or postoperatively

SYMPTOMATIC VERTEBRAL DISEASE

- Presentation—*vertebrobasilar insufficiency* = inadequate blood flow to posterior circulation of brain; symptoms may include daily or episodic attacks such as diplopia, ataxia, dizziness, falls, clumsiness
- Diagnosis
  - Duplex US—significant >60% stenosis, reversal of flow (retrograde) in the vertebral artery
  - CTA or MRA—assesses degree of stenosis or occlusion and location of lesion
  - Vertebral artery segments
    - V1—extraosseous from origin of the subclavian artery to C5 or C6 transverse foramen
    - V2—foraminal within bony canal from C6 to C2 transverse foramina
    - V3—extraspinal from C2 through foramen magnum to dura
    - V4—intracranial from atlantooccipital membrane to convergence of two vertebral arteries to from the basilar artery
- Treatment
  - Proximal versus distal disease
    - V1 and V3 segments can be accessed by open surgical approach; V2 and V4 are unable or rarely accessed
    - Proximal V1 segment—*vertebral artery transposition*: proximal vertebral artery is ligated above the stenosis near its origin and reimplanted onto the CCA or short bypass using saphenous vein to subclavian artery
    - Occluded V2 segment—*V1–V3 vertebral artery bypass* using saphenous vein or radial artery conduit; *carotid (CCA) to vertebral artery bypass using saphenous vein*; or *ECA (or occipital artery) transposition to V3 vertebral artery*

TABLE 12.2 Zones of the Neck

Zone of the Neck	Area Included	Neurovascular Structures	Other Structures	Surgical Considerations
I	Clavicles → cricoid cartilage	Innominate a, v CCA origin Subclavian a, v Vertebral a Brachial plexus	Trachea, esophagus, lung apex, thoracic duct	Challenging exposure due to clavicle, but possible; guarded prognosis
II[a]	Cricoid cartilage → angle of mandible	Carotid a Vertebral a Internal jugular v	Trachea, esophagus/ pharynx	More amenable to physical examination and surgical exploration; more easily accessible; more favorable prognosis
III	Angle of mandible → base of skill	Distal ICA Distal vertebral a	Pharynx	Not easily accessed for examination or direct exploration; location presents diagnostic and treatment challenges

[a]Most common.

a, Artery; *ICA,* internal carotid artery; v, vein.

- Open surgery versus endovascular
  - Comparable stroke and death rates with combined death/stroke rate ranges from 1% (proximal revascularization) to 4% (distal bypass)[40,41]
  - Surgery is more durable than endovascular repair; however, due to the limited number of high-volume centers with experienced surgeons, vertebral artery stenting has become more common
    - Open surgery has excellent long-term patency rate up to 90% at 10 years[42]
    - Vertebral angioplasty ± stenting is safe with high technical success but high rate of resteno-

sis, which ranges from 13% to 50% (based on small, single-center reviews)
- If both severe vertebrobasilar insufficiency and carotid disease, fix the carotid artery first to improve vertebrobasilar flow via collaterals
- Complications
  - Open surgery—thrombosis (1.4%), vagus and RLN injury (2%), Horner syndrome (8%–28%), lymphocele (4%), chylothorax (5%)[42]
  - Endovascular—in-stent restenosis, late stent fracture

REFERENCES

1. Virani SS, Alonso A, Benjamin EJ, et al. Heart disease and stroke statistics—2020 update: a report from the American Heart Association. *Circulation.* 2020;141(9):E139-E596. doi:10.1161/CIR.0000000000000757.
2. Petty GW, Brown RD, Whisnant JP, Sicks JRD, O'Fallon WM, Wiebers DO. Ischemic stroke subtypes: a population-based study of incidence and risk factors. *Stroke.* 1999;30(12):2513-2516. doi:10.1161/01.STR.30.12.2513.
3. De Weerd M, Greving JP, Hedblad B, et al. Prevalence of asymptomatic carotid artery stenosis in the general population: an individual participant data meta-analysis. *Stroke.* 2010;41(6):1294-1297. doi:10.1161/STROKEAHA.110.581058.
4. Piepoli MF, Hoes AW, Agewall S, et al. 2016 European guidelines on cardiovascular disease prevention in clinical practice. *Eur Heart J.* 2016;37(29):2315-2381. doi:10.1093/eurheartj/ehw106.
5. Dossabhoy S, Arya S. Epidemiology of atherosclerotic carotid artery disease. *Semin Vasc Surg.* 2021;34(1):3-9. doi:10.1053/j.semvascsurg.2021.02.013.
6. Barnett H, Taylor D, Haynes R, et al. Beneficial effect of carotid endarterectomy in symptomatic patients with high-grade carotid stenosis. *N Engl J Med.* 1991;325(7):445-453. doi:10.1056/NEJM199108153250701.
7. European Carotid Surgery Trialists' Collaborative Group. Randomised trial of endarterectomy for recently symptomatic carotid stenosis: final results of the MRC European Carotid Surgery Trial (ECST). *Lancet.* 1998;351(9113):1379-1387. doi:10.1016/S0140-6736(97)09292-1.
8. Walker MD, Marler JR, Goldstein M, et al. Endarterectomy for asymptomatic carotid artery stenosis. *JAMA.* 1995;273(18):1421-1428. doi:10.1001/jama.1995.03520420037035.
9. Halliday A, Mansfield A, Marro J, et al. Prevention of disabling and fatal strokes by successful carotid endarterectomy in patients without recent neurological symptoms: randomised controlled trial. *Lancet.* 2004;363(9420):1491-1502. doi:10.1016/S0140-6736(04)16146-1.
10. Skyler JS, Bergenstal R, Bonow RO, et al. Intensive glycemic control and the prevention of cardiovascular events: implications of the ACCORD, ADVANCE, and VA diabetes trials. *Diabetes Care.* 2009;32(1):187-192. doi:10.2337/dc08-9026.
11. Amarenco P, Kim JS, Labreuche J, et al. A comparison of two LDL cholesterol targets after ischemic stroke. *N Engl J Med.* 2020;382(1):9-19. doi:10.1056/nejmoa1910355.
12. Grundy SM, Stone NJ, Bailey AL, et al. 2018 AHA/ACC/AACVPR/AAPA/ABC/ACPM/ADA/AGS/APhA/ASPC/NLA/PCNA Guideline on the Management of Blood Cholesterol: Executive Summary: a report of the American College of Cardiology/American Heart Association Task Force on Clinical Practice Guidelines. *J Am Coll Cardiol.* 2019;73(24):3168-3209. doi:10.1016/j.jacc.2018.11.002.
13. Sillesen H, Amarenco P, Hennerici MG, et al. Atorvastatin reduces the risk of cardiovascular events in patients with carotid atherosclerosis: a secondary analysis of the stroke prevention by aggressive reduction in cholesterol levels (SPARCL) trial. *Stroke.* 2008;39(12):3297-3302. doi:10.1161/STROKEAHA.108.516450.
14. Baigent C, Sudlow C, Collins R, Peto R. Collaborative meta-analysis of randomised trials of antiplatelet therapy for prevention of death, myocardial infarction, and stroke in high risk patients. *Br Med J.* 2002;324(7329):71-86. doi:10.1136/bmj.324.7329.71.
15. Gent M, Beaumont D, Blanchard J, et al. A randomised, blinded, trial of clopidogrel versus aspirin in patients at risk of ischaemic events (CAPRIE). *Lancet.* 1996;348(9038):1329-1339. doi:10.1016/S0140-6736(96)09457-3.
16. Markus HS, Droste DW, Kaps M, et al. Dual antiplatelet therapy with clopidogrel and aspirin in symptomatic carotid stenosis evaluated using doppler embolic signal detection: the Clopidogrel and Aspirin for Reduction of Emboli in Symptomatic Carotid Stenosis (CARESS) trial. *Circulation.* 2005;111(17):2233-2240. doi:10.1161/01.CIR.0000163561.90680.1C.
17. AbuRahma AF, Avgerinos ED, Chang RW, et al. Society for Vascular Surgery clinical practice guidelines for management of extracranial cerebrovascular disease. *J Vasc Surg.* 2022;75(1S):4S-22S. doi:10.1016/j.jvs.2021.04.073.
18. Van Swieten JC, Koudstaal PJ, Visser MC, Schouten H, Van Gijn J. Interobserver agreement for the assessment of handicap in stroke patients. *Stroke.* 1988;19(5):604-607. doi:10.1161/01.STR.19.5.604.
19. Ricotta JJ, Aburahma A, Ascher E, Eskandari M, Faries P, Lal BK. Updated Society for Vascular Surgery guidelines for management of extracranial carotid disease: executive summary. *J Vasc Surg.* 2011;54(3):832-836. doi:10.1016/j.jvs.2011.07.004.
20. Arnold M, Perler BA. Carotid endarterectomy. In: Sidawy AN, Perler BA, eds. *Rutherford's Vascular Surgery and Endovascular Therapy.* 9th ed. Elsevier; 2019.

21. Schneider JR, Wilkinson JB, Rogers TJ, Verta MJ, Jackson CR, Hoel AW. Results of carotid endarterectomy in patients with contralateral internal carotid artery occlusion from the Mid-America Vascular Study Group and the Society for Vascular Surgery Vascular Quality Initiative. *J Vasc Surg.* 2020;71(3): 832-841. doi:10.1016/j.jvs.2019.05.040.

22. Lewis SC, Warlow CP, Bodenham AR, et al. General anaesthesia versus local anaesthesia for carotid surgery (GALA): a multicentre, randomised controlled trial. *Lancet.* 2008;372(9656): 2132-2142. doi:10.1016/S0140-6736(08)61699-2.

23. Yadav JS, Wholey MH, Kuntz RE, et al. Protected carotid-artery stenting versus endarterectomy in high-risk patients. *N Engl J Med.* 2004;351(15):1493-1501. doi:10.1056/nejmoa040127.

24. Gurm HS, Yadav JS, Fayad P, et al. Long-term results of carotid stenting versus endarterectomy in high-risk patients. *N Engl J Med.* 2008;358(15):1572-1579. doi:10.1056/NEJMOA0708028.

25. Mas JL, Chatellier G, Beyssen B, et al. Endarterectomy versus stenting in patients with symptomatic severe carotid stenosis. *N Engl J Med.* 2006;355(16):1660-1671. doi:10.1056/nejmoa061752.

26. SPACE Collaborative Group, Ringleb PA, Allenberg J, et al. 30 day results from the SPACE trial of stent-protected angioplasty versus carotid endarterectomy in symptomatic patients: a randomised non-inferiority trial. *Lancet.* 2006;368(9543): 1239-1247. doi:10.1016/S0140-6736(06)69122-8.

27. Ederle J, Dobson J, Featherstone RL, et al. Carotid artery stenting compared with endarterectomy in patients with symptomatic carotid stenosis (International Carotid Stenting Study): an interim analysis of a randomised controlled trial. *Lancet.* 2010;375(9719):985-997. doi:10.1016/S0140-6736(10)60239-5.

28. Brott TG, Hobson RW, Howard G, et al. Stenting versus endarterectomy for treatment of carotid-artery stenosis. *N Engl J Med.* 2010;363(1):11-23. doi:10.1056/nejmoa0912321.

29. Arya S, Pipinos II, Garg N, Johanning J, Lynch TG, Longo GM. Carotid endarterectomy is superior to carotid angioplasty and stenting for perioperative and long-term results. *Vasc Endovascular Surg.* 2011;45(6):490-498. doi:10.1177/1538574411407083.

30. Wang L, Kwolek CJ. Carotid artery stent/neck approach/difficult arch. In: Upchurch GR, Henke PK, eds. *Clinical Scenarios in Vascular Surgery.* 2nd ed. Wolters Kluwer; 2015.

31. Malas MB, Dakour-Aridi H, Wang GJ, et al. Transcarotid artery revascularization versus transfemoral carotid artery stenting in the Society for Vascular Surgery Vascular Quality Initiative. *J Vasc Surg.* 2019;69(1):92-103.e2. doi:10.1016/j.jvs.2018.05.011.

32. Kashyap VS, Schneider PA, Foteh M, et al. Early outcomes in the ROADSTER 2 study of transcarotid artery revascularization in patients with significant carotid artery disease. *Stroke.* 2020;51(9):2620-2629. doi:10.1161/STROKEAHA.120.030550.

33. Schermerhorn ML, Liang P, Eldrup-Jorgensen J, et al. Association of transcarotid artery revascularization vs transfemoral carotid artery stenting with stroke or death among patients with carotid artery stenosis. *JAMA.* 2019;322(23):2313-2322. doi:10.1001/jama.2019.18441.

34. Lee A, Guzman RJ. Recurrent carotid stenosis. In: Upchurch GR, Henke PK, eds. *Clinical Scenarios in Vascular Surgery.* 2nd ed. Wolters Kluwer; 2015.

35. Lal BK, Beach KW, Roubin GS, et al. Restenosis after carotid artery stenting and endarterectomy: a secondary analysis of CREST, a randomised controlled trial. *Lancet Neurol.* 2012; 11(9):755. doi:10.1016/S1474-4422(12)70159-X.

36. Malas M, Glebova NO, Hughes SE, et al. Effect of patching on reducing restenosis in the carotid revascularization endarterectomy versus stenting trial. *Stroke.* 2015;46(3):757-761. doi:10.1161/STROKEAHA.114.007634.

37. AbuRahma AF, Stone P, Deem S, Dean LS, Keiffer T, Deem E. Proposed duplex velocity criteria for carotid restenosis following carotid endarterectomy with patch closure. *J Vasc Surg.* 2009;50(2):286-291. doi:10.1016/j.jvs.2009.01.065.

38. AbuRahma AF, Jennings TG, Wulu JT, Tarakji L, Robinson PA. Redo carotid endarterectomy versus primary carotid endarterectomy. *Stroke.* 2001;32(12):2787-2792. doi:10.1161/hs1201.099649.

39. Arhuidese IJ, Faateh M, Nejim BJ, Locham S, Abularrage CJ, Malas MB. Risks associated with primary and redo carotid endarterectomy in the endovascular era. *JAMA Surg.* 2018;153(3): 252-259. doi:10.1001/jamasurg.2017.4477.

40. Ramirez CA, Febrer G, Gaudric J, et al. Open repair of vertebral artery: a 7-year single-center report. *Ann Vasc Surg.* 2012;26(1): 79-85. doi:10.1016/j.avsg.2011.09.001.

41. Berguer R, Flynn LM, Kline RA, Caplan L. Surgical reconstruction of the extracranial vertebral artery: management and outcome. *J Vasc Surg.* 2000;31(1):9-18. doi:10.1016/S0741-5214(00)70063-2.

42. Berguer R, Morasch MD, Kline RA, Sicard GA. Review of 100 consecutive reconstructions of the distal vertebral artery for embolic and hemodynamic disease. *J Vasc Surg.* 1998;27(5): 852-859. doi:10.1016/S0741-5214(98)70265-4.

OTHER RESOURCES

Audible Bleeding Podcast, Cerebrovascular VSITE review https://www.audiblebleeding.com/vsite-cerebrovascular/

CHAPTER 13

Thoracic Outlet Syndrome

KATHARINE L. McGINIGLE, MD, MPH and MORRIS SASSON, MD

DEFINITION AND EPIDEMIOLOGY

- Syndromes due to compression of the neurovascular structures crossing the thoracic outlet, commonly caused by anatomic anomalies, repetitive physical activities, and neck trauma
- Most patients present between 20 and 40 years old. Very rare in >65 years[1,2]
- Neurogenic thoracic outlet syndrome (nTOS): 95% of all cases. Venous TOS (vTOS): 2%–3% of cases. Arterial TOS (aTOS): 1% of cases[3]
- nTOS is more common in females (70%), but vTOS and aTOS have an equal sex distribution[1]
- aTOS is relatively more common in children and adolescents (~30% of cases)[4,5]
- Dominant arm involves the majority of cases (80%). Bilateral in ~20% of patients[1,6]

ANATOMY

See Fig 13.1.
- The borders of the thoracic inlet are comprised by the first thoracic vertebrae, the first rib, the costal cartilage of the first rib, and the superior edge of the manubrium
- The costoclavicular space is the most anteromedial aspect of the thoracic outlet. The anterior border is the subclavius muscle, the superior border is the clavicle, and the inferoposterior border is the first rib and anterior scalene muscle
  - It is traversed by the subclavian vein

- The scalene triangle is traversed by the subclavian artery and brachial plexus, between the anterior and middle scalene muscles. Cervical ribs can compress the plexus in this location. The anterior scalene muscle marks the anterior border, the middle scalene muscle is the posterior border, and the first rib makes up the inferior border of the triangle

Nerves

See Fig. 13.2.
- Phrenic nerve (C3 to C5): the only nerve that descends from lateral to the medial, anterior to the anterior scalene muscle and behind the subclavian vein. Provides innervation to the diaphragm
- Brachial plexus (C5 to T1): the nerve roots become three trunks in the scalene triangle. Provides sensation and motor innervation of the upper extremity
- Long thoracic nerve (C5 to C7): passes through the middle scalene muscle. Innervates the serratus anterior muscle
- Cervicodorsal sympathetic chain: along the posterior aspect of the ribs. A large stellate ganglion forms at the level of the first rib

Muscle Variations That Can Predispose Development of TOS

- Presence of scalene minimus muscle: most frequent variation. Courses between various nerve roots and inserts on the first rib
- Interdigitating muscle fibers between the scalene muscles or splitting of the anterior scalene muscle
- Congenital bands and ligaments: common to encounter a dense fascial band crossing over the origin of the T1 nerve root, underneath the first rib
- Thickened subclavius muscle tendon
- Pectoralis minor syndrome: caused by compression in the subcoracoid space. Compression between the muscle and ribs of the chest wall with shoulder hyperabduction. Coexists with nTOS up to 20% of the time, and is the cause of 75% of symptom persistence or recurrence after rib resection[7]

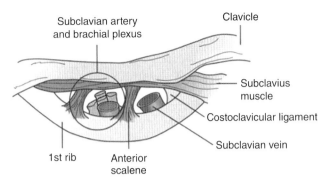

FIGURE 13.1 Thoracic outlet anatomy showing the relationship among the clavicle, first rib, scalene muscles, subclavian artery, vein, and brachial plexus. (From Sidawy AP, Perler, BA. *Rutherford's Vascular Surgery*. 9th ed. Elsevier; 2019.)

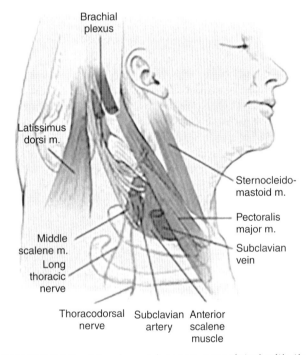

FIGURE 13.2 Muscles and nerves associated with the thoracic outlet. *m*, muscle. (From Sidawy AP, Perler, BA. *Rutherford's Vascular Surgery*. 9th ed. Elsevier; 2019.)

Skeletal Variations That Can Predispose Development of TOS

- Cervical rib: most common abnormality. Female to male ratio: 7:3. From the transverse process of C7 and may attach to the first rib. Found in <1% of the general population, 5%–20% in TOS patients[8]
- Clavicular or first rib anomalies: commonly hypoplastic or thickened after traumatic fractures

nTOS

Pathophysiology

- Commonly presents with a narrowed scalene triangle and after neck trauma/hyperextension injury (80% cases) or repetitive upper extremity activities
- Initial tears and swelling of the scalene muscle results in predominance of type 1 muscle fibers (slow-twitch) and fibrosis triggering compression of nerve roots

Symptoms

- Hand and arm pain, numbness, paresthesias, and weakness. Occipital headache and pain over the trapezius, neck, and shoulder are also seen
- Reproducible exacerbation of symptoms by activities that require elevation of the arm
- Raynaud phenomenon as a result of sympathetic nerve compression

Physical Exam

- Common to have tenderness over the scalene muscle, trapezius, and/or pectoralis minor with trigger points
- Provocative maneuvers[3]: helpful but not highly sensitive nor specific, with a high false-positive rate
  1. Elevated arm stress test *(Roos test)*: arms abducted at 90 degrees in external rotation, elbows flexed to 90 degrees, head in neutral position. Pain and paresthesia will develop when asked to open and close the hands for 3 minutes.
  2. Modified upper limb tension test *(Elvey test)*: abduct both arms to 90 degrees with elbows extended. Then dorsiflex both wrists. Symptoms are elicited on the ipsilateral side.
  3. *Adson test*: decrease in radial pulse when moving the upper extremity into an extended, abducted, and externally rotated position with the neck rotated and laterally flexed to the ipsilateral side while inhaling deeply. Fifty percent of normal individuals have a positive test.[9]

Workup

- Chest x-ray (CXR) to look for abnormal ribs
- Computed tomography (CT) or magnetic resonance imaging (MRI) sometimes used to rule out other anomalies that can be the source of compressive symptoms
- Electromyography (EMG) and nerve conduction studies: often negative or inconclusive. Useful to rule out other specific radiculopathy

- Anterior scalene muscle block: injection of the anterior scalene muscle with local anesthetic. Results in a change in configuration of the costoclavicular space, decompression of the thoracic outlet, and relief of symptoms. Helps select patients, high correlation between relief of symptoms and success of surgical treatment

Initial Nonsurgical Treatment

- Nonsteroidal antiinflammatory drugs (NSAIDs) and muscle relaxants
- Physical therapy (PT): individualized exercise program for 1–2 months with the goal to improve range of motion, relax, stretch, and strengthen the neck/shoulder musculature
  - Patients with residual or recurrent symptoms after improvement with PT will usually benefit from surgical decompression
- Scalene block with botulinum toxin injection: may decompress the thoracic outlet, but benefit limited to a few months and side effects preclude long-term use as definitive therapy

vTOS

- Also known as Paget-Schroetter syndrome or "effort thrombosis"
- *McCleery syndrome:* arm swelling or dilated superficial veins due to intermittent compression, without venous thrombosis

Pathophysiology

- vTOS is the result of repetitive overhead arm activities (throwing, swimming, weightlifting, house painting) causing compression of the subclavian vein between the subclavius tendon and the anterior scalene muscle within a narrowed costoclavicular space. May also have osteophytic degeneration and costochondral calcification
- The vein develops endothelial injury, fibrosis with subsequent luminal narrowing, with blood flow stasis and thrombosis
- Extensive venous collaterals are seen in chronic occlusion
- Up to 80% of patients will have narrowing of the contralateral subclavian vein with provocative maneuvers but bilateral thrombosis occurs in <15% of patients[2,10]

Symptoms

- Usually asymptomatic until the first thrombotic event. Acute episodes frequently preceded by intense physical activities. Dominant arm involved in most cases[6]

- Some patients may have a history of numbness and tingling from concomitant nerve compression
- Pulmonary embolism can complicate 10%–35% of patients with axillary and subclavian thrombosis[11]

Physical Exam

- >90% of patients present with edema (nonpitting), >70% with cyanosis, and >65% had aching pain with arm movement. Dilated superficial collateral veins can also be seen[2]

Workup

Duplex Ultrasound

- Study of choice for the initial diagnosis of upper extremity deep vein thrombosis (DVT)

Venogram

See Fig. 13.3.
- Aids in diagnosis, usually performed with the initial endovascular intervention—most commonly thrombolysis
- Intravascular ultrasound (IVUS) is also a very useful tool to accurately assess the degree of stenosis at the thoracic outlet
- Extensive collaterals indicate significance and chronicity of the occlusion

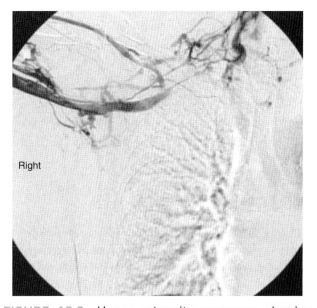

FIGURE 13.3 Upper extremity venogram showing occlusion of the right subclavian vein with multiple associated collaterals. (From Sidawy AP, Perler, BA. *Rutherford's Vascular Surgery*. 9th ed. Elsevier; 2019.)

CT Venogram

- Often not needed, but can be useful to characterize venous anatomy, compression from the first rib or cervical rib, and to rule out secondary causes of subclavian-axillary thrombosis: tumors, central catheters, pacemaker wires

  In patients with upper extremity DVT without clear indication of focal subclavian vein compression, it is important to rule out hypercoagulable states and hematologic pathology

Treatment

- Catheter-directed pharmacomechanical thrombolysis and balloon angioplasty is the initial management strategy for most patients presenting with acute thrombosis to restore luminal patency and improve symptoms
- Subclavian vein stenting without surgical outlet decompression has dismal results and should not be attempted[12]
- Anticoagulation decreases the risk of subclavian-axillary rethrombosis, and patients should be bridged perioperatively
- Outlet decompression followed by anticoagulation has a high rate of venous recanalization (>80%) even in chronic venous occlusion[13,14]
- Early surgical thoracic outlet decompression after thrombolysis decreases the risk of rethrombosis when compared with delayed decompression. Immediate outlet decompression followed by angioplasty is also acceptable but less commonly used
- Decompression involves first rib resection and external venolysis
- On-table venogram to evaluate the presence of residual vein stenosis after decompression, which may require balloon angioplasty and stenting after rib resection
- Open thrombectomy, patch angioplasty, or bypass is rarely required
- Surgical thoracic outlet decompression is not required in patients with chronically occluded deep veins who are asymptomatic due to circulatory compensation from collaterals

Central Venous Stenosis in End-Stage Renal Disease (ESRD) Patients

- Arteriovenous (AV) access–associated subclavian vein stenosis or occlusion is a commonly encountered situation
- Arteriovenous fistula (AVF) and arteriovenous graft (AVG) are frequently threatened by central venous stenosis or occlusion, and compression by the thoracic outlet plays a significant role in failure of the dialysis access
- Surgical decompression associated with open vein reconstruction, angioplasty, or stenting has shown >80% resolution of symptoms and salvage of the dialysis access[15,16]

- The surgical approach most commonly utilized in this situation is infraclavicular first rib resection or medial claviculectomy[15,16]

aTOS

Pathophysiology

- Rib abnormalities in almost all cases, with cervical ribs present in 60% of patients[1,8]
- Anomalies of the thoracic outlet producing subclavian arterial compression followed by poststenotic dilation, aneurysmal degeneration, and thrombus formation that leads to distal embolization

Symptoms

- Asymptomatic until arterial embolization occurs
- Pain, pallor, poikilothermia, pulselessness, paresthesia, and paralysis from forearm ischemia
- Microembolization to the hand and digital ischemia may also be seen

Physical Exam

- Bruit in the supraclavicular fossa and less commonly a palpable pulsatile mass
- Obliteration of the radial pulse with provocative maneuvers
- Fingers with pallor, cyanosis, mottling, petechiae, and gangrene

Workup

- In subacute, outpatient setting, duplex ultrasound looking for subclavian aneurysm, thrombus, turbulence, and elevated velocities. Imaging with the arm abducted is also recommended
- Computed tomography angiography (CTA) is currently the gold standard for diagnosis of >30% stenosis in abduction compared with adduction as well as poststenotic dilation[17]
- Magnetic resonance angiography (MRA) has low sensitivity with high false-negative rates
- Diagnostic angiography performed when thrombolysis or additional surgical planning is needed. Best at demonstrating embolic occlusion of distal small arteries

Treatment

- Asymptomatic patients with mild arterial compression do not require surgical treatment

- All symptomatic patients require surgical thoracic outlet decompression, subclavian artery repair, and possibly distal revascularization
- Supraclavicular approach is the preferred method; an additional infraclavicular exposure may be required for vascular reconstruction pending the extent of the poststenotic aneurysmal degeneration
- Prosthetic grafts have shown higher patency rates than great saphenous vein (GSV) conduits when subclavian artery reconstruction is needed (>95% at 5 years for polytetrafluoroethylene [PTFE])[18,19]
- In patients with acute embolization and a threatened limb, an embolectomy can be performed through the supraclavicular exposure or through a separate distal arm incision
- In chronic embolization, a distal bypass may be required
- Recurrence of aTOS is very rare after adequate outlet decompression and arterial reconstruction

SURGICAL APPROACHES FOR THORACIC OUTLET DECOMPRESSION

- Involves resection of the first rib and cervical rib, if present
- Initial surgical success and symptomatic improvement in >80%–90% of patients[20,21]

Transaxillary Approach

- Lateral decubitus position with a beanbag and axillary roll
- The extremity is placed in a stockinette and extended 90 degrees
- A transverse incision is made just above the inferior aspect of the hairline
- The avascular space over the chest wall is entered
- The subclavian vein, anterior scalene muscle, subclavian artery, and inferior nerve root are dissected
- The intercostal muscle fibers and middle scalene muscle along the lateral aspect of the rib are freed up
- The anterior scalene and subclavius muscles are divided and excised
- The first rib is resected close to the sternum and as far posterior as possible
- The wound is filled with fluid and a Valsalva maneuver performed to test for an air leak. A drain/chest tube is placed if needed

Advantage

- Less field of operative dissection required, cosmetically better for some

Disadvantage

- Incomplete exposure and inability to perform a complete anterior/middle scalenectomy and neurolysis. Limited when vascular reconstruction is needed

Supraclavicular Approach

- Semi-Fowler position with a transverse shoulder roll, head is extended and rotated to the opposite side. The extremity is prepped and wrapped in a stockinette
- Transverse incision is made 2 cm above the clavicle and lateral to the sternocleidomastoid muscle. Subplatysmal flaps are created. The scalene fat pad is retracted laterally and lymphatics are carefully tied to prevent postoperative lymph leak
- The anterior scalene muscle is mobilized, divided off the first rib and then excised, while identifying and preserving the phrenic nerve, which lies anterior to the muscle. Immediately posterior to the anterior scalene muscle is where the subclavian artery is encountered
- The brachial plexus and the middle scalene muscle are dissected and the long thoracic nerve is identified and protected. The middle scalene muscle is divided from its attachment to the first rib, avoiding injury to the long thoracic nerve on the posterior aspect of the muscle. The first rib is freed from its attachments to the intercostal and scalene muscle and then divided just proximal to the vertebra and medially close to the sternum
- The subclavian vein and brachial plexus are dissected free from any surrounding fibrosis
- The wound is filled with fluid and a Valsalva maneuver performed to test for an air leak. A drain/chest tube is placed if needed

Advantage

- Most common approach and known surgical exposure for most surgeons. Wider exposure of the thoracic outlet allows complete scalenectomy and neurolysis. Easier to perform vascular reconstructions

Disadvantage

- Removal of the anteromedial portion of the first rib is more difficult. Control of the vessels centrally may require a second infraclavicular incision

Infraclavicular Approach

- A transverse incision is made over the anterior surface of the first rib from the lateral border of the manubrium to the deltopectoral groove

- The first rib is exposed by splitting the pectoralis major in the direction of its fibers
- The subclavius muscle is divided from the superior aspect of the first rib
- The anterior scalene, middle scalene, and intercostal muscle attachments to the first rib are dissected and freed up
- The first rib is resected at the edge of the sternum and posteriorly as far as possible
- The subclavian vein can be repaired if needed
- The wound is filled with fluid and a Valsalva maneuver performed to test for an air leak. A drain/chest tube is placed if needed

Advantage

- Used mostly for vTOS. Adequate approach to perform a vein patch if needed
- As a secondary incision in aTOS for distal vascular control and bypass

Disadvantage

- Only the anterior half of the first rib is excised

Pectoralis Minor Release

- May be performed as an isolated procedure or in addition with a standard TOS decompression
- Incision is made in the deltopectoral groove and the pectoralis minor tendon is divided at its insertion on the coracoid process

POSTOPERATIVE CARE

- CXR to evaluate for pneumothorax or pleural effusion
- Small pneumothorax or effusions can be observed. If large, may need a chest tube
- Pain control: long-acting local anesthetic commonly used. A combination of NSAIDs, opioids, and muscle relaxants for the initial few weeks is required
- If a closed suction drain or chest tube was placed, it is removed when the output is minimal or pneumothorax resolves, usually before discharge
- PT is resumed as soon as possible after the first week. The goal is to restore movement and function of the shoulder, extremity, and cervical spine

- Patients advised to avoid excessive lifting or repetitive movements. Also avoid upper extremity muscle strain and activities that produce pain
- Long-standing symptoms of nTOS may improve but not completely resolve after surgery and months of PT may be required. Support and reassurance during the recovery and rehabilitation are critical
- In vTOS, patients with subclavian vein thrombosis or if venoplasty was required, anticoagulation is recommended for 3 months after surgery, similar to a provoked DVT. A duplex is performed to reevaluate for adequate venous recanalization
- If venous or arterial reconstruction or bypass was required, duplex surveillance is usually performed in 3- to 6-month intervals the first year

COMPLICATIONS

- Nerve injury: brachial plexus palsy can occur secondary to stretching and retraction. Usually temporary and will improve within weeks to months
  - Transaxillary has a lower risk
- Pneumothorax: if the pleural cavity is entered, a drain can be placed in the operating room and can usually be removed within 24–48 hours. A larger-bore chest tube may be required for a larger pneumothorax or effusion
- Diaphragmatic paralysis: secondary to phrenic nerve dysfunction from retraction or injury, occurs in 10% of patients.[1] Most are asymptomatic, but can develop shortness of breath if underlying chronic lung disease or strenuous exercise
  - Treated with diaphragm plication if needed
- Lymphatic leak: not uncommon to have a small leak. Most will resolve within days to weeks with conservative management and drainage. High-volume leaks (especially from the thoracic duct on the left side) may require nothing by mouth, total parenteral nutrition, and drainage for 1–2 weeks
- Vascular injuries during TOS decompression are rare but can be life-threatening. Prompt vascular control and repair is needed
- Recurrence of symptoms: majority within 2 years after surgery. Most cases occur due to incomplete resection of the anterior segment of the first rib. The scalene muscle is commonly found attached to the brachial plexus in many recurrent cases. Reoperation through a different approach is usually indicated. Reoperations are associated with a higher risk of nerve and vascular injury[1,22]

REFERENCES

1. Sidawy AP, Perler BA. *Rutherford's Vascular Surgery*. 9th ed. Elsevier; 2019.
2. Urschel HC, Razzuk MA. Paget-Schroetter syndrome: what is the best management? *Ann Thorac Surg*. 2000;69(6):1663-1668.
3. Sanders RJ, Hammond SL, Rao NM. Diagnosis of thoracic outlet syndrome. *J Vasc Surg*. 2007;46(3):601-604.
4. Maru S, Dosluoglu H, Dryjski M, Cherr G, Curl GR, Harris LM. Thoracic outlet syndrome in children and young adults. *Eur J Vasc Endovasc Surg*. 2009;38(5):560-564.
5. Chang K, Graf E, Davis K, Demos J, Roethle T, Freischlag JA. Spectrum of thoracic outlet syndrome presentation in adolescents. *Arch Surg*. 2011;146(12):1383-1387.
6. Jones MR, Prabhakar A, Viswanath O, et al. Thoracic outlet syndrome: a comprehensive review of pathophysiology, diagnosis, and treatment. *Pain Ther*. 2019;8(1):5-18.
7. Ambrad-Chalela E, Thomas GI, Johansen KH. Recurrent neurogenic thoracic outlet syndrome. *Am J Surg*. 2004;187(4):505-510.
8. Weber AE, Criado E. Relevance of bone anomalies in patients with thoracic outlet syndrome. *Ann Vasc Surg*. 2014;28(4):924-932.
9. Plewa MC, Delinger M. The false-positive rate of thoracic outlet syndrome shoulder maneuvers in healthy subjects. *Acad Emerg Med*. 1998;5(4):337-342.
10. Adelman MA, Stone DH, Riles TS, Lamparello PJ, Giangola G, Rosen RJ. A multidisciplinary approach to the treatment of Paget-Schroetter syndrome. *Ann Vasc Surg*. 1997;11(2):149-154.
11. Sajid MS, Ahmed N, Desai M, Baker D, Hamilton G. Upper limb deep vein thrombosis: a literature review to streamline the protocol for management. *Acta Haematol*. 2007;118(1):10-18.
12. Urschel HC Jr, Patel AN. Paget-Schroetter syndrome therapy: failure of intravenous stents. *Ann Thorac Surg*. 2003;75(6):1693-1696.
13. Doyle A, Wolford HY, Davies MG, et al. Management of effort thrombosis of the subclavian vein: today's treatment. *Ann Vasc Surg*. 2007;21(6):723-729.
14. Chang KZ, Likes K, Demos J, Black JH III, Freischlag JA. Routine venography following transaxillary first rib resection and scalenectomy (FRRS) for chronic subclavian vein thrombosis ensures excellent outcomes and vein patency. *Vasc Endovascular Surg*. 2012;46(1):15-20.
15. Glass C, Dugan M, Gillespie D, Doyle A, Illig K. Costoclavicular venous decompression in patients with threatened arteriovenous hemodialysis access. *Ann Vasc Surg*. 2011;25(5):640-645.
16. Wooster M, Fernandez B, Summers KL, Illig KA. Surgical and endovascular central venous reconstruction combined with thoracic outlet decompression in highly symptomatic patients. *J Vasc Surg Venous Lymphat Disord*. 2019;7(1):106-112.e3.
17. Moriarty JM, Bandyk DF, Broderick DF, et al. ACR appropriateness criteria imaging in the diagnosis of thoracic outlet syndrome. *J Am Coll Radiol*. 2015;12:438-443.
18. Schneider DB, Azakie A, Messina LM. Management of vascular thoracic outlet syndrome. *Chest Surg Clin N Am*. 1999;9:781-802.
19. Druy EM, Trout HH III, Giordano JM, Hix WR. Lytic therapy in the treatment of axillary and subclavian vein thrombosis. *J Vasc Surg*. 1985;2(6):821-827.
20. Sanders RJ, Hammond SL, Rao NM. Thoracic outlet syndrome: a review. *Neurologist*. 2008;14(6):365-373.
21. Sanders RJ. Results of the surgical treatment for thoracic outlet syndrome. *Semin Thorac Cardiovasc Surg*. 1996;8(2):221-228.
22. Phillips WW, Donahue DM. Reoperation for persistent or recurrent neurogenic thoracic outlet syndrome. *Thorac Surg Clin*. 2021;31(1):89-96.

CHAPTER 14

Acute Upper and Lower Limb Ischemia

PRANAVI RAVICHANDRAN, MD

- Acute limb ischemia (ALI) is defined as a sudden decrease in arterial perfusion of less than 2 weeks, duration that threatens limb viability
- It is a surgical emergency, in which the promptness of clinical recognition and treatment greatly influences outcomes
- ALI represents a morbid condition that is often indicative of significant comorbidity
  - ALI is associated with a high rate of limb loss, need for reintervention, and a 1-year mortality rate of up to 20%

ETIOLOGY

- A growing proportion of ALI is thrombotic in origin, relating to local atherosclerosis or failed vascular reconstructions
  - Patient with this acute-on-chronic presentation can present late (within days)
- Embolic ALI is often more abrupt and severe (presenting within hours)

Embolic

- **Common features:** often abrupt and severe presentation due to the involvement of relatively normal native arteries without well-established collaterals
- Lodge at bifurcations where arterial diameters naturally narrow (e.g., common femoral artery [CFA] and popliteal

in the lower extremities, and the brachial bifurcation in the arm)
- **Cardiogenic** (>80% of embolic ALI)—*often platelet-rich, organized, white-surface appearance*
  - Afib (accounts for ⅔ of cardiogenic emboli)
  - Other cardiogenic sources: myocardial infarction (MI), ventricular aneurysm, valvular heart disease, endocarditis, paradoxical embolus, myxoma
- **Vascular**—*thromboembolism or atheroembolism arising from upstream arterial disease*
  - Proximal aneurysm
  - Proximal atherosclerosis

Thrombotic

- **Common features:** possibly a more gradual and delayed presentation, with an often-abnormal contralateral limb examination, and preceding peripheral arterial disease symptoms such as claudication or prior revascularization
- **Potential causes of thrombosis**;
  - Preexisting atherosclerosis
  - Prior vascular reconstruction (e.g., bypass graft or stent occlusion)
  - Peripheral aneurysms
  - Aortic/arterial dissection
  - Nonatherosclerotic occlusive disease (e.g., popliteal entrapment, adventitial cyst disease)
  - Hypercoagulability (e.g., heparin-induced thrombocytopenia and thrombosis (HITT), malignancy, thrombocythemia)
  - Low-flow state
  - Vasospasm

Trauma/Iatrogenic

- Penetrating and blunt trauma may be complicated by ALI secondary to direct or indirect arterial injury (refer to Chapter 22 to review traumatic vascular injuries)
- Wire/catheter manipulation of atherosclerotic major vessels or aortic thrombus resulting in atheroembolic or thromboembolic ischemia
- Intraarterial drug or particulate injection
- Traumatic or iatrogenic aortic or arterial dissections

PRESENTATION

- The severity of presentation can be heterogenous and is dependent on the acuity and extent of arterial occlusion, the presence of collaterals, and the duration of ischemia
- The of ALI reflect the manifestations of ischemic nerve, skin, and muscle injury

The Rutherford Society for Vascular Surgery (SVS) classification system offers a clinical grading tool for the assessment of ALI. It classifies limbs as either viable, threatened, or irreversibly ischemic, and guides clinical management (PMID 9308598):

Stage	Description/Prognosis	FINDINGS Sensory Loss	Muscle Weakness	DOPPLER SIGNALS Arterial	Venous
I. Viable	Not immediately threatened; includes acute-onset claudication	None	None	Audible	Audible
IIa. Marginally threatened	Salvageable with *prompt* revascularization	Minimal (toes) or none	None	(Often) Inaudible	Audible
IIb. Immediately threatened	Salvageable with *immediate* revascularization	More than toes, associated with rest pain	Mild–moderate	(Usually) Inaudible	Audible
III. Irreversible	Major tissue loss or permanent nerve damage inevitable; primary amputation often required	Profound anesthesia	Profound paralysis (rigor)	Inaudible	Inaudible

Primary Amputation

- Roughly 10% of patients will present with a nonviable limb, characterized by terminal skin changes (skin blistering; nonblanching staining indicative of capillary disruption), muscle paralysis or rigor, and profound anesthesia
- In Rutherford III ALI, revascularization is not only futile but it also poses significant systemic risk to the patient. A patient-centered approach to management, consisting of primary amputation or palliative/supportive care, is most appropriate
- It is important to be clear on what interventions are not feasible and why (e.g., revascularization not offered due to a nonviable limb, or a moribund patient for whom complex revascularization confers prohibitively high risk)
- Amputations performed in the setting of ALI are generally more proximal than in critical limb ischemia (CLI) due to calf muscle involvement
  - In some situations, partial inflow revascularization may be undertaken to facilitate above-knee amputation (AKA) in a patient with multilevel acute occlusive disease

TREATMENT

- Patients presenting with ALI are started on therapeutic IV anticoagulation at the time of presentation in order to reduce thrombus propagation and/or further embolism, and for its added antiinflammatory effect

- For mild cases manifesting with nonthreatening signs and symptoms, anticoagulation alone may be most appropriate
- Computed tomography angiography (CTA) imaging, which provides helpful anatomic information to guide treatment, should be performed first when possible; however, this should not delay revascularization, particularly in those patients with sensory and motor deficits (grade IIb ischemia)
- As with many other areas of vascular surgery, open and endovascular approaches both have a role in the management of ALI
  - Complementary armamentarium for the management of this acutely threatening condition in complex patients depends on multiple factors, including the severity of ischemia, the etiology and extent of arterial occlusion, the general medical status of the patient, therapy-related risk profiles, and resource availability

Open Surgery

- Immediate open surgery is generally favored in:
  - Imminently threatened limb (grade IIb) with prolonged ischemia—catheter-directed thrombolysis (CDT) often requires 12–72 hours, which cannot be tolerated in cases of prolonged, severe ischemia on presentation
  - Ischemic symptoms >2 weeks—poorer outcomes with CDT after 14 days
  - Suprainguinal thromboembolic disease

- History and physical consistent with embolic disease in an easily accessible vessel
- Trauma
- Infected graft
- Interventions range from simple balloon catheter thromboembolectomy under local anesthetic for embolic ALI to more complex reconstructions (e.g., bypass) in the setting of in situ arterial disease
- While the technique of vascular reconstruction is similar to that used in patients with CLI, the immediate and long-term outcomes are generally poorer in the setting of ALI
- Success may be evident in the setting of discrete embolus retrieval with excellent backbleeding, palpable distal pulses, and brisk capillary refill
- Completion angiography is of high utility in gauging the completeness of revascularization, particularly in complex ALI reconstructions

Open Surgery Adjuncts

- Completion angiography
- Over-the-wire embolectomy to facilitate selective guidance into distal vessels
- Intraoperative arterial thrombolytic instillation for residual thrombus inaccessible to balloon catheter, or nonreflow with persistent ischemia—bleeding complications from intraoperative arterial tissue plasminogen activator instillation with control of inflow are rare

Catheter-Directed Thrombolysis

- A CDT-first approach may be considered in:
  - Grade IIa ALI of <14-day duration resulting from thrombosis of a native artery or graft
  - Acute embolic ALI that is not accessible to open embolectomy or where surgery is deemed too high risk
  - Acute popliteal artery aneurysm (PAA) thrombosis with absent runoff—*as a stage to bypass repair in most patients*
  - Grade IIb ALI in a comorbid patient with increased surgical risk, particularly when mechanical adjuncts are available
- There is no role of systemic intravenous thrombolysis in the treatment of ALI
  The primary advantages of CDT over open surgery include:
- Avoiding complex open surgery in a high-risk patient
- Local anesthetic
- Accurate angiographic imaging with the ability to perform directed endovascular therapy
- May facilitate open surgery—*CDT can be followed by open surgery, whereas the reverse is often not feasible*
  Improved recanalization of small outflow vessels that are not amenable to balloon catheter passage.

Limitations and Complications of CDT (PMID 14514841)

- General guidelines do *not* recommend CDT for acute-onset claudication or symptoms >14 days
- The time needed for successful CDT (often 12–72 h) precludes its use in patients with prolonged and severe ischemia
- Theoretically, decreased effectiveness in the setting of embolic occlusion arising from mature, well-organized thrombus or atheromatous debris—*though trial data suggest efficacy of CDT in embolic disease*
- Bleeding complications occur—*proportional to intensity and duration of thrombolytic therapy*
  - Most often access-site related, which may be managed with sheath upsizing or repositioning, and may be reduced with ultrasound-guided access
  - Major bleeding can occur in up to 10% of patients
  - Intracranial hemorrhage risk is 2%
- Distal embolization is common during CDT—*usually managed with continued CDT, catheter repositioning, or mechanical adjuncts*
- Catheter-related iatrogenic injury (e.g., arterial dissection, pseudoaneurysm, embolization)
- Allergy—*rare*

Contraindications to CDT

Generally, CDT is contraindicated in patients with a bleeding diathesis or a high-risk anatomic lesion that may bleed.

Contraindications to Pharmacological Thrombolysis (PMID 17223489)

Absolute Contraindications
1. Established cerebrovascular event within 2 months
2. Active bleeding diathesis
3. Recent gastrointestinal bleeding within 10 days
4. Neurosurgery (intracranial, spinal) within 3 months
5. Intracranial trauma within 3 months

Relative Major Contraindications
1. Cardiopulmonary resuscitation within 10 days
2. Major nonvascular surgery or trauma within 10 days
3. Uncontrolled hypertension >180 mm Hg systolic or >110 mm Hg diastolic
4. Puncture of a noncompressible vessel
5. Intracranial tumor
6. Recent eye surgery

Relative Minor Contraindications
1. Hepatic failure, particularly those with coagulopathy
2. Bacterial endocarditis
3. Pregnancy
4. Diabetic hemorrhagic retinopathy

Predictors of Success With CDT

- The ability to cross the occlusion with a guidewire is the most powerful predictor of CDT success—*it reflects the "freshness" of the thrombus and allows for desirable catheter placement within the thrombus*
- The presence of an inciting lesion after thrombus clearance that may be treated via endovascular or surgical means
- Some proposed predictors of CDT failure include diabetes, multisegment arterial occlusion, smoking

Monitoring

- Most centers will monitor serial complete blood count (CBC), coagulation profiles, urine output, and renal function, alongside clinical signs and symptoms for the duration of CDT, particularly focused on identifying signs of occult bleeding and worsening ischemia
- Fibrinogen levels every 6 hours
  - Levels that drop >50% of baseline or <100 mg/dL have been used by some authors as a threshold to lower or stop CDT infusions due to suspected bleeding risk

Thrombolytic Agent

- Recombinant human tissue plasminogen activator (rt-PA) is the most used thrombolytic agent for CDT in North America (refer to Chapter 4 to review thrombolytic agents)
- The Surgery versus Thrombolysis for Ischemia of the Lower Extremity (STILE) trial and other comparative studies have found similar clinical outcomes with rt-PA and urokinase (UK)
- Streptokinase has largely been abandoned due to immunogenicity and increased bleeding risk

Concurrent Heparinization

- Full-dose heparinization was found to be associated with an increased bleeding risk in the Thrombolysis or Peripheral Arterial Surgery (TOPAS) trial and other series
- Many will use a low-dose heparin infusion coaxially within the indwelling sheath during CDT, with the goal of preventing presheath thrombosis

Duration

- Typically, patients receive CDT over a period of 24–48 hours, with serial angiography every 6–12 hours

CDT adjuncts

- Percutaneous mechanical thrombectomy (PMT) devices may complement CDT by accelerating thrombus clearance and reducing the duration and dose of thrombolytic therapy
- Devices may assist via rapid thrombus debulking or by improving lytic penetration
- As with standard CDT, identified residual lesions that are implicated in the acute thrombotic event should be subsequently treated via endovascular or surgical means, with improved outcomes compared with patients without an identified and treatable inciting lesion

Categories of Percutaneous Mechanical Thrombectomy Devices Include

1. Aspiration catheters—*the size of retrievable thrombus fragments is proportional to the distal catheter diameters; improved efficacy with fresh clot and large-bore catheters*
2. Ultrasound-accelerated thrombolysis—*high-frequency, low-intensity ultrasound energy delivery to disaggregate fibrin strands, potentiating the penetration and action of thrombolytic agents*
3. Hydrodynamic/rhyolitic thrombectomy—*high-pressure saline jets create a relative vacuum at the tip of the catheter, promoting thrombus fragmentation and aspiration via the Venturi effect*
4. Rotational—*rotating blades or propellers macerate thrombus*
5. Mixing—*double-balloon catheter system confines the thrombolytic agent within a vessel, paired with intervening rotational thrombectomy*

Data comparing the relative efficacy and safety of these devices are lacking. Potential limitations and complications of PMT include:
- Increased embolization risk
- Hemolysis and hemoglobinuria
- Limited use in smaller vessels
- High cost

Surgery Versus CDT

- Three major landmark trials comparing CDT and open surgery for the treatment of ALI were published in the 1990s (Rochester, STILE, and TOPAS)

The relevance to contemporary practice is likely reduced due to advancements in endovascular techniques and devices, presumed lower-risk thrombolytic regimens, and an older patient population with increased comorbidities.

RANDOMIZED CONTROL TRIALS COMPARING CDT VS. SURGICAL REVASCULARIZATION

Study	Patients	Duration of Ischemia	Lytic Agent	Amputation-Free Survival at 1 year		Major Bleeding at 30 days	
				CDT	Surgery	CDT	Surgery
"Rochester" Ouriel et al. (1994) (PMID 8201703)	114	<7 days	UK	75%	53%	10%	2%

Notable findings and study features:
- Similar cumulative limb salvage rates, but increased mortality observed in the surgery group (predominantly due to in-hospital cardiopulmonary complications)
- CDT was observed to be equally effective in embolic and thrombotic ALI

| "STILE" The STILE Investigators (1994) (PMID 8092895) | 393 (112 with <14-day ALI) | <6 months | UK or rt-PA | <14-day ALI subgroup: 84.7% *Overall:* 82.9% (at 6 months) | <14-day ALI subgroup: 62.5% *Overall:* 82.3% | 5.6% | 0.7% |

Notable findings and study features:
- Mostly CLI patients; did not include embolic ALI
- Composite clinical outcome of death, ongoing/recurrent ischemia, major amputation, and major morbidity
- No difference in efficacy and safety of rt-PA vs. UK
- Study prematurely halted due to higher incidence of composite primary outcome in the CDT group, mainly due to treatment failure with persistent ischemia and major morbidity including hemorrhage
- Subgroup analysis of patients with <14 days of ALI symptoms noted improved clinical outcomes with CDT vs. surgery, particularly in patients with occluded bypass grafts
- Acute graft occlusion <14 day had best outcomes form CDT vs. surgery

| "TOPAS" Ouriel et al. (1998) (PMID 9545358) | 544 | <14 days | UK | 65% | 70% | **11.8%** | **5.1%** |

Notable findings and study features:
- 85% thrombotic ALI; >50% of all patients presented with an occluded bypass graft
- Similar 1-year amputation-free survival between groups, and a significant reduction in the need for surgical procedures in the CDT group (551 open procedures in the surgery group at 6 months, vs. 315 in the CDT group)
- Among patients with CDT, those with bypass grafts had better clinical outcomes and rates of clot dissolution
- Early abolishing of concomitant therapeutic heparin due to increased bleeding complications

- Comparable limb salvage, amputation, or death between CDT and surgery groups at 6 months and 1 year
- There appears to be an increased risk of embolization and bleeding complications with CDT compared with surgery at 30 days
- Patients receiving CDT underwent fewer subsequent invasive procedures
  - Despite a likely increased risk of bleeding events with CDT, this does not translate to an increase in overall morbidity and mortality, with a comparable amputation-free survival at 1 year

ACUTE BYPASS GRAFT OCCLUSIONS

- A significant proportion of the patients included in the landmark CDT versus surgery trials were patients with ALI secondary to acute bypass graft occlusion

- Secondary patency and limb salvage rates are low, particularly if the initial bypass was constructed for CLI or ALI, and if acute graft occlusion occurs early (within 30 days of construction)
- An acutely occluded bypass graft without limb-threatening symptoms (e.g., recurrent claudication or a resolved ulcer) may be managed conservatively
- The poor prognosis following acute bypass graft occlusion informs the recommendation to monitor and intervene on threatened grafts to promote primary assisted patency and prevent morbid occlusions
- Categorizing acute bypass graft occlusions by conduit type (venous vs. prosthetic) and timing (early vs. late relative to initial bypass construction) assists with identifying likely etiological factors and guiding optimal management—which includes surgical thrombectomy, thrombolysis, revision or redo arterial reconstruction, and/or endovascular interventions

- Following both thrombectomy and thrombolysis, identification and treatment of an underlying inciting lesion is an important predictor of revascularization durability
- The same criteria for CDT are applicable in the setting of ALI secondary to acute bypass graft occlusion: CDT is reserved for patients with symptoms <14 days, with less severe ischemia who can therefore tolerate prolonged CDT treatment, and without any contraindications to pharmacologic thrombolytic therapy
- CDT success is also relatively higher in prosthetic grafts than vein grafts, though similar relative outcomes are also seen with open thrombectomy and likely reflect the unique vulnerability of venous conduits to intimal injury from thrombosis and subsequent luminal instrumentation during recanalization

Timing of Acute Bypass Graft Occlusion	Etiology	Implications for Treatment
Early <30 days	Technical factors*—inadequate inflow/outflow, clamp injury, anastomotic stenosis/flap, graft kinking or extrinsic compression, poor vein conduit quality or sustained endothelial injury, arteriovenous fistulas Vasospasm Low-flow state Hypercoagulability Graft thrombogenicity—prosthetic grafts can present with acute thrombosis without underlying structural abnormalities	• Open thrombectomy and revision of the underlying technical issue is most often performed • CDT outcomes are less favorable in early graft occlusion compared with more established grafts • CDT for early prosthetic graft occlusions yields more favorable results than vein grafts, but must be weighed against the high success, relative safety, and cost-effectiveness of straightforward early synthetic graft thrombectomy ± revision • Useful intraoperative adjuncts include completion angiography, intraarterial vasodilatory medications, etc.
Late >30 days	Neointimal hyperplasia (intermediate, 30 days–1 year) Progressive atherosclerosis (>1 year)—affecting inflow, outflow, and/or conduit Conduit or anastomotic degeneration	• A CDT-first approach, followed by endovascular or surgical treatment of the identified inciting lesion, is a common approach (in suitable patients without profound and prolonged ischemia on presentation, and symptoms <14 days) • Open thrombectomy remains favorable for prosthetic graft occlusions, often paired with concurrent revision of the distal anastomosis (a common site for intimal hyperplasia secondary to compliance mismatch) • CDT performs better in acutely occluded grafts that have been patent for >1 year • Redo surgery is often more involved for late occlusions (e.g., interposition or redo bypass is frequently required)

ACUTE AORTOILIAC OCCLUSION

- Acute aortoiliac occlusion (AAIO) may occur secondary to in situ thrombosis (atherosclerosis, aneurysm), aortic dissection, aortic graft occlusion, or saddle embolus
- Presenting features may include bilateral lower extremity sensorimotor deficits, mottling, general malaise, acute kidney injury only use
- AAIO is more acutely life-threatening than infrainguinal acute occlusive disease, with poorer outcomes attributable to delayed diagnosis, concomitant renovisceral compromise, and profound IRI. Treatment is dependent on etiology and presentation and may include thromboembolectomy (with adjunctive angiographic guidance), in situ or extraanatomic bypass, and CDT and stent grafting in select cases

POPLITEAL ANEURYSMS AND ALI

- PAAs comprise 70% of peripheral aneurysms
- Largely degenerative in nature, occur mostly in men, and are associated with concomitant abdominal aortic aneurysmal disease
- PAAs are most often complicated by thromboembolism, which can result in severe ALI
- Acute PAA occlusion is associated with a high rate of limb loss, due in part to concomitant tibiopedal occlusion that is frequently present
- Prophylactic repair of asymptomatic PAAs is recommended to avoid thromboembolic complications and limb loss. Criteria for elective repair include a diameter >2 cm in fit patients, or smaller aneurysms with thrombus and evidence of tibial embolization

The feasibility of urgent bypass surgery for ALI secondary to PAA thrombosis is greatly impacted by the presence or absence of suitable outflow vessels on presentation.

Occluded PAA, patent outflow vessel in imaging	→	Bypass surgery
Occluded PAA, no outflow vessel seen, Rutherford I or IIa ischemia	→	CDT with the objective of restoring an outflow vessel suitable for bypass construction
Occluded PAA, no outflow vessel seen, severe ischemia with sensorimotor deficits	→	Open thromboembolectomy of distal popliteal or tibial arteries, possible pedal outflow, intraarterial lytic adjuncts, bypass construction

- In the elective setting, endovascular stent graft repair of PAAs may be considered in elderly, comorbid patents, without a suitable conduit, and with widely patent tibiopedal outflow

FOLLOW-UP POST-ALI REVASCULARIZATION

- Evaluate for (± treat) embolic source, hypercoagulability
- Usual surveillance of vascular reconstruction (favor closer surveillance due to generally poorer patency in the setting of ALI)
- Screen for concomitant aneurysmal disease in the case of acute PAA occlusion
- Optimize and monitor cardiovascular risk factors—*ALI patients are prone to repeated major cardiovascular events leading to readmissions, reintervention, and early mortality*
- Anticoagulation—*limited data regarding the role of therapeutic anticoagulation post thrombotic ALI perfusion; individualized regimen informed by anatomic and patient factors:*
  - Cardioembolic disease or implicated hypercoagulability resulting in ALI in the absence of underlying arterial abnormality
  - Some secondary patency benefit following prosthetic graft occlusion (particularly in the absence of a treated inciting lesion)

ACUTE UPPER LIMB ISCHEMIA

- ALI of the upper extremities is less common
- Predominantly cardioembolic in origin, affects generally older patients, and is associated with a lower rate of limb loss than lower extremity ALI
- The associated all-cause mortality still approaches 20% due to underlying cardiovascular disease
Other causes of acute upper extremity ischemia:
- Noncardiogenic embolism—*proximal atherosclerosis or aneurysmal disease*
- Progressive local atherosclerosis—*uncommon*

- Trauma—*blunt and penetrating injuries;* ± concomitant brachial plexus or individual upper extremity nerve injury (see Chapter 22 to review traumatic vascular injuries)
- Arterial thoracic outlet syndrome (TOS) (see Chapter 13 to review TOS)
- Iatrogenic traumatic arterial access
- Aortic dissection
- Arteritis
- Inadvertent intraarterial drug injection
  - Preoperative imaging is recommended, unless cardioembolic occlusion is obvious by history and examination, the limb is immediately threatened, and inflow proximal pulses are palpable (proximal brachial or axillary pulses)

Surgical management: *typically, good long-term results with upper extremity thromboembolectomy and bypass surgery*
- Brachial embolectomy—*may be performed under local anesthetic transverse versus longitudinal versus S-shaped antecubital incision;* ± intraoperative angiogram to confirm restoration of flow or interrogate ongoing signs of ischemia; intraarterial lysis or vasodilatory medications for persistent palmar or digital vessel occlusion
- Bypass—*e.g., humeral fracture with proximal brachial artery injury and occlusion,* managed with axillary-distal brachial bypass with saphenous vein
CDT:
- Transfemoral access (risk of cranial embolic disease) versus proximal brachial access
- Particular role in primary or persistent distal palmar and digital thrombosis
- ± vasodilatory or prostaglandin infusion

ISCHEMIA-REPERFUSION INJURY AND COMPARTMENT SYNDROME

- Restoration of flow to ischemic tissues can lead to a paradoxical acceleration of tissue injury leading to severe local and systemic effects
- The severity of IRI is often proportional to the burden of ischemic injury present at the time of revascularization
- It is mediated by increased production of reactive oxygen species, an influx of inflammatory cells, and the systemic washout of accumulated toxic metabolites, which activate intra-and extracellular pathways that lead to severe metabolic, thrombotic, and inflammatory changes
Manifestations include:
  - Myocardial stunning
  - Reperfusion arrhythmias
  - Renal failure
  - Multiorgan failure
  - Acute respiratory distress syndrome only use
  - Tissue edema and compartment syndrome (CS)
- The severity of IRI is presumably decreased with milder forms of initial ischemic injury, and a more gradual rate of reperfusion

Renal injury

- Acute renal failure can occur in the setting of IRI via multiple mechanisms, including acute tubular necrosis (ATN) caused by myoglobinuria. This can manifest as post-reperfusion (or pre- in the case of severe, advanced ischemia) tea-colored urine, elevated creatine kinase (CK), and a positive urine myoglobin assay
- Treatment includes aggressive hydration, alkalinization of the urine (i.e., bicarbonate infusion), and targeting the source of myoglobin (e.g., urgent fasciotomy for CS, or early amputation of a nonsalvageable limb)

Compartment Syndrome

- CS is a serious complication post ALI revascularization that poses a significant risk to the limb and to the patient
- It is precipitated by IRI-mediated tissue edema within the confines of the fascial compartments of the limb

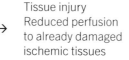

Edema Post-IRI tissue edema → Increased compartmental pressure Progressively elevated pressures constrained by the fascial compartments leading to impaired capillary flow → Tissue injury Reduced perfusion to already damaged ischemic tissues → Irreversible muscle necrosis and nerve dysfunction without immediate surgical decompression + Myoglobinuria with subsequent acute renal failure

- Postreperfusion CS is rare in the upper extremities
- The *anterior compartment* of the lower limb is most vulnerable, with new peroneal nerve dysfunction (impaired dorsiflexion) serving as an ominous late sign of the condition
- Deep posterior compartment involvement is less common, but most consequential with respect to limb viability
  Other signs and symptoms of CS include:
- Worsening pain
- Pain on passive stretch (i.e., with passive ankle plantar and dorsiflexion)
- Paresthesias—*sensory changes may occur early and progress to irreversible profound anesthesia*
- Motor dysfunction—*late finding with poor prognosis of recovery*
- Tense, tender compartments on palpation
- Loss of distal pulses or Doppler signals
  - CS is primarily diagnosed clinically and is particularly confounded by concomitant signs/symptoms of

preceding or progressive ischemic injury in patients with ALI
- Delays in diagnosis and treatment will lead to irreversible muscle and nerve injury in a matter of hours. Therefore many will advocate for prophylactic four-compartment lower leg fasciotomy following reperfusion in patients presenting with severe and prolonged ischemia
- Objective intracompartmental pressure measurements of >30 mm Hg or within 30 mm Hg of the diastolic blood pressure only use are diagnostic of CS, but not commonly used in this setting
Profound or Prolonged ischemia → Prophylactic fasciotomy post reperfusion for ALI
- Complications of fasciotomy in these patients are primarily related to wound complications, infection, and bleeding. There are many approaches to wound closure, including delayed primary skin closure, negative pressure wound therapy, "shoelace" suturing, or skin graft coverage

SUGGESTED READINGS

Björck M, Earnshaw JJ, Acosta S, et al. Editor's Choice - European Society for Vascular Surgery (ESVS) 2020 clinical practice guidelines on the management of acute limb ischaemia. *Eur J Vasc Endovasc Surg.* 2020;59(2):173-218.

Darwood R, Berridge DC, Kessel DO, Robertson I, Forster R. Surgery versus thrombolysis for initial management of acute limb ischaemia. *Cochrane Database Syst Rev.* 2018;8(8):CD002784. PMID 30095170.

Farber A, Angle N, Avgerinos E, et al. The Society for Vascular Surgery clinical practice guidelines on popliteal artery aneurysms. *J Vasc Surg.* 2022;75(1S):109S-120S. PMID 34023430.

Norgren L, Hiatt WR, Dormandy JA, et al. Inter-society consensus for the management of peripheral arterial disease (TASC II). *J Vasc Surg.* 2007;45:S5-S67. PMID 17223489.

Ouriel K, Shortell CK, DeWeese JA, et al. A comparison of thrombolytic therapy with operative revascularization in the initial treatment of acute peripheral arterial ischemia. *J Vasc Surg.* 1994;19:1021-1030. PMID 8201703.

Ouriel K, Veith FJ, Sasahara A.; TOPAS Investigators. A comparison of recombinant urokinase with vascular surgery as initial treatment for acute arterial occlusion of the legs. *N Engl J Med.* 1998;338:1105-1111. PMID 9545358.

Results of a prospective randomized trial evaluating surgery versus thrombolysis for ischemia of the lower extremity: the STILE trial. *Ann Surg.* 1994;220:251-268. PMID 8092895

Rutherford RB, Baker JD, Ernst C, et al. Recommended standards for reports dealing with lower extremity ischemia: revised version. *J Vasc Surg.* 1997;26(3):517-538. PMID 9308598.

Working Party on Thrombolysis in the Management of Limb Ischemia. Thrombolysis in the management of lower limb peripheral arterial occlusion—a consensus document. *J Vasc Interv Radiol.* 2003;14(9 Pt 2):S337-S349. PMID 14514841.

CHAPTER 15

Chronic Peripheral Arterial Disease

BARATH BADRINATHAN, MD

ETIOLOGY AND RISK FACTORS

- Peripheral arterial disease (PAD) is estimated to affect 8–12 million US Americans and more than 200 million worldwide
- Not all patients who have PAD are symptomatic
- Risk factors include cigarette smoking, age >65, or <65 with risk factors for atherosclerosis, diabetes mellitus, end-stage renal disease, hypertension, hyperlipidemia, and physical inactivity

SYMPTOMS

Symptoms of PAD depend on the extent and level of affected arteries in the lower extremities.

- **Claudication**—cramping pain that starts after walking a specific distance. Symptoms abate with a period of rest. This pattern is reproducible. Claudication occurs due to inadequate oxygen delivery to match the metabolic demand of the affected muscular bed
- **Rest pain**—foot pain at rest that is exacerbated while lying flat. The pain improves with the foot in the dependent position. Patients report improvement when the affected foot is dangled off the side of the bed at night
  - Rest pain occurs due to inadequate oxygen delivery to match the basal metabolic requirement of the foot
  - Rest pain is considered chronic limb-threatening ischemia (CLTI), and mandates a revascularization procedure

- **Tissue loss**—this is the end-stage manifestation of CLTI and usually starts after a minor trauma to the toes/foot
  - This can be a small abrasion or a small wound that worsens after a nail clipping
  - Tissue loss may or may not be accompanied with pain—you would expect that rest pain would precede this stage. However, in patients with severe diabetic peripheral neuropathy, the diminished sensation can lead to progression of wounds without pain
  - Superimposed infection is common with these ischemic ulcerations; this makes management much more challenging and is associated with a higher risk of limb loss

DIAGNOSTIC EVALUATION

- A thorough history is mandatory in evaluating vascular patients. This should include (but is not limited to) past medical and surgical history, allergies, and evaluation of cardiovascular risk factors
- All extremity pulses should be assessed (femoral, popliteal, dorsalis pedis [DP], posterior tibial, brachial, radial, and ulnar). The abdomen should be palpated for any aneurysms. The presence or absence of Doppler signals in the lower extremity should be discerned
- Pay attention to any skin changes, hair growth pattern on the legs, and any wounds on the feet. Pedal wounds should thoroughly be examined to discern ulcer depth and to evaluate for infection
- **Consider differential diagnoses:**
  - Spinal stenosis, radiculopathy, gout, peripheral neuropathy, myopathy, arthritis, complex regional pain syndrome
- **Noninvasive physiologic testing**—this is the first diagnostic step used for chronic PAD
  - Usually referred to as pulse volume recordings (PVRs), which is a blanket term that comprises four specific sets of objective data: pulse volume recordings, ankle brachial index (ABI), segmental pressures, and Doppler
  - Helps validate or refute physical examination findings that may differ between examiners. They are also used for long-term surveillance of PAD
- **PVRs**—these waveforms represent the change in volume of the limb with each pulse, at the specific level of the limb being studied

- **ABI**—this is represented as a ratio between the highest systolic pressure obtained at each ankle (DP or [PT]) and the highest systolic pressure obtained on either arm
- Toe pressures and toe brachial index (TBI) should also be obtained
  - Normal ABI is 0.9–1.3. Above 1.3 is unreliable due to vessel calcification. In this situation, evaluation of the waveforms and arterial duplex can be helpful
  - Normal TBI is >0.65
  - An absolute toe pressure of <30 mm Hg has a poor healing potential
- **Segmental pressures**—these are systolic pressures taken at the high thigh, low thigh, calf, ankle, foot, and toe levels. The values are used to compare with the contralateral limb at the same level and to compare the pressure drop-off between the level above and below
- **Doppler**—a graphic representation of the audible signals of a continuous-wave Doppler at different levels of the lower extremity. It will show you a monophonic, biphasic, or triphasic waveform
- **Other noninvasive physiologic testing** can include transcutaneous oximetry and skin perfusion pressure if the ABI, TBI, and segmental pressures are not reliable (e.g., calcified vessels)
- **Noninvasive imaging**
  - **Arterial duplex ultrasound**—this is the first imaging modality that should be utilized. It helps quantify degree of stenosis across a lesion from velocity shifts
    - It is also helpful in identifying whether the tibial vessels are patent
  - **Computed tomography angiography (CTA)**—very useful in imaging the large vessels, including aorta, iliac, common femoral, profunda, superficial femoral artery (SFA), and popliteal arteries
    - CTA is particularly useful if the patient *does not* have a palpable femoral pulse, as it helps characterize aortoiliac and common femoral lesions
    - A disadvantage is that CTA is not considered adequate to assess patency of tibial vessels, as well as a large bolus of contrast is necessary and this may not be feasible in patients with renal insufficiency along with the extra radiation
  - **Magnetic resonance angiography**—not particularly useful to image arteries, as it tends to overestimate the degree of stenosis
- **Invasive imaging**—arteriography is traditionally considered the gold standard imaging modality. However, *diagnostic* arteriography has largely been replaced by CTA due to widespread CT availability, its noninvasive nature, and excellent image quality
  - If planning an open tibial/distal bypass, diagnostic arteriography is helpful in determining an adequate distal tibial target. CTA is not adequate to image tibial vessels
  - In patients with renal insufficiency, excellent quality images can be obtained with arteriography using significantly less iodinated contrast than what is used

for a CTA. A diagnostic arteriogram can be performed with CO_2, and as little as 20 mg/mL of contrast, compared with 100–120 mg/mL (350–400 mg/mL) used for CTA
- Angiography also gives the ability to intervene at the same time (angioplasty, atherectomy, stenting)
  - Arteriography being performed for CLTI patients should include dedicated images of the ankle and the foot

CLASSIFICATION

Classification systems for PAD can be based on multiple factors including patients' symptomatology (e.g., Rutherford classification), physical examination and physiologic studies (e.g., WIfI classification), or anatomic level involved (e.g., Inter-Society Consensus for the Management of Peripheral Arterial Disease [TASC], Global Anatomic Staging System [GLASS]).
- **Rutherford classification**
  - Class I—claudication, mild
  - Class II—claudication, moderate
  - Class III—claudication, severe
  - Class IV—rest pain
  - Class V—tissue loss, minor (limited to toes)
  - Class VI—tissue loss, major (proximal to metatarsophalangeal joint)
- **WIfI classification**
  - Wound, Ischemia, and Foot Infection
  - Each of these categories is assigned a grade based on physical examination and physiologic testing. Combining these scores helps estimate risk of amputation at 1 year, and helps determine the benefit of revascularization as it corresponds to the severity of the threatened limb (Tables 15.1 through 15.4)
- **Important points:**
  - The Society for Vascular Surgery (SVS) recommends use of a classification staging system to guide clinical management in CLTI with use of evidence-based revascularization
  - With increasing wound class, the risk of amputation increases
  - An infected wound with worse pressure indices (i.e., higher grade of ischemia) is more likely to require revascularization for limb salvage
  - A foot infection category of 3 has a high risk of amputation regardless of the other categories

TREATMENT

Medical Management

- Evaluate and treat cardiovascular risk factors
- All patients must be on antiplatelet therapy

TABLE 15.1   **Wound Grade (WIfI Classification)**

Grade	Ulcer	Gangrene	Notes
0	None	None	Rest pain without tissue loss
1	Small, shallow ulcer in distal foot	None, or limited to distal phalanx	Minor tissue loss that is salvageable with simple digital amputation of 1 or 2 digits
2	Exposed bone, joint, or tendon without heel involvement	Gangrene involves digits only	Needs 3+ digits amputated or TMA
3	Extensive and full-thickness ulceration involving forefoot/midfoot/heel	Extensive full-thickness necrosis involving more than just the digits	Complex wound reconstruction required, or nontraditional TMA (Charcot, Lisfranc)

TMA, Transmetatarsal amputation; *WIfI,* wound, ischemia, and foot infection.

TABLE 15.2   **Ischemia Grade (WIfI Classification)**

Grade	Ankle Brachial Index	Ankle Systolic Pressure (mm Hg)	Toe Pressure (mm Hg)
0	≥0.80	>100	≥60
1	0.6–0.79	70–100	40–59
2	0.4–0.59	50–70	30–39
3	≤0.39	<50	<30

WIfI, Wound, ischemia, and foot infection.

TABLE 15.3   **Foot Infection Grade (WIfI Classification)**

Grade	Signs	Notes
0	No signs of infection	
1	Local infection—skin/subQ only	At least *two* of these should be present: • Swelling/induration • Erythema ≤2 cm • Pain or tenderness • Warmth • Purulent discharge
2	Local infection of skin/subQ with erythema >2 cm; or deeper infections	Abscess, osteomyelitis, etc. *without* systemic signs present
3	Local infection *with* SIRS	SIRS criteria: • Temperature >38°C or <36°C • HR >90 beats/min • RR >20 or $Paco_2$ <32 mm Hg • WBC >12 or <4 μ/L

HR, Heart rate; *RR,* respiratory rate; *SIRS,* systemic inflammatory response syndrome; *subQ,* subcutaneous; *WBC,* white blood cell; *WIfI,* wound, ischemia, and foot infection.

- Aspirin 81 + 2.5 mg BID rivaroxaban has been shown to decrease cardiovascular events and lower extremity ischemic events in patients with CLTI
- Do not use therapeutic anticoagulation as the treatment for atherosclerosis in CLTI. Anticoagulation may be considered after all medical management and prior surgical interventions have been unsuccessful
- All CLTI patients should be on moderate- to high-intensity statin therapy
- Treat hypertension with a systolic blood pressure goal of <140 mm Hg, diastolic blood pressure goal of <90 mm Hg
- For patients with diabetes, hemoglobin A_{1c} (HbA_{1c}) goal should be <7%. Metformin should be the primary hypoglycemic agent. Hold metformin 24 hours prior to, and up to 48 hours after using iodinated contrast agents
- Smoking cessation should be aggressively pursued and discussed at every visit

Treatment of Claudication

- The natural history of claudication is *not* critical limb ischemia
- Approximately only 4% of patients with claudication will progress to critical limb ischemia
  - Thus treatment of claudication centers on maximizing medical management and optimizing cardiovascular risk factors (see earlier Medical Management section)
- If the claudication is deemed *lifestyle-limiting* despite smoking cessation and maximizing medical therapy, then revascularization can be considered on an individual basis
- Claudication typically involves a lesion at one arterial level, and an endovascular approach is commonly attempted first. In some cases, a femoral endarterectomy may need to be included
- In the case of aortoiliac disease, if endovascular attempts fail, open surgical reconstruction can be pursued with an aortobifemoral bypass

TABLE 15.4   **SVS WIfI Clinical Limb Stage**

	Ischemia – 0				Ischemia – 1				Ischemia – 2				Ischemia – 3			
W-0	1	1	2	3	1	2	3	4	2	2	3	4	2	3	3	4
W-1	1	1	2	3	1	2	3	4	2	3	4	4	3	3	4	4
W-2	2	2	3	4	3	3	4	4	3	4	4	4	4	4	4	4
W-3	3	3	4	4	4	4	4	4	4	4	4	4	4	4	4	4
	fI-0	fI-1	fI-2	fI-3	fI-0	fI-1	fI-2	fI-3	fI-0	fI-1	fI-2	fI-3	fI-0	fI-1	fI-2	fI-3

Clinical stages: *1,* very low risk; *2,* low risk; *3,* moderate risk; *4,* high risk. *SVS,* Society for Vascular Surgery; *WIfI: W,* wound; *I,* ischemia; *fI,* foot infection.

- It is important to note that even if there is evidence of a hemodynamically significant tibial stenosis, this should not be treated if the symptoms are purely claudication
- Tibial intervention is considered an "outflow" procedure and should be reserved for CLTI patients (usually tissue loss)

Treatment of Rest Pain

- Rest pain is a form of CLTI. In addition to maximum medical management, revascularization is required to preserve the limb
- Rest pain usually correlates with lesions at multiple arterial levels. However, due to the chronicity of PAD in these patients, they tend to have a robust network of collaterals in the lower leg that have developed over time
- An "inflow" procedure alone will often resolve symptoms. Increasing the blood supply into the limb proximally will improve oxygen delivery to the tissues below, utilizing the collaterals already in place in the lower limb
  - It is acceptable to perform an inflow procedure at the index operation, and then follow the patient thereafter to see if their symptoms resolve. If they do not, then further revascularization to perform an outflow procedure can be considered
  - An inflow procedure can consist of a femoral endarterectomy with extension across the origin of the profunda to perform a profundaplasty. This may need to be combined with an iliac angioplasty/stent placement if there is a hemodynamically significant (>50%) stenosis at this level

Treatment of Tissue Loss

- For tissue loss, both inflow and outflow procedures are required to restore direct in-line flow to the foot. An ischemic ulceration is end-stage PAD where basal perfusion is not adequate to support a viable limb
- In patients with tissue loss, a 50% or greater stenosis at any arterial level requires treatment as it is considered a hemodynamically significant stenosis

- In *average-risk* CLTI patients, endovascular-first or open-first approaches are dictated by the severity of the limb threat, the anatomic pattern of disease, and availability of an autologous conduit
- In *high-surgical risk* CLTI patients, attempt an endovascular approach first. This usually involves extensive endovascular reconstruction with employment of advanced endovascular techniques (see n section). This may also be the case for average-risk surgical patients who do not have an autogenous conduit available for bypass
  - A hybrid endovascular + open approach may also be utilized in the appropriate setting (e.g., common femoral artery [CFA]/profunda femoris artery [PFA] endarterectomy with patch angioplasty ± retrograde iliac angioplasty stenting ± antegrade SFA/popliteal angioplasty or stenting + tibial angioplasty)

Advanced Endovascular Techniques for CLTI

- *SAFARI*—Subintimal Arterial Flossing with Antegrade-Retrograde Intervention. This technique is useful when attempted antegrade recanalization happens in a subintimal plane with failure to reenter the true lumen distally. In this situation, retrograde ultrasound-guided access can be obtained in the target distal vessel (SFA, popliteal, or tibial artery), and a wire is advanced retrograde in a subintimal plane. The subintimal planes are connected from above and below, and the channel is angioplastied ± stented to allow for in-line flow
- *Pedal access* in the DP or PT can also be obtained in a similar fashion with the wire staying in the true lumen as it is advanced retrograde. This retrograde wire can be snared from above, usually within the ipsilateral SFA or popliteal artery. This establishes through-and-through intraluminal access, and angioplasty can be performed over this wire from either the antegrade or retrograde approach
  - Once interventions are complete, direct manual pressure is held to achieve hemostasis over the pedal access site

- Pedal access should be reserved for high–surgical risk patients who would not tolerate a tibial/pedal bypass, or those who do not have adequate autologous conduit to complete the surgical bypass. This is due to the risk of damaging the distal target/outflow vessel from endovascular instrumentation, which would otherwise result in a successful surgical bypass
- Caution should always be taken when the patient has only a single-vessel runoff to the foot

Surgical Bypass in CLTI

- The proximal anastomosis is usually performed at the common femoral level (or proximal SFA if limited conduit length)
- The distal target can be the above-knee popliteal, below-knee popliteal, or a tibial artery (anterior tibial, posterior tibial, peroneal) based on patency revealed by angiogram. The distal target should be the most proximal healthy vessel you can sew to, which will establish in-line flow to the foot
- A continuous segment of autologous vein should be the first choice of conduit. If no vein is available, and no endovascular options available, a nonautologous conduit may be used (e.g., polytetrafluoroethylene, Dacron, CryoVein [Artivian])
- Preoperative vein mapping should image bilateral great saphenous vein (GSV) and small saphenous vein (SSV). The vein diameter must be at least 3 mm as veins smaller than this have a high bypass failure rate. The upper extremities can also be vein mapped in the case of insufficient lower extremity veins. A spliced venous conduit comprised of a combination of upper and lower extremity veins may have to be used if a single-vein segment is not long enough. The cephalic vein is typically used if vein is needed from the upper extremity. While the basilic vein can be used as well, there are reports of aneurysmal degeneration over time
- The vein conduit can be used in the reversed or nonreversed fashion (with valvulotomy), without significant difference in patency
- In some cases (usually femorotibial bypass), inadequate length autologous vein may have to be spliced with a prosthetic conduit to complete the bypass. In these situations, the prosthetic conduit should be sewn to the inflow vessel proximally, with the distal target receiving the venous end of the spliced conduit
  - On the target vessel, a vein patch can be sewed on and the distal anastomosis can be sewn to the vein patch (Linton patch; Miller cuff; Taylor patch; St. Mary's boot)
- In patients with severe tibial disease, a pedal bypass may be the only option for limb salvage. The distal target here is usually the DP artery or posterior tibialis as the ankle
  - This pattern of disease is frequently seen in patients with diabetes and end-stage renal patients where the

tibial vessels are primarily involved and otherwise nonreconstructible
- The inflow vessel can be any vessel proximally that will provide in-line flow to the foot; however, the shorter the bypass conduit, the better the patency
- The ideal pedal bypass will establish in-line flow to the foot using a single segment of GSV, with adequate soft tissue coverage over the distal anastomosis
- After open surgical reconstruction, perform intraoperative completion imaging (angiography and/or duplex ultrasound) to identify and correct technical defects at the initial operation

Management of Common Femoral and Profunda Disease

- In CLTI patients with >50% CFA and/or profunda stenosis, perform endarterectomy with patch angioplasty. If the patient has tissue loss, an additional revascularization further distally will usually be required
- In high-risk patients, consider endovascular treatment of CFA/PFA disease. However, avoid placing stents in the CFA or the origin of the PFA

The Role of Amputations

- Offered to high-risk surgical candidates, nonviable limbs, nonambulatory patients
- Major amputations are below-knee amputation (BKA) and above-knee amputation (AKA)
- Digit, ray, and transmetatarsal (TMA) amputations can be offered in combination with revascularization in order to preserve as much of the foot as possible. If more than two digit ray amputations are necessary, consider TMA, especially when the first digit is involved
- Consider a revascularization procedure (open or endovascular) to help heal the distal most amputation possible
- In nonambulatory patients who require a major amputation, the recommendation should be for AKA instead of BKA. Contractures develop in patients who are nonambulatory, causing flexion at the knee and development of pressure ulcerations on the posterior aspect of the BKA stump. These patients will ultimately require revision to AKA

TRIALS

- **BASIL trial**—Bypass versus Angioplasty in Severe Ischemia of the Leg trial
  - The only published prospective, multicenter, randomized controlled trial that has compared endovascular versus open surgery for treatment of chronic PAD
  - The endovascular group had a higher early failure rate than the surgical group, with a significant portion of endovascular patients requiring bypass surgery

- At 6 months, the two groups had a similar amputation-free survival; bypass with vein conduit had better amputation-free survival in the long term
- In addition, it was found that the outcome of bypass surgery for patients who have a failed angioplasty had worse outcomes than those who underwent bypass first
- Conclusion—patients who have an expected survival >2 years should undergo the bypass-first approach if they have a usable autologous conduit. Those who have an expected survival of <2 years should undergo endovascular therapy first as they will not survive long enough to fully realize the benefit of having a surgical bypass
- **STILE trial**—Surgery versus Thrombolysis for Ischemia of the Lower Extremity trial
  - Prospective randomized controlled trial; however, it specifically focused on evaluating surgery vs. thrombolysis for lower limb ischemia caused by nonembolic graft or native vessel occlusion
  - The authors concluded that surgical revascularization in patients with <6 months of ischemia is more effective and safer than catheter-directed thrombolysis
  - 30-day outcomes were similar, but 28% of thrombolysis patients had failure of therapy, requiring surgical treatment
  - Patients with acute ischemia (<14 days) had better amputation-free survival and shorter hospital stays when treated with thrombolysis. However, patients with chronic ischemia (>14 days) had better outcomes with surgical revascularization
- **BEST-CLI trial**—The Best Endovascular Versus Surgical Therapy in Patients With Critical Limb Ischemia trial
  - Ongoing prospective, multicenter, multinational, multispecialty, randomized controlled trial started in 2007 to compare treatment efficacy, functional outcomes, cost-effectiveness, and quality of life for 2100 patients with critical limb ischemia
  - Designed to compare endovascular versus single-segment GSV surgical bypass to treat CLTI. The surgical group is further divided into those who undergo GSV versus prosthetic conduit use. The study has also been stratified to address key issues, such as outcomes for tissue loss versus rest pain, as well as anatomic variables

PRACTICAL POINTS

- Determine if any urgent/emergent procedures need to be performed, prior to considering revascularization. A patient who is septic from an infected wound needs definitive source control before revascularization
- Once the patient is stable, then consider if they are an acceptable candidate for limb salvage

- If patients are nonambulatory or have an unsalvageable limb, primary amputation or palliation should be recommended. If they are ambulatory yet have numerous medical comorbidities that portend high surgical risk, they may not be candidates for revascularization
- Some high-risk patients will still be candidates for endovascular therapy due to its minimally invasive nature without the need for general anesthesia. However, these high-risk patients who are unable to lay flat for an extended period of time (i.e., severe chronic obstructive pulmonary disease [COPD], severe back pain, etc.) may not be candidates for any type of revascularization
- The patient is average surgical risk if their anticipated periprocedural mortality is <5% and estimated 2-year survival is >50%
- The patient is considered high surgical risk if their anticipated periprocedural mortality is ≥5% or estimated 2-year survival is ≤50%
- In patients *without* a palpable femoral pulse, start with a CTA if renal function permits
- In patients *with* palpable femoral pulses, consider proceeding to angiogram + intervention without a CTA
- In patients with multiple prior revascularizations (e.g., at different facilities without available records), a full set of noninvasive studies, including physiologic testing, arterial duplex, and CTA, is helpful to discern anatomy and the status of previously attempted interventions before embarking on another one
- For patients undergoing endovascular intervention for CLTI, who are also considered acceptable candidates for surgical bypass, obtain vein mapping prior to the endovascular intervention. If the endovascular intervention is challenging despite your attempt at revascularization, a surgical bypass is a good option if suitable vein is available to use as a conduit

POSTOPERATIVE CARE

- After revascularization, excellent wound care must continue until all wounds are healed
- Mechanical offloading for pedal wounds is a primary component of postoperative care in CLTI patients
- Poor attention to wounds despite revascularization will invariably lead to a suboptimal result
- Continue to encourage smoking cessation after undergoing lower extremity revascularization
- Continue best medical therapy to manage cardiovascular risk factors, including antiplatelet therapy, statin, adequate management of hypertension and diabetes
- Consider dual antiplatelet therapy (DAPT) aspirin + clo·pid·o·grel in patients who had an infrainguinal bypass with a prosthetic conduit for 6–24 months to help maintain graft patency

- Consider DAPT (aspirin + clopidogrel) in patients who had lower extremity endovascular interventions for a period of at least 1 month. In patients who require repeated endovascular interventions, consider DAPT for 1–6 months
- Therapeutic anticoagulation after lower extremity bypass is typically reserved for patients whose bypass grafts thrombose despite being on DAPT, and an anatomic/technical etiology is ruled out
- Surveillance after surgical/percutaneous intervention can be accomplished with arterial duplex ultrasound at 1, 3, 6, and 12 months after bypass
- Surveillance should continue for at least 2 years postoperatively. If abnormalities are noted, surveillance should be done at a shorter time interval
  - An ABI decrease of ≥ 0.15 is considered significant in patients with a bypass graft and should be evaluated further (typically with duplex ultrasound). This is especially true if the patient complains of recurrent symptoms or if there is a change in the pulse examination
  - Intervention should be offered if arterial duplex ultrasound of a bypass graft shows *peak systolic velocity (PSV)* >300 cm/s and PSV ratio >3.5. These findings are consistent with a stenosis of 70% or greater
  - If duplex shows low-velocity flow in a bypass graft (<45 cm/s), this is consistent with impending bypass graft failure and intervention should be offered

COMPLICATIONS

- **Percutaneous access site complications**
  - Retroperitoneal hematoma if percutaneous access is above the inguinal ligament. Can also manifest as a groin hematoma or a pseudoaneurysm (PSA) if adequate percutaneous closure or direct manual pressure was inadequately utilized postprocedure
  - *Direct manual pressure*—20–30 minutes can resolve some PSAs. There is less likelihood that this will resolve if the patient is on anticoagulation, or if the PSA neck is >2 mm
  - *Ultrasound-guided compression*—direct pressure on the PSA neck using image guidance throughout the compression time. Effectiveness will depend on adequate visualization of the PSA, patient body habitus, and whether the patient is on anticoagulation

- *Ultrasound-guided thrombin injection*—percutaneous injection of thrombin into the PSA cavity. This helps thrombose the PSA. Higher likelihood of success if PSA neck is ≤ 2 mm in diameter. Complications include thrombosis of the native artery or distal embolization of thrombin, leading to limb ischemia
- *Surgical repair*—this typically involves a femoral cutdown in the operating room, with direct suture repair of the arterial access site, and evacuation of hematoma from the PSA cavity. This usually requires one or two sutures to achieve hemostasis
- **Lower extremity graft infection**
  - More common when prosthetic bypass grafts are used compared with vein conduits
  - The femoral wound is especially susceptible to wound dehiscence and infection due to its location over a joint that transmits constant flexion/extension forces to the wound
  - Most common bacteria to infect prosthetic grafts are *Staphylococcus aureus*; however, *S. epidermis* and gram-negative bacterial infections have increased in frequency. Gram-negative infections are particularly virulent and are associated with a higher incidence of anastomotic dehiscence and arterial rupture, due to the production of endotoxins that can disrupt the integrity of the vessel
  - Safest way to manage an infected graft would be to excise the entire graft and repair the proximal and distal anastomotic sites with a vein patch. This might be sufficient in someone in whom the initial indication was claudication. However, in CLTI, a revascularization procedure still needs to be performed due to the threatened limb
    - Excision of the entire graft with debridement of the infected/devitalized tissue should be performed. Then, an extra-anatomic bypass can be performed by tunneling the new graft away from the infected sites. This can be done in a staged fashion after intravenous antibiotics and wound care have treated the majority of the infection
    - In patients who are systemically ill from the graft infection, life must be prioritized over limb

In some cases, graft salvage can be attempted when the infection is localized to one portion of the graft. The wound can be thoroughly irrigated and debrided, covered with a sartorius muscle flap with negative wound pressure therapy. This is in addition to culture-driven antibiotic therapy.

SUGGESTED READINGS

Abu Dabrh AM, Steffen MW, Asi N, et al. Bypass surgery versus endovascular interventions in severe or critical limb ischemia. *J Vasc Surg.* 2016;63(1):244 253.e11.

Abu Dabrh AM, Steffen MW, Asi N, et al. Nonrevascularization-based treatments in patients with severe or critical limb ischemia. *J Vasc Surg.* 2015;62(5):1330-1339.e13.

Almasri J, Adusumalli J, Asi N, et al. A systematic review and meta-analysis of revascularization outcomes of infrainguinal chronic limb-threatening ischemia. *J Vasc Surg.* 2018;68(2):624-633.

Bradbury AW, Adam DJ, Bell J, et al. Bypass versus Angioplasty in Severe Ischaemia of the Leg (BASIL) trial: analysis of amputation free and overall survival by treatment received. *J Vasc Surg.*

2010;51(suppl 5):18S-31S. Erratum in: *J Vasc Surg.* 2010; 52(6):1751. Bhattachary, V [corrected to Bhattacharya, V].

Conte MS, Bradbury AW, Kolh P, et al. Global vascular guidelines on the management of chronic limb-threatening ischemia. *J Vasc Surg* 2019;69(suppl 6):3S-125S.

Conte MS. Challenges of distal bypass surgery in patients with diabetes: patient selection, techniques, and outcome. *J Vasc Surg.* 2010;52:96S-103S.

Mills JL Sr, Conte MS, Armstrong DG, et al. The Society for Vascular Surgery Lower Extremity Threatened Limb Classification System: risk stratification based on wound, ischemia, and foot infection (WIfI). *J Vasc Surg.* 2014;59:220-234.e1-2.

Pomposelli FB Jr, Jepsen SJ, Gibbons GW, et al. Efficacy of the dorsal pedal bypass for limb salvage in diabetic patients: short-term observations. *J Vasc Surg.* 1990;11:P745-P752.

Results of a prospective randomized trial evaluating surgery versus thrombolysis for ischemia of the lower extremity. The STILE trial. *Ann Surg.* 1994;220(3):251-266; discussion 266-268.

Spinosa DJ, Harthun NL, Bissonette EA, et al. Subintimal arterial flossing with antegrade-retrograde intervention (SAFARI) for subintimal recanalization to treat chronic critical limb ischemia. *J Vasc Interv Radiol.* 2005;16(1):37-44.

CHAPTER 16

Diabetic Foot and Wound Care

KEVIN MANGUM, MD, PhD, and KATHERINE GALLAGHER, MD

EPIDEMIOLOGY

- Cumulative incidence of foot ulcers is 6%–7% annually. Higher incidence in Medicare recipients, US veterans, and diabetics
- Approximately 5%–10% of diabetic patients have had a foot ulcer previously
- Lifetime risk of developing foot ulcer in diabetic patient is 25%
- Nonhealing diabetic wounds are the leading cause of amputation in the United States and of the roughly $200 billion spent annually on diabetic complications, one-third of this cost burden is spent on peripheral wounds
- Sequelae of diabetic foot ulcers (DFUs) include infection, ischemia, amputation, and death

PATHOGENESIS

- Etiology of DFUs is a combination of peripheral neuropathy, pathobiomechanics, and may occur with or without peripheral vascular disease
  - Peripheral neuropathy—results from metabolic and ischemic changes to nerve fibers causing sensory, motor, and autonomic neuropathy. Requires early detection and treatment to prevent ulcers
    - **Sensory:** large and small fiber neuropathy—small fiber symptoms include burning, tingling, and electric sensation; large fiber symptoms include numbness and tingling
      - Result in loss of protective sensation that normally cue patient they may develop injury to their foot so they do not avoid the source (pressure, cut, infection)
    - **Autonomic:** due to increased symptomatic tone in lower extremity. Leads to small vessel ischemia and change in soft tissue turgor, which creates skin fissures that predispose to ulcers
      - Can result in Charcot foot
    - **Motor:** leads to muscle atrophy, joint laxity, bony misalignment, and foot deformity. Intrinsic muscle atrophy, leading to imbalance between opposing muscle groups (e.g., flexors and extensors)
      - Can result in hammer toe and *hallux abductovalgus* (metatarsophalangeal [MTP] joints dislocate, muscle imbalance causes toes to contract, pushes head of metatarsals through bottom of foot bunion)
      - Abnormal prominence of bones pushing into the ground or footwear lead to erosion, callus and/or pressure - all leading to ulceration (especially if insensate)
  - Biomechanics—stiffening of soft tissue, ligaments, tendons, and joint capsules results in limited range of motion and shifting of pressure points (sagittal plane and shear/frontal direction), thereby contributing to ulcer development
    - Conservative treatments: offloading shoes, boots, braces, casts
    - Surgical treatments: tendon rebalancing or lengthening, bony correction, amputation
  - Ischemia—peripheral artery disease (PAD) in diabetics is a major cause of amputation. It is imperative to treat underlying PAD to improve tissue perfusion and wound healing
    - Angiosomes give insight into the artery involved in a specific tissue distribution. Goal of surgery when possible is to revascularize the artery involved in the angiosome containing the wound to improve healing
    - Ischemic ulcers should not be debrided until revascularization is performed due to possibility of creating a larger nonhealing wound
    - When assessing level of amputation, it is crucial to know the level of perfusion that is adequate for healing
    - Generally, an absolute toe pressure >50 mm Hg is sufficient for healing a toe amputation

SIGNS/SYMPTOMS OF DISEASE

- Clinical presentation of DFUs may include pain (if no significant neuropathy or ischemia), cellulitis, purulence, induration, tenderness, necrosis

- May present with hallux valgus (bunions), hammer/claw toes, and Charcot arthropathy
- DFUs can progress to infection with systemic signs of fever, malaise, nausea, tachycardia, hyperglycemia, and leukocytosis
- If left untreated, diabetic foot infections may lead to sepsis

DIAGNOSTIC EVALUATION

- First diagnostic test should include arterial-brachial indices (ABIs)/toe brachial indices (TBIs) in patient with DFU to determine the presence and degree of ischemia as well as assess risk of amputation and potential improvement after revascularization
- Toe pressures <30 mm Hg have a high risk of amputation without revascularization
  - Toe pressures have a higher sensitivity for identifying PAD in diabetic patients than ankle pressures or ABIs due to noncompressible, calcified tibial vessels
- **Society for Vascular Surgery WIfI classification system**—used to predict 1-year amputation risk and benefit from revascularization; based on staging within three classification areas: wound, ischemia, and foot infection
  - Wound—0: no ulcer and no gangrene; 1: small ulcer and no gangrene; 2: deep ulcer and gangrene limited to toes; 3: extensive ulcer or extensive gangrene
  - Ischemia—0: toe pressure >60 mm Hg; 1: 40–59 mm Hg; 2: 30–39 mm Hg; 3: <30 mm Hg
  - Foot Infection (based on Infectious Diseases Society of America [IDSA]/International Working Group on the Diabetic Foot [IWGDF] criteria)—0: noninfected; 1: mild (<2 cm cellulitis); 2: moderate (>2 cm cellulitis/purulence); 3: severe (systemic response/sepsis)
- Infection can be graded according to IDSA and IWGDF classification systems:
  - Grade 1—uninfected without signs or symptoms of infection
  - Grade 2—mild, infection is confined to skin and subcutaneous tissue with 2 or more of the following: purulence, erythema, tenderness, warmth, and induration
  - Grade 3—moderate, infection extends beneath subcutaneous tissue with 1 or more of the following: cellulitis extending >2 cm from wound, lymphangitic streaking, spread beneath superficial fascia, deep tissue abscess, gangrene, involvement of muscle, tendon, joint, or bone; patient is clinically well with overall normal labs
  - Grade 4—severe, local infection with signs of systemic involvement/toxicity, including fevers, chills, hypothermia, tachycardia, hypotension, confusion, vomiting, leukocytosis (white blood cells [WBCs] >12,000 μ/L), acidosis, hyperglycemia, azotemia, tachypnea

Treatment

- Prevention strategies to avoid injury (e.g., offloading shoes and orthotics)
- Aggressive wound care and antibiotics
- If clinical signs of moderate or severe foot infection, should undergo operative drainage and debridement of underlying soft tissue involvement or amputation if indicated
  - Debridement involves removing surrounding tissue and any eschar at wound base until healthy, viable, vascularized tissue is encountered
- If there are signs of wet gangrene and/or sepsis, patient should undergo guillotine amputation of involved limb to obtain source control with subsequent formalization based on the initial level of amputation
- Elective amputation
  - About 20% of moderate to severe infections require amputation

Complications

- Infection
  - Acute and chronic infections are common in the diabetic foot and must be appropriately treated
  - Acute infection typically occurs through seeding of bacteria via a puncture wound
  - Most often polymicrobial but can also be monomicrobial
  - Most commonly Staphylococcus (especially methicillin-resistant *Staphylococcus aureus* [MRSA]) or *Streptococcus*
  - Aerobic gram-negative bacilli (*Escherichia coli* and *Pseudomonas*) are frequently involved
  - Anaerobes seen in ischemic or necrotic tissue
  - Fungal and yeast infections make up about 25% of chronic wounds
  - Osteomyelitis is found in a significant number of diabetics who require amputation (20% of diabetics outpatient; 67% of diabetics inpatient)
  - Wound that probes to bone is diagnostic of osteomyelitis
  - Treatment includes intravenous antibiotics ± amputation/source control. Complete treatment with antibiotics alone is difficult because many bacteria form biofilms, which need to be mechanically disrupted
- Dry gangrene
- Wet gangrene
  Follow-up
- Daily self-diabetic foot examinations to identify ulcers, callus, injuries, or signs of infection
- Based on mode of intervention (e.g., revascularization)

SUGGESTED READINGS

Kim PJ, Lavery LA. Chapter 115: Diabetic foot abnormalities and their management. In: *Rutherford's Vascular Surgery and Endovascular Therapy*. Elsevier 2022; 1527-1535.e3.

Mills JL, Sr, Conte MS, Armstrong DG, et al. The society for vascular surgery lower extremity threatened limb classification system: risk stratification based on Wound, Ischemia, and foot Infection (WIfI) J Vasc Surg. 2014;59(1):220-34.e2.

Zhan LX, Branco BC, Armstrong DG, Mills JL Sr. The Society for Vascular Surgery lower extremity threatened limb classification system based on Wound, Ischemia, and foot Infection (WIfI) correlates with risk of major amputation and time to wound healing. J Vasc Surg. 2015 Apr;61(4):939-44.

CHAPTER 17

Major Amputation

ADAM BARAKA, BS, and LUKE BREWSTER, MD, PhD

EPIDEMIOLOGY

- Foot ulcers and amputation are most common in patients with diabetes mellitus (DM), uninsured, Black, and Hispanic patients
- Cost for minor amputation is ~$45,000 and major is ~$66,000 (>75% is *after* the actual amputation—hospital, medical practitioners, rehabilitation, reoperations, adaptive devices). Thus focus must be on prevention[1]
Multidisciplinary limb salvage programs have shown decreased amputation rates in reports from around the world.

Incidence

- ~150,000 amputations per year in the United States.[2] A report from 1997 found nearly 70% of all amputations were in diabetics
- The ratio of below-knee amputation (BKA) to above-knee amputation (AKA) should approach 2:1
- 5-year mortality rates are similar to advanced malignancies:[3]
  - 30-day all-cause mortality is *now* near 8.6%—worse for AKA versus BKA (16.5% vs. 5.7%). Older series reported ~20%–30%[4]
  - 1- and 3-year mortality rates are as high as 48% and 71%, respectively
- Highest mortality risk factor is chronic kidney disease (CKD)/dialysis

- Decreased 15-year trend of amputation by 45% in Medicare patients[5]
- Venous thromboembolism (VTE) has been shown to affect over 10% of patients in the 2 months following amputation (The National Institute for Health and Care Excellence [NICE] Guidelines suggest low-molecular-weight heparin [LMWH] for >7 days post amputation)

Etiology and Risk Factors

- The most common causes of major amputation are:
  (1) Infection (often in diabetic patients) $\pm$ peripheral arterial disease (PAD)
  (2) Nonhealing diabetic foot ulcers or recalcitrant osteomyelitis
  (3) Chronic limb-threatening ischemia (CLTI)
  (4) Less common: trauma and cancer.
- DM is associated with 70%–80% of all lower extremity amputations. DM increases likelihood for amputation 30 times, more likely to be amputated young, all with an earlier mortality[6]
- DM alone has a higher risk of major amputation versus PAD alone[7]
- Increased incidence of PAD in diabetics over older than age 65 (30% vs. the 12%–20% of general US population)

Ethnicity

- Fourfold differences in amputation risk among Medicare beneficiaries are recognized between Black Americans and other racial/ethnic groups, with Black patients more likely to undergo amputation even after similar revascularization procedures and risk adjustment[8]

MODIFYING FACTORS THAT DECREASE RISK OF AMPUTATION

- Optimal medical therapy including moderate and high-intensity stain use decreases risk of amputation[9,10]

Signs and Symptoms

Vascular Indications for Amputations

- Critical limb ischemia without revascularization or with poor risk/benefit ratio due to general medical condition/revascularization options
- Multidisciplinary wound care for critical limb ischemia improves amputation survival compared with standard wound care of inconsistent providers[11]
- Refractory myoglobinemia after ischemia reperfusion injury in acute limb ischemia leading to multisystem organ failure
- Primary amputation or palliation to those with limited life expectancy, poor functional status (e.g., nonambulatory), or an unsalvageable limb (after shared decision making) (Global Vascular Guidelines for CLTI[12]

RELATIVE CONTRAINDICATIONS TO PERFORMING AMPUTATION

- Advanced comorbidities and frailty may benefit from palliative care or palliative wound care, instead of major amputation[13,14]

DIAGNOSTIC EVALUATION: HEALING POTENTIAL AND FUNCTION

Vascular examination and healing potential:
- Low ambulation rate due to slow wound healing,[9,10] chronic pain, imbalance, and falls[3,8,11]
- BKAs in untreated vascular patients may have delayed wound healing with prolonged debilitation prior to prosthesis fit, or worse, a need to revise the BKA to an AKA[9,10]
- Popliteal Doppler signal predicts >90% success for BKA
- Toe pressure <40 mm Hg associated with decreased forefoot healing
- Transcutaneous oxygen pressure (TcPo$_2$ mm Hg) >40% suggests good wound healing
- Infection, deep vein thrombosis (DVT) prophylaxis, and nutritional status (albumin >3.5 gm/dL) will also affect ability to heal

Rehabilitation Potential

- Nonweight bearing is essential for forefoot wounds to heal
- BKA requires extension of knee and better distal perfusion of extended limb
- AKAs preferred when BKA healing outcomes are predicted to be poor (due to noncompliance in healthcare or ambulatory difficulty)

- Nonmodifiable predictors of postoperative ambulation such as nonambulatory status prior to amputation, end-stage renal disease (ESRD), and the inability to participate in rehabilitation lead to low rates of ambulation after major amputation[11]

Treatment Pearls

- Vascular examination: pulse above the level of amputation is the best predictor of healing
- Guillotine amputation with staged reconstruction: reduces wound infection rate in patients with gross infection (e.g., diabetic foot)
- Regional anesthesia may lead to decreased complications compared with general anesthesia
- Peripheral nerve blockade may improve analgesia after major amputation (either transprocedural block with long-acting local or postprocedure infusions)
- Evaluate for hardware prior to incision. May require special tools or removal of orthopedic hardware "hidden" in the bone

Toe and Foot Amputations

- Absolute systolic toe pressure >45 mm Hg has the highest success rate for healing a wound and/or toe amputation[15]
- The phalanx itself can be taken if the base of the toe is healthy with no signs of infection
- In general, ray amputations are performed for ischemic toe(s)
  - A "tennis racket" incision is made to circumferentially take the toe as well as the head of the metatarsal
  - The vertical incision on the metatarsal allows for a nontension closure

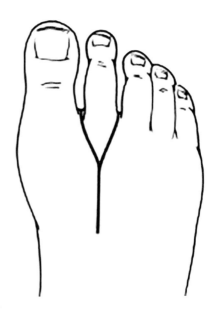

- Great toe amputations will have the vertical incision along the medial aspect of the foot rather than the dorsum of it
- Transmetatarsal amputation: through the metatarsal bones and leaving a plantar flap to bring to the dorsal aspect of the foot
- Lisfranc amputation: resection of the entire metatarsal bones at the tarsometatarsal joint
- Chopart amputation: leaving only the talus and calcaneus bones
  - The more proximal the foot amputation, the more energy expenditure for balance
  - Sometimes a BKA allows for better function due to better prosthetics
- Consider thrombotic microangiopathy (TMA) in CLTI patients requiring more than two digital ray amputations (Global Vascular Guidelines for CLTI[12]
- Bone viability from biopsy of margin has conflicting studies due to interobserver reliability (<70%) for which its use is institution-dependent[16]
- Yes, there are toe prosthetics (aesthetics and better shoe-fitting)

TCPo₂

In 1972, Huch[17] reported the use of heated (45°C) Clark electrodes (platinum cathode was covered with a semipermeable membrane) as a practical method to monitor skin surface (transcutaneous) po₂. These instruments were first applied clinically to monitor O_2 in neonates during and after delivery. TcPo₂ is a *metabolic* test requiring ~35 minutes to get a reading.

Normal value is ~60 mm Hg. Vasoconstriction (cold room, smoking, coffee, pain, anxiety) will artificially lower results. Studies have not been consistent for which there are proponents and detractors, making its use mostly institution-associated.

PROXIMAL AMPUTATIONS

- BKA
  - Minimal inflow is considered to be a widely patent profunda femoris
  - TcPo₂ >40 is ideal for healing BKA. Less than 20 has highest failure,[18] but a 2012 metaanalysis showed no significant correlation for successful amputation[19] = no rigid adaptation of this technique)
  - Anterior incision one hand's breadth below the tibial condyle
  - Posterior flap needs the gastrocnemius fascia to be long enough to bring anterior. Sometimes the soleus needs to be cut back to minimize the thickness to close
    - 12–15 cm proximal incision (as long "as possible" for better-fitting prosthetic)
    - One-third to one-half the circumference of the proximal leg

- Posterior flap should be as long as possible to have a tension-free suture line to anterior fascia
- Fibula should then be cut higher than tibia (rongeur/saw)
- Bevel anterior tibia to avoid pressure/skin necrosis
- Both nerves ligated and cut under tension to be covered by muscle/fascia
- Myodesis of the soleus fascia to the tibia is sometimes done for young patients to "secure" a muscle cushion to the bone—presumably to improve prosthesis fitting/support
- Two stage (guillotine followed by completion) is best for healing if there is infection (lower risk of reinfection and revision)[20]
- Through-knee amputation
  - Fish-mouth incision for closure
  - Keep the patella. Remove the femoral condyles to make less bulbous
  - Not preferred over AKA with a prosthetic as it leaves a longer-than-the-other-side lever (knee) after installing prosthetic[21]
- AKA
  - As long as possible with adequate muscle closure for amputation fitting
  - Fish-mouth incision is traditional *but* not critical—flaps can be created according to available/viable skin/muscle
    - Length of incision should be half the diameter of the thigh
  - Adductor magnus myodesis can be performed to eliminate hip contracture
  - Higher amputation risk versus BKA (see earlier)
  - Energy consumption during ambulation is 50%–100% higher than BKA
  - Only 10% will use a prosthetic
  - Higher primary healing rate compared with BKA

COMPLICATIONS

BKA has a higher revision rate than AKA (~5%).[3–5]
- Phantom limb pain: burning, throbbing, stabbing, and sharp, presents in 67% of patients at 6 months, and 50% of patients at 5–7 years,[10,11] risk factors include female gender, upper extremity amputation, bilateral amputations, and preamputation pain[22]
- ESRD: when compared with non–dialysis-dependent CKD and normal renal function, is associated with an increased risk of death and shorter long-term survival rates after limb amputation[23]
- Neuroma: inflammatory response at the end of an exposed nerve leading to hyperalgesia, worse when compressed (unable to use prosthetic). Thought to be prevented by using absorbable suture on nerve, ensuring nerve is covered by muscle (or enveloping it and securing the muscle to it). Risks favoring it: previous chronic pain, infection in region, leaving long segment of nerve. No hard evidence

- May need revision with resection and muscle flap coverage of the terminal nerve
- Successful peripheral nerve block confirms diagnosis (possible benefit with RFA)

FUTURE DIRECTIONS IN AMPUTATION CARE

- Incorporating neural operations into the amputation operation
- Regenerative peripheral nerve interface (RPNI) incorporates muscle patches onto the peripheral nerves from the amputated limb, effective operation for relieving pain from neuromas shown in two clinical trials[24,25]

- Successfully pilot tested in healthy, high-functioning individuals[12,13]
- Reestablishing quasi-normal muscle tension relationships into the amputation operation
- Agonist-antagonist myoneural interface (AMI)
  - Similar normal muscular tension preventing fibrofatty degeneration and allowing for improved prosthesis fitting
  - Improved residual limb health with ambulation rate of 75%
  - Posterior mountainous flap provides durable soft tissue coverage leading to residual limb health
- Ewing amputation (EA): incorporates both RPNI and AMI into the BKA operation[26]

REFERENCES

1. Boulton AJ, Vileikyte L, Ragnarson-Tennvall G, Apelqvist J. The global burden of diabetic foot disease. *Lancet.* 2005; 366(9498):1719-24.
2. Molina CS, Faulk JB. *Lower Extremity Amputation.* StatPearls; 2022.
3. Barnes JA, Eid MA, Creager MA, Goodney PP. Epidemiology and risk of amputation in patients with diabetes mellitus and peripheral artery disease. *Arterioscler Thromb Vasc Biol.* 2020;40:1808-1817.
4. Aulivola B, Hile CN, Hamdan AD, et al. Major lower extremity amputation: outcome of a modern series. *Arch Surg.* 2004; 139(4):395-9.
5. Goodney PP, Tarulli M, Faerber AE, Schanzer A, Zwolak RM. Fifteen-year trends in lower limb amputation, revascularization, and preventive measures among medicare patients. *JAMA Surg.* 2015;150:84-86.
6. Dillingham TR, Pezzin LE, Shore AD. Reamputation, mortality, and health care costs among persons with dysvascular lower-limb amputations. *Arch Phys Med Rehabil.* 2005;86:480-486.
7. Chery J, Semaan E, Darji S, Briggs WT, Yarmush J, D'Ayala M. Impact of regional versus general anesthesia on the clinical outcomes of patients undergoing major lower extremity amputation. *Ann Vasc Surg.* 2014;28:1149-1156.
8. Creager MA, Matsushita K, Arya S, et al. Reducing nontraumatic lower-extremity amputations by 20% by 2030: time to get to our feet: a policy statement from the American Heart Association. *Circulation.* 2021;143:e875-e891.
9. Arya S, Khakharia A, Binney ZO, et al. Association of statin dose with amputation and survival in patients with peripheral artery disease. *Circulation.* 2018;137:1435-1446.
10. Chung J, Timaran DA, Modrall JG, et al. Optimal medical therapy predicts amputation-free survival in chronic critical limb ischemia. *J Vasc Surg.* 2013;58:972-980.
11. Chung J, Modrall JG, Ahn C, Lavery LA, Valentine RJ. Multidisciplinary care improves amputation-free survival in patients with chronic critical limb ischemia. *J Vasc Surg.* 2015;61:162-169.
12. Conte MS, Bradbury AW, Kolh P, et al. Global vascular guidelines on the management of chronic limb-threatening ischemia. *J Vasc Surg.* 2019;69:3S-125S.e40.
13. Kwong M, Curtis EE, Mell MW. Underutilization of palliative care for patients with advanced peripheral arterial disease. *Ann Vasc Surg.* 2021;76:211-217.
14. Barshes NR, Gold B, Garcia A, Bechara CF, Pisimisis G, Kougias P. Minor amputation and palliative wound care as a strategy to avoid major amputation in patients with foot infections and

severe peripheral arterial disease. *Int J Low Extrem Wounds.* 2014;13:211-219.
15. Apelqvist J, Castenfors J, Larsson J, Stenström A, Agardh CD. Prognostic value of systolic ankle and toe blood pressure levels in outcome of diabetic foot ulcer. *Diabetes Care.* 1989;12:373-8.
16. Schmidt BM, McHugh JB, Patel RM, Wrobe JS. Prospective analysis of surgical bone margins after partial foot amputation in diabetic patients admitted with moderate to severe foot infections. *Foot Ankle Spec.* 2019;12(2):131-7.
17. Huch R, Marburg F.D.U. Quantitative Continuous Measurement of Partial Oxygen Pressure on the Skin of Adults and New-Born Babies. *Pflugers Arch.* 1972;337:185-198.
18. Nishio H, Minakata K, Kawaguchi A, et al. Transcutaneous oxygen pressure as a surrogate index of lower limb amputation. *Int Angiol.* 2016;35(6):565-57.
19. Arsenault KA, Al-Otaibi A, Devereaux PJ, Thorlund K, Tittley JG, Whitlock RP. The use of transcutaneous oximetry to predict healing complications of lower limb amputations: a systematic review and meta-analysis. *Eur J Vasc Endovasc Surg.* 2012;43(3):329-36.
20. Tisi PV, Than MM. Type of incision for below knee amputation. Cochrane *Database Syst Rev.* 2014;2014(4):CD003749.
21. Geertzen JHB, de Beus MC, Jutte PC, Otten E, Dekker R. What is the optimal femur length in a trans-femoral amputation? A mixed method study: scoping review, expert opinions and biomechanical analysis. *Med Hypotheses.* 2019;129:109238.
22. Ahuja V, Thapa D, Ghai B. Strategies for prevention of lower limb post-amputation pain: a clinical narrative review. *J Anaesthesiol Clin Pharmacol.* 2018;34:439-449.
23. Meyer A, Griesbach C, Maudanz N, Lang W, Almasi-Sperling V, Rother U. Influence of end-stage renal disease on long-term survival after major amputation. *Vasa.* 2020;49:317-322.
24. Hoyt BW, Gibson JA, Potter BK, Souza JM. Practice patterns and pain outcomes for targeted muscle reinnervation: an informed approach to targeted muscle reinnervation use in the acute amputation setting. *J Bone Joint Surg Am.* 2021;103:681-687.
24. Kemper SWP, Kung TA. Regenerative peripheral nerve interfaces for the treatment of painful neuromas in major limb amputees. Technical report 30, September 30, 2019. Contract No. 2018.W81XWH-17-1-0641. *Defense Technical Information Center;* 2019. https://apps.dtic.mil/sti/citations/AD1088470
25. Tuffaha S. Surgical treatments for neuroma pain in amputees (STOCAP). *Johns Hopkins University;* April 1, 2021. NCT04204668.
26. Carty M. Somatotopic configuration of distal residual limb tissues in lower extremity amputations. *Brigham and Women's Hospital;* December 15, 2017. NCT03374319

CHAPTER 18

Visceral Artery Aneurysms

MANUEL GARCIA-TOCA, MD, MS

SPLENIC ARTERY ANEURYSM (SAA)

- Most common of the splanchnic artery aneurysms, accounting for nearly 60%. Incidence of 0.78% in the general population
- Affects females at a ratio of 4:1 over males

Diagnosis

- *Computed tomography angiography (CTA) is the initial diagnostic tool of choice for SAAs,* magnetic resonance angiography (MRA) for patients with suspected SAAs and preexisting renal insufficiency; arteriography when noninvasive studies have not sufficiently demonstrated the status of relevant collateral blood flow and endovascular intervention is planned

Treatment

- Treatment may appropriately involve open surgical, endovascular, or laparoscopic intervention methods, depending on the patient's anatomy and underlying clinical condition
- *Emergent* intervention for ruptured SAAs
- Nonruptured splenic artery *pseudoaneurysms* of any size in patients of acceptable risk
- Nonruptured splenic artery true aneurysms of any size in women of childbearing age

- Nonruptured splenic artery true aneurysms >3 cm, with a demonstrable increase in size or associated symptoms in patients of acceptable risk
- The splenic artery does not routinely require preservation or revascularization. However, when treating a distal SAA adjacent to the hilum of the spleen consider open surgical techniques, including splenectomy, given concern for the possibility of end-organ ischemia, including splenic infarction and pancreatitis
- In pregnant women with SAA, treatment decisions should be individualized regardless of size, and the potential morbidity to both the mother and fetus should be considered
- Patients undergoing SAA embolization or ligation may be at risk for splenic loss and should receive pneumococcal, meningococcal, and *Haemophilus influenzae* type b vaccinations
- After endovascular intervention for SAAs, periodic surveillance with CTA, ultrasound (US), or MRA to assess for the possibility of continued risk of aneurysm growth

Observation

- Small (<3 cm), stable asymptomatic splenic artery true aneurysms or those in patients with significant medical comorbidities or limited life expectancies
- Annual surveillance with computed tomography (CT) or US to assess for growth in size

Screening

- Screening of other intraabdominal, intrathoracic, intracranial, and peripheral artery aneurysms

RENAL ARTERY ANEURYSM (RAA)

- RAAs occur in approximately 0.1% of the population
- Pregnancy has been associated with increased risk and rates of rupture
- Recent estimates suggest a median annualized growth rate of 0.06–0.6 mm

Diagnosis

- *CTA is the initial diagnostic tool of choice for RAAs*, MRA for patients with suspected RAAs and preexisting renal insufficiency and radiation risks; arteriography for preoperative planning and to delineate better distal renal artery branches and when endovascular intervention is planned. Non–contrast-enhanced MRA is best suited to children and women of childbearing potential or those who have contraindications to CTA or MRA contrast materials

Treatment

- Treatment may appropriately involve open surgical, endovascular, or laparoscopic methods of intervention, depending on the patient's anatomy and underlying clinical condition
- Treatment for aneurysm size >3 cm, for noncomplicated RAA of acceptable operative risk
- Emergent intervention for any size RAA resulting in patient symptoms or rupture
- Treatment regardless of size, in patients of childbearing potential with noncomplicated RAA of acceptable operative risk
- Treatment regardless of size, in patients with medically refractory hypertension and functionally important renal artery stenosis
- Open surgical reconstructive techniques for the elective repair of most RAAs in patients with acceptable operative risk
- Ex vivo repairs and autotransplantation for complex distal branch aneurysms over nephrectomy when it is technically feasible
- Endovascular techniques for the elective repair of anatomically appropriate RAAs to include stent-graft exclusion of main RAAs in patients with poor operative risk and embolization of distal and parenchymal aneurysms
- Completion imaging after open surgical reconstruction for RAA, before hospital discharge, by way of axial imaging with CTA or MRA or arteriography in select cases, and long-term follow-up with surveillance imaging

Observation

- Small (<3 cm), stable asymptomatic RAA or those in patients with significant medical comorbidities or limited life expectancies
- Annual surveillance imaging until two consecutive studies are stable; after that, it may be extended to every 2–3 years

Screening

- Female patients of childbearing age with RAA for fibromuscular dysplasia with a focused history and one-time axial imaging study (CTA or MRA) to assess cerebrovascular, mesenteric, and iliac artery dysplasia

CELIAC ARTERY ANEURYSM (CAA)

- Represent 4% of all splanchnic aneurysms; found concomitantly with other visceral aneurysms in 40% of cases and with aortic aneurysms 20% of the time

Diagnosis

- *CTA is the initial diagnostic tool of choice for CAAs*, MRA for patients with preexisting renal insufficiency and radiation risks, arteriography when there is insufficient information on relevant collateral blood flow (superior mesenteric artery, gastroduodenal artery, and other relevant collateral circulation)

Treatment

- Treatment may appropriately involve open surgical or endovascular methods of intervention, depending on the patient's anatomy and underlying clinical condition
- Treatment of nonruptured celiac artery pseudoaneurysms of any size in patients of acceptable operative risk
- Treatment of nonruptured celiac artery true aneurysms >2 cm, with a demonstrable increase in size or associated symptoms in patients of acceptable risk
- In patients with ruptured CAA discovered at laparotomy, consider treatment with ligation if there is sufficient collateral circulation to the liver and the liver is not cirrhotic
- After endovascular intervention for CAAs, patients need periodic surveillance with appropriate imaging studies to assess for the possibility of endoleak or aneurysm reperfusion

Observation

- Small (<2 cm), stable asymptomatic CAAs or those in patients with significant medical comorbidities or limited life expectancy
- Annual surveillance with CTA scans to assess for growth in size

Screening

- Patients with CAAs for other arterial aneurysms

GASTRIC AND GASTROEPIPLOIC ARTERY ANEURYSMS

Diagnosis

- *CTA is the initial diagnostic tool of choice*, MRA, for patients with preexisting renal insufficiency and radiation risks

Treatment

- Treatment of *all* gastric artery and gastroepiploic artery aneurysms of any size
- Endovascular embolization for first-line treatment of gastric artery and gastroepiploic artery aneurysms
- Postembolization surveillance every 1–2 years with axial imaging to assess for vascular remodeling and evidence of aneurysm reperfusion

Screening

- Abdominal axial imaging to screen for concomitant abdominal aneurysms
- CTA (or MRA) of the head, neck, and chest for those patients with segmental arterial mediolysis
- Interval surveillance (12–24 months) with axial imaging (CTA or MRA) in cases of segmental medial arteriolysis

HEPATIC ARTERY ANEURYSM (HAA)

- The hepatic artery is the second most common location of splanchnic aneurysm formation
- 75%–80% localized in the extrahepatic vasculature; 63% are in the common hepatic artery and 28% in the right hepatic artery
- The male/female ratio is 3:2

Diagnosis

- CTA is the diagnostic tool of choice, MRA for patients preexisting renal insufficiency and radiation risks, *mesenteric* angiography for preoperative planning, if there is not sufficient information of relevant collateral blood flow

Treatment

- Treatment may appropriately involve open surgical or endovascular methods of intervention, depending on the patient's anatomy and underlying clinical condition

Indications for Treatment

- All hepatic artery pseudoaneurysms, regardless of cause, should be repaired as soon as the diagnosis is made, given the high propensity of rupture
- All symptomatic HAAs regardless of size
- Asymptomatic patients without significant comorbidity, with true HAA, is >2 cm or enlarges >0.5 cm/year
- In patients with significant comorbidities, repair if HAA *is* >5.0 cm
- Repair of HAA in patients with vasculopathy or vasculitis, regardless of size
- Repair of all HAA patients with positive blood cultures
- In patients with extrahepatic aneurysms, open and endovascular techniques to maintain liver circulation. *Endovascular-first approach* to all HAAs if anatomically feasible
- In patients with intrahepatic aneurysms, perform coil embolization of the affected artery. In patients with large intrahepatic aneurysms, resection of the involved lobe of the liver is recommended to avoid significant necrosis

Screening

- One-time screening CTA or MRA of the head, neck, and chest in patients with nonatherosclerotic causes of HAA

Observation

- Annual follow-up with CT for patients with asymptomatic HAA <2 cm

SUPERIOR MESENTERIC ARTERY ANEURYSM (SMAA)

- SMAA most commonly results from an infectious cause or dissection; the superior mesenteric artery is the most common site of infection outside of the aorta

Diagnosis

- *CTA is the initial diagnostic tool of choice.* Mesenteric angiography to delineate anatomy in preoperative planning for SMAA repair

Treatment

- Treatment may appropriately involve open surgical or endovascular methods of intervention, depending on the patient's anatomy and underlying clinical condition
- *Repair* all true SMAAs and pseudoaneurysms as soon as the diagnosis is made *regardless of size*

- Careful observation of SMAA because of *dissection* unless refractory symptoms develop
- Recommended an endovascular-first approach to all SMAAs if it is anatomically feasible

Screening

- Abdominal axial imaging to screen for concomitant intraabdominal aneurysms in patients who did not have CTA at the time of diagnosis
- Annual CTA to observe postsurgical patients

JEJUNAL, ILEAL, AND COLIC ARTERY ANEURYSMS

- Extremely rare, anecdotally reported in the literature

Diagnosis

- *CTA* is the diagnostic tool of choice, MRA for patients with preexisting renal insufficiency and radiation risks

Treatment

- Treatment with endovascular methods of intervention for ruptured cases and all mesenteric branch vessel pseudoaneurysms of any size
- Elective intervention for jejunal and ileal artery aneurysms >2 cm in maximal diameter and for all colic artery aneurysms
- Open surgical ligation or aneurysm excision for cases of jejunal, ileal, and colic artery aneurysms when laparotomy is being considered for hematoma evacuation or bowel assessment for viability
- Endovascular embolization for cases of jejunal, ileal, and colic artery aneurysms
- Medical treatment of nonruptured, asymptomatic ileal, jejunal, and colic artery aneurysms *associated with polyarteritis nodosa*
- *Repair* all true SMAAs and pseudoaneurysms as soon as the diagnosis is made *regardless of size*
- Careful observation of SMAA because of *dissection* unless refractory symptoms develop
- Recommended an endovascular-first approach to all SMAAs if it is anatomically feasible

Screening

- Screening all patients with jejunal, ileal, and colic artery aneurysms for vasculitis with routine inflammatory markers

- Abdominal axial imaging to screen for concomitant abdominal aneurysms
- One-time screening CTA of the head, neck, and chest for those patients with segmental arterial mediolysis

Surveillance

- Interval surveillance (12–24 months) with axial imaging for cases of segmental medial arteriolysis to monitor rapid arterial transformation and to monitor regression in cases of polyarteritis nodosa
- Postembolization surveillance every 1–2 years with axial imaging to assess for vascular remodeling and evidence of aneurysm reperfusion

PANCREATICODUODENAL ARTERY ANEURYSM (PDAA) AND GASTRODUODENAL ARTERY ANEURYSM (GDAA)

- Celiac artery occlusive disease has been implicated in true GDAA and PDAA
- Associated also with pancreatic pathology or trauma
- The male/female ratio is 4:1

Diagnosis

- *CTA* is the diagnostic tool of choice in patients who are thought to have GDAA and PDAA
- In patients in whom celiac stenosis is suspected, we suggest further workup with *duplex US* to determine if the stenosis is hemodynamically significant
- *MRA* for patients with preexisting renal insufficiency and radiation risks

Treatment

All patients with noncomplicated GDAA and PDAA of acceptable operative risk, treatment is recommended no matter the size of the aneurysm because of the risk of rupture (Fig. 18.1)

- Coil embolization as the treatment of choice in patients with intact and ruptured aneurysms
- In cases where coil embolization is not feasible, covered stenting or stent-assisted coil embolization is a treatment option. Transcatheter embolization with liquid embolic agents and flow-diverting, multilayered stents are treatment options in selected cases of GDAA and PDAA
- *Treatment* with open surgical reconstruction if needed to preserve flow

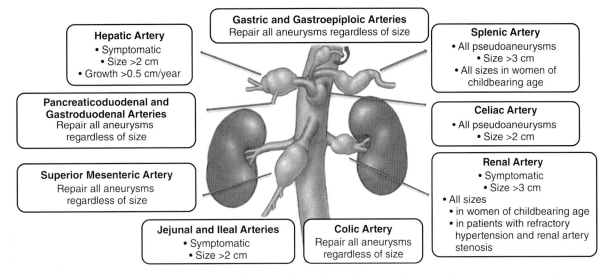

FIG. 18.1 Society for Vascular Surgery clinical practice guidelines on the management of visceral aneurysms. (From Chaer RA, Abularrage CJ, Coleman DM, et al. The Society for Vascular Surgery clinical practice guidelines on the management of visceral aneurysms. *J Vasc Surg.* 2020;72(1S):3S-39S.)

- Treatment with celiac artery reconstruction in patients with concomitant stenosis or occlusion

Screening

- Patients with median arcuate ligament syndrome, with CTA or duplex US

Surveillance

- Postembolization surveillance with axial imaging to assess for vascular remodeling and evidence of aneurysm reperfusion

SUGGESTED READINGS

Chaer RA, Abularrage CJ, Coleman DM, et al. The Society for Vascular Surgery clinical practice guidelines on the management of visceral aneurysms. *J Vasc Surg.* 2020;72(1S):3S-39S.

Carroccio A, Jacobs TS, Faries P, et al. Endovascular treatment of visceral artery aneurysms. *Vasc Endovascular Surg.* 2007;41(5):373-382.

DeCarlo C, Mohebali J, Dua A, Conrad MF, Mohapatra A. Morbidity and mortality associated with open repair of visceral aneurysms. *J Vasc Surg.* 2022;75(2):632-640.e2.

Fankhauser GT, Stone WM, Naidu SG, et al. The minimally invasive management of visceral artery aneurysms and pseudoaneurysms. *J Vasc Surg.* 2011;53(4):966-970.

Tulsyan N, Kashyap VS, Greenberg RK, et al. The endovascular management of visceral artery aneurysms and pseudoaneurysms. *J Vasc Surg.* 2007;45(2):276-283; discussion 283.

Stanley JC, Fry WJ. Pathogenesis and clinical significance of splenic artery aneurysms. *Surgery.* 1974;76(6):898-909.

Saba L, Anzidei M, Lucatelli P, Mallarini G. The multidetector computed tomography angiography (MDCTA) in the diagnosis of splenic artery aneurysm and pseudoaneurysm. *Acta Radiol.* 2011;52(5):488-498.

Carr SC, Mahvi DM, Hoch JR, Archer CW, Turnipseed WD. Visceral artery aneurysm rupture. *J Vasc Surg.* 2001;33(4):806-811. Available at: https://www.jvascsurg.org/article/S0741-5214(01)04103-9/fulltext.

Ejstrud P, Hansen JB, Andreasen DA. Prophylaxis against pneumococcal infection after splenectomy: a challenge for hospitals and primary care. *Eur J Surg.* 1997;163(10):733-738.

Stanley JC, Rhodes EL, Gewertz BL, Chang CY, Walter JF, Fry WJ. Renal artery aneurysms. Significance of macroaneurysms exclusive of dissections and fibrodysplastic mural dilations. *Arch Surg.* 1975;110(11):1327-1333.

Klausner JQ, Lawrence PF, Harlander-Locke MP, et al. The contemporary management of renal artery aneurysms. *J Vasc Surg.* 2015;61(4):978-984.

Shanley CJ, Shah NL, Messina LM. Uncommon splanchnic artery aneurysms: pancreaticoduodenal, gastroduodenal, superior mesenteric, inferior mesenteric, and colic. *Ann Vasc Surg.* 1996;10(5):506-515.

CHAPTER 19

Renal Artery Occlusive Disease

THEODORE G. HART, MD, and MICHAEL D. SGROI, MD

CHAPTER OUTLINE

EPIDEMIOLOGY

- Prevalence of renal artery stenosis on duplex is 6.8% in asymptomatic patients older than 65 years screened with duplex ultrasound[1]
- Associated with increasing age, low high-density cholesterol levels, and increasing systolic blood pressure in screening[1]
- Higher-risk cohorts, such as those with aortoiliac occlusive disease, coronary artery disease, and new-onset dialysis have a 20%–40% prevalence[2-4]
- Bilateral lesions seen in 12.5% during screening,[1] up to 50% in autopsy series[5]
- Hypertension (HTN) in adults is not synonymous with renal artery stenosis; 50% of patients with normal duplex on screening have HTN[1]
- A pediatric patient with HTN is pathognomonic for renovascular HTN[6]

ETIOLOGY

Pathophysiology

- A comprehensive review of renal physiology is beyond the scope of a Vascular Surgery In-Training Examination (VSITE) review. However, fundamental conceptual knowledge of renal physiology is sometimes tested directly or through pharmacology
- The lack of significant collateralization to the kidney as a whole makes it sensitive to ischemia and loss of function through glomerular collapse and tubular necrosis[7]

Renin-Angiotensin-Aldosterone System

- The renin-angiotensin-aldosterone system regulates blood pressure through its impact on renal sodium and water excretion
- The kidneys are the body's primary source of circulating renin, which is secreted in response to decreased perfusion pressure
  - Renin has enzymatic activity to cleave angiotensinogen from the liver into angiotensin I
  - Pulmonary and renal endothelial cells use angiotensin-converting enzyme (ACE) to cleave angiotensin I to angiotensin II[8]
- Angiotensin II leads to arteriolar vasoconstriction and increased tone in the efferent arterioles, direct fluid retention through enhancement of sodium reabsorption and stimulation of aldosterone secretion by the adrenal cortex, as well as indirectly through stimulation of antidiuretic hormone secretion and promotion of thirst[9]
- Aldosterone is secreted by the adrenal gland in response to angiotensin II and increased plasma K^+ concentration and similarly functions to mediate renal sodium reabsorption and volume expansion[10]

Physiologic Changes of Occlusive Disease

- Renal artery stenosis leads to a decrease in the perfusion pressure sensed in the afferent arteriole and release of renin[8]
- This leads to vasoconstriction, which raises the glomerular filtration rate (GFR) through action on the efferent arterioles as well as fluid retention mediated by the renin-angiotensin-aldosterone system, resulting in increased volume expansion[9,10]
- In unilateral renal artery stenosis, the contralateral kidney will adapt to limit the volume expansion through compensatory natriuresis. Solitary kidney patients and patients with bilateral renal artery stenosis are at risk for more severe Goldblatt volume-dependent renovascular HTN[9,10]
- ACE inhibitors limit the vasoconstriction in the efferent arterioles and may demonstrate a decrease in the GFR that is profound in the setting of bilateral renal artery stenosis[11]

Atherosclerosis

- Most common reason by far for stenting referrals[12]
- Usually ostial and contiguous with aortic plaque; however, can affect main artery and/or smaller intraparenchymal branches as well

Fibromuscular Dysplasia

- Usually main artery and branches with series of stenoses
- Medial fibroplasia is the most common pathologic subtype with theses stenoses appearing angiographically as a "string of beads"[13]

Other Etiologies

- Dissection (spontaneous, traumatic, or periprocedural) which can manifest as narrowing or thrombosis of the main renal artery or branches[11]
- Rarer causes include congenital syndromes such as renal artery hypoplasia and midaortic syndromes or inflammatory arteritis
- Renal artery embolus and nonembolic renal artery thrombosis and renal vein thromboses are additional relevant clinical presentations[14]

SIGNS/SYMPTOMS

- HTN, classically resistant to multiple agents
- Hypertensive crisis, especially in the setting of unrecognized or poorly treated advanced renovascular HTN
- Decreased renal function, mild to significant ischemic nephropathy
- Incidental imaging finding
- Peripheral edema
- Abdominal bruit
- Diminished pulses consistent with systemic atherosclerotic disease

DIAGNOSTIC EVALUATION

Laboratory

- Blood chemistries, diabetic screening, urinalysis, and electrolytes, and can expand significantly to investigate for other rare etiologies in the differential, such as primary hyperaldosteronism or pheochromocytoma when suspected clinically[11]

Imaging

The gold standard diagnostic imaging is digital subtraction angiography (DSA) but has limitations relative to other modalities given its invasive nature and lack of three-dimensional visualization

- Renal duplex ultrasound is the preferred primary methodology for screening and following renal artery stenosis given its noninvasive and reproducible nature
  - The aorta and each renal artery are evaluated segmentally through the level of the kidney parenchyma in a fasting state[15]
- Criteria for a hemodynamically significant renal artery stenosis (>60%) can vary by laboratory but peak systolic velocity (PSV) criteria of >180 cm/s in the main renal artery or renal artery to aortic PSV ratio (RAR) of >3.5 are common thresholds[15]
- The resistive index (RI) measured as $(PSV - EDV)/PSV$ helps to identify intrinsic renal disease with normal values <0.8,[16] where EDV is end-diastolic velocity

Cross-sectional imaging with computed tomographic angiography (CTA) or magnetic resonance angiography (MRA) is highly accurate and detailed. The consequences of gadolinium contrast for MRA in patients with estimated GFR (eGFR) <30 mL/min as well as the radiation and contrast required for CTA should be taken into account when ordering[17]

- Nuclear medicine studies such as ACE inhibitor renography are utilized to help distinguish renovascular and essential HTN[18]

TREATMENT

- Medical treatment is the mainstay of treatment for atherosclerotic renal artery stenosis. However, there remain several important clinical scenarios to recognize and intervene
- Severe HTN refractory to medical management with three or more agents including a diuretic, ischemic nephropathy, or significant decline in eGFR <45 mL/min in the setting of bilateral renal artery stenosis or solitary kidney, or cardiac disturbance syndromes such as flash pulmonary edema or acute coronary syndrome with severe HTN[19]
- A lower threshold for treatment is also appropriate for children with renovascular HTN and in the setting of fibromuscular dysplasia (FMD) with unsatisfactory control of HTN as the results often offer significant improvement[11]
- Acute renal vein thrombosis is extremely rare in adults but can lead to resultant renal ischemia. Treatment is anticoagulation with thrombectomy or thrombolysis reserved for propagation despite anticoagulation, thrombosis of a solitary kidney or bilateral kidneys, renal failure, or refractory severe symptoms[14]

Medical

- Smoking cessation and risk factor modification along with aspirin and statin unless a specific contraindication exists[20]

- Treatment of HTN including ACE inhibitors or angiotensin receptor blockers (ARBs) given the pathophysiology as well as thiazide diuretics, calcium channel blockers, or beta blockers are first-line therapies. Patients often require multiple agents[21]
- Target blood pressure is 140/90 mm Hg in nondiabetic patients, 130/80 mm Hg if diabetes or renal insufficiency[21]

Open

- Appropriate in younger patients of suitable risk and when anatomic limitations to a durable result for endovascular therapy exist[22]
- Preferred methods are direct repair with aortorenal bypass, endarterectomy, or reimplantation
- There are also indirect repair options of splanchnic-renal bypass such as the hepatorenal or splenorenal bypass
- Ex vivo reconstruction is appropriate in reconstructions that require complex branch exposure or reconstruction[22]
- Bypass conduit options include autologous saphenous vein, autologous hypogastric artery, which is preferred in children, and synthetic grafts[22]
- Endarterectomy is suitable for classic ostial disease as well as in patients with concomitant mesenteric disease and a large coral reef plaque
  - This is approached through a larger trap door endarterectomy in the aorta after sufficient mobilization of branch vessels to effectively evert the plaque[23]
- Large open series generally report an 85% curative or improved blood pressure response, with nearly two thirds of patients demonstrating an improvement in renal function[24]

Endovascular

- Several randomized clinical control trials demonstrate a lack of evidence for revascularization when compared to best medical therapy. This has resulted in the stringent criteria to offer intervention
- In appropriately selected patients, primary angioplasty is the recommended endovascular management for FMD
- Primary endoluminal stenting is the recommended management for ostial atherosclerotic disease[25]
- In patients with bilateral renal artery stenosis, start with percutaneous transluminal angioplasty (PTA) and stenting of the most severe side. If HTN does not resolve, then can come back to stent the contralateral side
  - Balloon expandable stent is preferred
    - More radial force
    - More accurate deployment
    - ~0.5 cm of stent into the aorta to treat the ostial portion of the lesion

Clinical Trials

CORAL Trial

- 947 participants with atherosclerotic renal artery stenosis, systolic HTN on two or more agents, or chronic kidney disease randomized to medical therapy or renal artery stenting plus medical therapy followed for adverse cardiovascular or renal events[26]
- Median follow-up of 43 months did not demonstrate any significant difference between the treatment groups[26]

ASTRAL Trial

- 806 participants randomized to medical therapy or medical therapy plus revascularization followed up for primary outcome of renal function and secondary outcomes of blood pressure and adverse cardiovascular events and mortality[27]
- Median follow-up of 36 months did not demonstrate significant differences between the groups, but it was noted 23 patients had complications related to their interventions[27]

STAR Trial

- 140 patients with creatinine clearance less than 80 mL/min randomized to stent and medical treatment or medical treatment only followed up for primary endpoint of 20% or greater decrease in creatinine clearance and secondary endpoints of cardiovascular morbidity and mortality[28]
- During 2-year follow-up, no significant differences were seen in the primary endpoint; however, there were several serious procedural complications in the stent group[28]

RADAR Trial

- Viewing the inclusion criteria of the above trials as liberal, sought to enroll 300 patients but was terminated after enrolling 86 patients and demonstrating no difference[29]
- Randomized trials in angioplasty and stenting of the renal artery: tabular review of the literature and critical analysis of their results[30]
  - Review of all the literature on renal artery stenting
  - Explains the flaws and biases seen in the above trials
  - PTA alone has a 50% restenosis rate at 3 months. This is why stenting is recommended
  - Pooled data of endovascular revascularization compared with open surgical revascularization demonstrate an improved outcome with open repair in long-term renal function and management in HTN
  - Finding the optimal patient with a potentially reversible renovascular etiology for HTN and renal dysfunction continues to be elusive

COMPLICATIONS

- Postoperative stenosis or thrombosis rates in large open series are reported as 3%–4%, suggesting excellent patency outcomes[31]
- Mortality in isolated open renal arterial interventions in experienced centers is less than 2%, but rises when combined with aortic repair and visceral repairs[31]
- Endovascular complications include bleeding, access complications, dissection, contrast nephropathy as well as restenosis and thrombosis[25]

POSTOPERATIVE FOLLOW-UP

- Treated patients require lifelong surveillance with duplex ultrasound to evaluate for patency of intervention and restenosis
- Blood pressure and renal function should be closely monitored and considered in concert with evidence of anatomic recurrence
- Restenosis is often treated by endovascular means[32]

REFERENCES

1. Hansen KJ, Edwards MS, Craven TE, et al. Prevalence of renovascular disease in the elderly: a population-based study. *J Vasc Surg.* 2002;36(3):443-451.
2. Miralles M, Corominas A, Cotillas J, Castro F, Clara A, Vidal-Barraquer F. Screening for carotid and renal artery stenoses in patients with aortoiliac disease. *Ann Vasc Surg.* 1998;12(1):17-22.
3. Jean WJ, al-Bitar I, Zwicke DL, Port SC, Schmidt DH, Bajwa TK. High incidence of renal artery stenosis in patients with coronary artery disease. *Cathet Cardiovasc Diagn.* 1994;32(1):8-10.
4. Wu YW, Lin MS, Lin YH, Chao CL, Kao HL. Prevalence of concomitant atherosclerotic arterial diseases in patients with significant cervical carotid artery stenosis in Taiwan. *Int J Cardiovasc Imaging.* 2007;23(4):433-439.
5. Schwartz CJ, White TA. Stenosis of renal artery: an unselected necropsy study. *Br Med J.* 1964;2(5422):1415-1421.
6. Lawson JD, Boerth R, Foster JH, Dean RH. Diagnosis and management of renovascular hypertension in children. *Arch Surg.* 1977;112(11):1307-1316.
7. Textor SC. Pathophysiology of renal failure in renovascular disease. *Am J Kidney Dis.* 1994;24(4):642-651.
8. Tobian L. Relationship of juxtaglomerular apparatus to renin and angiotensin. *Circulation.* 1962;25:189-192.
9. Kobori H, Nangaku M, Navar LG, Nishiyama A. The intrarenal renin-angiotensin system: from physiology to the pathobiology of hypertension and kidney disease. *Pharmacol Rev.* 2007;59(3):251-287.
10. Williams GH. Aldosterone biosynthesis, regulation, and classical mechanism of action. *Heart Fail Rev.* 2005;10(1):7-13.
11. Rickey AK, Geary RL. Chapter 125: Renovascular disease: pathophysiology, epidemiology, clinical presentation, and medical management. In: Sidaway AN, Perler BA, eds. *Rutherford's Vascular Surgery.* 9th ed. Saunders/Elsevier; 2019:1663-1674.
12. Ruchin PE, Baron DW, Wilson SH, Boland J, Muller DW, Roy PR. Long-term follow-up of renal artery stenting in an Australian population. *Heart Lung Circ.* 2007;16(2):79-84.
13. Avgerinos E, Schneider PA, Chaer RA. Chapter 142: Fibromuscular dysplasia. In: Sidaway AN, Perler BA, eds. *Rutherford's Vascular Surgery.* 9th ed. Philadelphia, PA: Saunders/Elsevier; 2019:1870-1890.
14. Velazquez-Ramirez G, Corriere MA. Chapter 129: Renovascular disease: acute occlusive and ischemic events. In: Sidaway AN, Perler BA, eds. *Rutherford's Vascular Surgery.* 9th ed. Saunders/Elsevier; 2019:1704-1713.
15. Motew SJ, Cherr GS, Craven TE, Travis JA, Wong JM, Reavis SW, Hansen KJ. Renal duplex sonography: main renal artery versus hilar analysis. *J Vasc Surg.* 2000;32(3):462-469; 469-471.
16. Radermacher J, Chavan A, Schäffer J, et al. Detection of significant renal artery stenosis with color Doppler sonography: combining extrarenal and intrarenal approaches to minimize technical failure. *Clin Nephrol.* 2000;53(5):333-343.
17. Wagner B, Drel V, Gorin Y. Pathophysiology of gadolinium-associated systemic fibrosis. *Am J Physiol Renal Physiol.* 2016;311(1):F1-F11.
18. Geyskes GG, de Bruyn AJ. Captopril renography and the effect of percutaneous transluminal angioplasty on blood pressure in 94 patients with renal artery stenosis. *Am J Hypertens.* 1991;4(12 Pt 2):685S-689S.
19. Textor SC, McKusick MM. Renal artery stenosis: if and when to intervene. *Curr Opin Nephrol Hypertens.* 2016;25(2):144-151.
20. Anderson JL, Halperin JL, Albert NM, et al. Management of patients with peripheral artery disease (compilation of 2005 and 2011 ACCF/AHA guideline recommendations): a report of the American College of Cardiology Foundation/American Heart Association Task Force on Practice Guidelines. *Circulation.* 2013;127(13):1425-1443.
21. James PA, Oparil S, Carter BL, et al. 2014 evidence-based guideline for the management of high blood pressure in adults: report from the panel members appointed to the Eighth Joint National Committee (JNC 8). *JAMA.* 2014;311(5):507-520.
22. Benjamin ME, Hansen KJ. Chapter 126: Renovascular disease: open surgical treatment. In: Sidaway AN, Perler BA, eds. *Rutherford's Vascular Surgery.* 9th ed. Philadelphia, PA: Saunders/Elsevier; 2019:1675-1686.
23. DeRubertis BG, Jabori SO, Quinones-Baldrich W, Lawrence PF. Retroperitoneal trapdoor endarterectomy for paravisceral "coral-reef" aortic plaque. *Vasc Endovascular Surg.* 2012;46(6):487-491.
24. Cherr GS, Hansen KJ, Craven TE, et al. Surgical management of atherosclerotic renovascular disease. *J Vasc Surg.* 2002;35(2):236-245.
25. Edwards, MS, Cooper CJ. Chapter 127: Renovascular disease: endovascular treatment. In: Sidaway AN, Perler BA, eds. *Rutherford's Vascular Surgery.* 9th ed. Philadelphia, PA: Saunders/Elsevier; 2019:1687-1695.
26. Cooper CJ, Murphy TP, Cutlip DE, et al; CORAL Investigators. Stenting and medical therapy for atherosclerotic renal-artery stenosis. *N Engl J Med.* 2014;370(1):13-22.

27. ASTRAL Investigators, Wheatley K, Ives N, Gray R, et al. Revascularization versus medical therapy for renal-artery stenosis. *N Engl J Med.* 2009;361(20):1953-1962.

28. Bax L, Woittiez AJ, Kouwenberg HJ, et al. Stent placement in patients with atherosclerotic renal artery stenosis and impaired renal function: a randomized trial. *Ann Intern Med.* 2009; 150(12):840-848, W150-W151.

29. Zeller T, Krankenberg H, Erglis A, et al.; RADAR Investigators. A randomized, multi-center, prospective study comparing best medical treatment versus best medical treatment plus renal artery stenting in patients with hemodynamically relevant atherosclerotic renal artery stenosis (RADAR) - one-year results of a pre-maturely terminated study. *Trials.* 2017;18(1):380.

30. Escobar GA, Campbell DN. Randomized trials in angioplasty and stenting of the renal artery: tabular review of the literature and critical analysis of their results. *Ann Vasc Surg.* 2012;26(3): 434-442.

31. Benjamin ME, Hansen KJ, Craven TE, et al. Combined aortic and renal artery surgery. A contemporary experience. *Ann Surg.* 1996;223(5):555-565; discussion 565-567.

32. Davies MG, Saad WA, Bismuth JX, Peden EK, Naoum JJ, Lumsden AB. Outcomes of endoluminal reintervention for restenosis after percutaneous renal angioplasty and stenting. *J Vasc Surg.* 2009;49(4):946-952.

CHAPTER 20

Mesenteric Ischemia

KRISHNA MARTINEZ-SINGH, MD, and KARTHIKESHWAR KASIRAJAN, MD

INTRODUCTION

- **Mesenteric ischemia:** occurs when metabolic demands of the intestines are not met due to a decrease in blood flow to the mesenteric circulation
- Two types: *acute* and *chronic*
- Acute mesenteric ischemia is from four different etiologies:
  - Arterial embolism
  - Arterial thrombosis
  - Nonocclusive mesenteric ischemia
  - Mesenteric venous thrombosis

ACUTE MESENTERIC ISCHEMIA DUE TO ARTERIAL EMBOLISM OR THROMBOSIS

Incidence: acute mesenteric ischemia is relatively rare and accounts for only 0.1% of hospital admissions.

Etiology

- **Risk factors** for atherosclerosis are often the underlying etiology for the occlusion
  - Advanced age, smoking, hypertension, hyperlipidemia, diabetes, chronic renal failure, and cardiac disease
- **Embolic occlusion:** often a thrombotic cardiac source due to cardiac arrhythmias (atrial fibrillation), prosthetic valves, ventricular aneurysms, prior myocardial infarction, or other valvular disorders
- Embolism is the most common etiology (50%), followed by in situ thrombosis in underlying atherosclerotic lesions (25%), followed by other less common etiologies (vasculitis, dissection, and aneurysms)

Presentation

- **Early:** benign abdominal examination (pain out of proportion to examination)
  - Presenting symptoms: vomiting, diarrhea, and hematochezia
  - Many patients may have a classic triad of *pain*, *bowel emptying* (vomiting/diarrhea), and *embolic source* (atrial fibrillation)
- **Late:** acute abdomen
  - Tenderness, guarding, and rebound are often late findings indicating transmural bowel infarct with a worse prognosis

Diagnosis

A high index of clinical suspicion is vital for the prompt diagnosis of acute mesenteric ischemia

- **Laboratory markers:** elevated leukocyte count, lactic acid, D-dimer, and base excess are helpful indicators but are not highly sensitive or specific
- **Radiographic diagnosis:** the most commonly used and reliable test is computed tomogram angiography (CTA)
  - Highly sensitive (94%) and specific (95%)
  - **Findings:** arterial occlusion, signs of bowel ischemia (bowel wall thickening and/or enhancement, ascites, portal venous gas), or perforation (free air)
- **Superior mesenteric artery (SMA):** most prone to embolic occlusion due to the large diameter and acute angle of origin

Management

- **Immediate resuscitation** is key to improved outcomes
  - Tissue perfusion should be maximized immediately with adequate *fluid resuscitation and supplemental oxygen*
  - Prioritize volume resuscitation over use of vasopressors
- **Broad-spectrum antibiotics** should be administered to counteract bacterial translocation from the compromised mucosal barrier
- **Anticoagulation** with unfractionated heparin should be initiated once imaging studies confirm the diagnosis

- **Endovascular management**: in the absence of clinical or imaging signs of bowel ischemia endovascular therapy is gaining popularity, especially for patients who are elderly and fragile. While not shown superior survival vs. open and 1/3 still require bowel resection, endo does offer some benefits and can involve:
  - Percutaneous techniques include thrombolysis, percutaneous mechanical thrombectomy, and balloon angioplasty with or without stenting
  - In a review consisting of 28 articles and 1110 patients comparing open surgical versus endovascular techniques for the management of acute mesenteric ischemia, outcomes were superior for the endovascular group. The endovascular group had lower cardiac/pulmonary complications, wound infection, and multisystem organ failure
  - In another study of 679 patients, the endovascular group had shorter length of stay (12.9 vs. 17.1 days), lower mortality (24.9% vs. 39.3%), and less need for bowel resection (14.4% vs. 33.4%)
- **Open management**: in the presence of bowel ischemia, laparotomy with damage control surgery is mandatory for survival. Open treatment has a similar survival and allows for concomitant open exploration/resection of bowel
  - In patients undergoing laparotomy, *open surgical thrombectomy/embolectomy* may also be performed
  - **Mesenteric bypass** may be required in patients with acute in situ thrombosis from underlying atherosclerotic lesions
  - **Retrograde percutaneous techniques** of the exposed vessels have also been performed with good outcomes (retrograde open mesenteric stenting)
  - **Initial revascularization** is recommended before bowel resection to minimize loss of bowel
  - **Damage control** involves resection of frankly nonviable bowel and leaving the abdomen open for a second look in the first 48 hours (Figs. 20.1 and 20.2)
    - Short bowel syndrome can occur when less than 200 cm of small bowel is spared, requiring the use of long-term total parenteral nutrition

  Predictors of mortality: advanced age, renal failure, associated organ failure, and presence and length of bowel necrosis were all independent predictors of mortality.
- Plasma lactate level of >*2.7 mmol/L* at initial presentation was also an independent predictor of mortality
- Most studies continue to reveal a high mortality in patients presenting with acute mesenteric ischemia, often exceeding 60% in the first 30 days

CHRONIC MESENTERIC ISCHEMIA

Due to the abundant collateral flow between vessels supplying the foregut (celiac axis), midgut (SMA), and the hindgut (inferior mesenteric artery and internal iliac arteries),

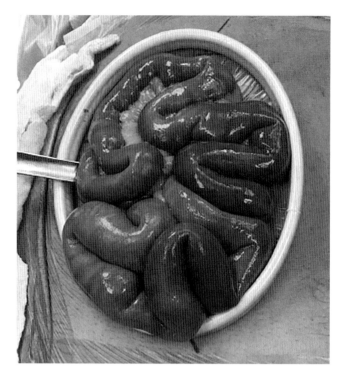

FIG. 20.1   Ischemic bowel on laparotomy prior to revascularization.

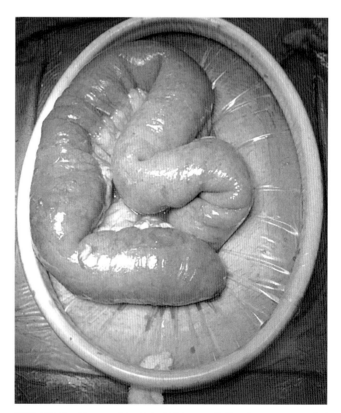

FIG. 20.2   Second look in 24 hours following successful endovascular revascularization.

patients may not have symptoms until at least two of the major vessels have significant stenosis (>70%) or occlusion. The small intestines can tolerate up to a 75% overall reduction in blood flow with minimal symptoms.

Incidence: accounts for fewer than 1 in 1000 hospital admissions for abdominal pain.
- Strong female predominance with typical atherosclerotic risk factors

Etiology

- Significant associated *cardiovascular risk factors,* such as hyperlipidemia, hypertension, renal failure, and diabetes, resulting in *atherosclerosis* and subsequent stenosis of the mesenteric vessels
- Most patients are elderly and are smokers
- Prior myocardial infarction, coronary stents, peripheral arterial disease, or strokes are also frequent comorbidities
- Less frequent causes include vasculitis, fibromuscular dysplasia, and radiation

Presentation

Most patients have a long history of *postprandial abdominal pain, weight loss,* and *"food fear."*
- Many experience early satiety, bloating, diarrhea, nausea, and vomiting after eating
- Some may not complain of typical postprandial pain, as they have learned to eat small meals to avoid abdominal discomfort
- Patients with significant atherosclerotic risk factors, especially with prior cardiac or peripheral arterial procedures, who appear cachectic should have imaging studies to rule out mesenteric occlusive disease

Diagnosis

A high index of suspicion is required for early diagnosis
- Initial diagnosis can often be made with a *duplex ultrasound*
  - High sensitivity (72%–100%) and specificity (94%–98%) when diagnosing SMA stenosis of >70%
  - **Duplex criteria**:
    - *Celiac:* peak systolic velocity (PSV) >200 cm/s, end-diastolic velocity (EDV) >55 cm/s; reversed hepatic/splenic arterial flow
    - *SMA:* PSV >275 cm/s, EDV >45 cm/s
- **CTA** to confirm the diagnosis
  - CTA is considered the gold standard
  - Diagnosis is straightforward when clinical symptoms correlate with *multivessel* disease
  - When *single-vessel* disease is present, other causes for abdominal pain will need to be ruled out, often requiring an upper endoscopy and colonoscopy

Treatment

Revascularization is required to eliminate or decrease symptoms and to prevent the development of acute mesenteric ischemia that is highly fatal.
- **Endovascular therapy:** largely replaced open surgical techniques as the preferred method for revascularization in most centers around the country (Figs. 20.3 and 20.4)
  - *Covered stents* are being used with increasing frequency compared with bare metal stents as they are associated with a lower rate of restenosis
  - In a recent study involving 225 patients (197 vessels with bare metal stents and 67 vessels with covered stents), covered stents were associated with lower rates of restenosis, symptom recurrence, and reintervention
    - Contraindicated if jejunal branches or middle colic covered. SVS guidelines also recommend covered stents as first line
- **Open revascularization:** antegrade or retrograde bypass using synthetic conduits
  - *Retrograde bypass:* typically from the right common iliac artery (inflow) to the SMA. This allows for the fastest open bypass (easy access to inflow and outflow). Must have a "lazy S" configuration when created off the left iliac and a "lazy C" from the right to avoid kinking/occlusion
  - *Antegrade bypass:* supraceliac aorta (inflow) to the celiac and SMA using a bifurcated graft. Compared to retrograde, has shorter trajectory (and presumably

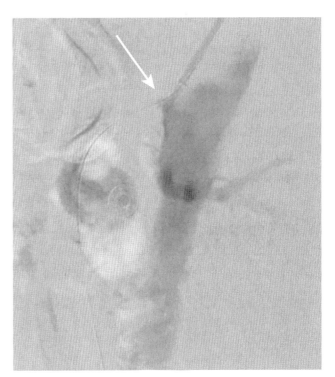

FIG. 20.3 Acute-on-chronic occlusion of superior mesenteric artery. *Arrow* points to stump of superior mesenteric artery with wire across the occlusion.

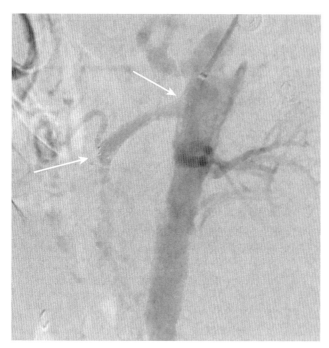

FIG. 20.4   Recanalization of occluded superior mesenteric artery with stent and angioplasty.

better patency by being antegrade), "hides" the inflow/outflow for cases of intraperitoneal spillage, and the exposure takes longer
- Celiac limb can be placed at the axis or the common hepatic artery
- The SMA limb may be tunneled retropancreatic to land on the proximal SMA, or through the mesocolon to land on the mid-distal SMA
  - Mesenteric endarterectomy is done via trapdoor aortotomy, usually via retroperitoneal approach. Especially good for coral-reef aortas where the aorta also has calcific stenosis
- In a metaanalysis comparing endovascular (209 patients) with open surgical techniques (360 patients), the endovascular group had a lower in-hospital complication rate but a higher recurrence at 3 years

ACUTE MESENTERIC VENOUS THROMBOSIS

Incidence: due to its rarity, knowledge surrounding true incidence and prevalence is limited.
- In a recent study from Italy the overall incidence was 3.8 per 100,000 in males and 1.7 per 100,000 in females. It accounts for about 5%–10% of all cases of mesenteric ischemia

Etiology

- **Cirrhosis:** in patients with cirrhosis, a systemic hypercoagulable condition is often present

- Other local factors that may be present include *malignancy, intraabdominal infection, trauma,* or *surgery* (splenectomy)

Presentation

Mild to severe abdominal pain and fever
- Pain out of proportion to physical findings
- **Poor prognostic indicators:** clinical signs of peritonitis, elevated lactic acid and white blood cell count, imaging evidence of ascites, ischemic bowel, and extension of thrombus into superior mesenteric vein or smaller tributaries

Diagnosis

Multiphasic abdominal computed tomography venogram (CTV) is currently the gold standard in evaluating the portal-venous mesenteric system.
- Can identify ischemic bowel, cirrhosis, or hepatocellular carcinoma that may be associated with acute portal vein thrombosis
- Oral contrast often obscures vasculature and is best avoided
- Magnetic resonance imaging is also gaining popularity due to absence of radiation and greater sensitivity in detecting malignancy
- Ultrasound with Doppler is commonly used for follow-up imaging
  - Sensitivity of 89%–93% and specificity of 92%–99%
  - Obesity, ascites, bowel gas, and operator experience may limit accuracy

Treatment

Goal of treatment is to prevent thrombus propagation, promote recanalization, and avoid bowel ischemia.
- **Anticoagulation** remains the cornerstone of therapy and should be initiated on diagnosis
  - Initial therapy with low-molecular-weight heparin (LMWH) or unfractionated heparin is preferred
- If and when clinical and laboratory markers improve and patient can tolerate oral intake, oral anticoagulation is recommended
  - Recent data on use of direct oral anticoagulants (DOACs) in noncirrhotic acute mesenteric venous thrombosis are promising
  - A minimum treatment duration of 6 months is recommended
  - Complete recanalization with anticoagulation is noted in 40%–45% of patients
- **Surgical intervention:** indicated with worsening clinical examination, laboratory, or imaging studies
  - *Endovascular therapy:* percutaneous access to the mesenteric and portal veins is most commonly obtained

via transjugular intrahepatic portal shunt (TIPS) or via direct hepatic or transsplenic approaches

- Lytic agents or mechanical thrombectomy devices can be used for thrombus removal
- *Open surgical therapy:* bowel resection is indicated for cases of venous gangrene with subsequent bowel ischemia. Also, provides direct access to the mesenteric vessels or portal vein
- Patients with no cirrhosis or underlying malignancy should also have an extensive hypercoagulable workup after the acute phase

NONOCCLUSIVE MESENTERIC ISCHEMIA (NOMI)

Incidence: accounts for ~20% of all cases of mesenteric ischemia.

Etiology: seen in critically ill patients with *low cardiac output* with prolonged intestinal vasoconstriction.
- Patients are frequently in shock with multisystem organ failure and on vasopressors

Diagnosis

Diagnosis is often challenging as patients are frequently sedated and on a ventilator.
- **Indicators of NOMI:** abdominal distention, undiagnosed sepsis, and progressive lactic acidosis
- **CTA** is often the diagnostic imaging of choice, as other causes for abdominal sepsis would need to be excluded at the same time
  - CTA findings would not typically demonstrate a frank obstruction but irregularities of intestinal branches of the SMA suggestive of spasm and impaired filling of the intramural vessels

Treatment

Primary therapy is to *address the underlying medical condition* causing the low flow state and discontinuing vasopressors if possible.
- Catheter-directed infusion of vasodilators directly into the SMA has demonstrated some benefit in patients who can tolerate it
  - Commonly used agents: prostaglandin E_1 (alprostadil), papaverine, and nitroglycerin

MEDIAN ARCUATE LIGAMENT SYNDROME

Incidence: true incidence and prevalence of this condition is unknown.
- More common in females (4:1) and ages 30–50 years

Etiology

Clinical syndrome associated with compression of the celiac artery by the median arcuate ligament (MAL).
- **MAL:** fibrous band that bridges diaphragmatic crura
- Celiac artery compression *increases* with expiration, resulting in intestinal ischemia
- Irritation of celiac plexus can also be a source of symptoms—affects antral motility
- The true etiology and the syndrome itself remain a subject of debate

Presentation

Abdominal pain, vomiting, weight loss, and postprandial or exercise-induced abdominal pain and abdominal bruit that amplifies with expiration

Diagnosis

Typically a diagnosis of exclusion; all imaging studies should be performed on inspiration and expiration.
- **Duplex ultrasound** is the first-line recommended study
  - One study concluded that a deflection angle >50 degrees and expiratory PSV of >350 cm/s are associated with an 83% sensitivity, 100% sensitivity, and 100% positive predictive value for diagnosis of median arcuate ligament syndrome (MALS)
- **CTA** may be used to aid in diagnosis
  - Focal narrowing of proximal celiac artery with characteristic "hooked" appearance (differentiates from atherosclerosis)
- **Dynamic angiography,** historically, is considered the gold standard of diagnosis (>50% stenosis of the celiac artery)
- **Gastric exercise tonometry (GET):** measures partial pressure of carbon dioxide from anaerobic respiration
  - Positive study is 76% sensitive and 92% specific for diagnosis of intestinal ischemia
- Positive response to celiac plexus block may predict good response to surgical decompression and celiac ganglionectomy

Treatment

- **Endovascular therapy:** angioplasty or stenting is *contraindicated*; stents will be subject to extrinsic forces and may fracture or thrombose
- **Open surgical management:** mainstay of therapy; involves release of the MAL with decompression of the celiac artery and wide ganglionectomy
  - *Laparoscopic* or *robotic* options
  - Persistent stenosis following decompression can be treated with aortoceliac bypass or celiac patch angioplasty

SUGGESTED READINGS

Beaulieu RJ, Arnaoutakis KD, Abularrage CJ, Efron DT, Schneider E, Black JH III. Comparison of open and endovascular treatment of acute mesenteric ischemia. *J Vasc Surg.* 2014;59(1):159-164.

Cai W, Li X, Shu C, et al. Comparison of clinical outcomes of endovascular versus open revascularization for chronic mesenteric ischemia: a meta-analysis. *Ann Vasc Surg.* 2015;29(5):934-940.

Goodall R, Langridge B, Onida S, Ellis M, Lane T, Davies AH. Median arcuate ligament syndrome. *J Vasc Surg.* 2020;71(6):2170-2176.

Oderich GS, Erdoes LS, Lesar C, et al. Comparison of covered stents versus bare metal stents for treatment of chronic atherosclerotic mesenteric arterial disease. *J Vasc Surg.* 2013;58(5):1316-1323.

Zhao Y, Yin H, Yao C, et al. Management of acute mesenteric ischemia: a critical review and treatment algorithm. *Vasc Endovascular Surg.* 2016;50(3):183-192.

CHAPTER 21

Vascular Access

VICTORIA J TEODORESCU, MD, MBA, RVT, and KARTHIK BHAT, MD

ACCESS CREATION

Initiation of Hemodialysis

- Patients with advanced renal disease should ideally be under the care of a nephrologist and will be educated in all modalities of renal replacement therapy once estimated glomerular filtration rate (eGFR) reaches 30 mL/min/1.73^2
- If the patient chooses hemodialysis (HD), evaluation of vascular anatomy is undertaken in order to identify an appropriate vein for an arteriovenous fistula (AVF)
  - The vein then should be protected with no intravenous (IV) lines and limited phlebotomy in that arm. If possible, a vein in the nondominant arm is preferred
- Placement of AVF will ideally occur prior to the initiation of dialysis to allow a sufficient amount of time so that the fistula may mature
  - Referral to the surgeon for AVF should be made when eGFR falls to 15–20 mL/min/1.73^2
- Evaluation prior to access creation includes a detailed history and physical examination
- Performance of a complete pulse examination is necessary as well as blood pressure measurements of both upper extremities
  - A pressure difference >20 mm Hg between the two arms indicates there may be significant subclavian or axillary artery disease
  - Performing an Allen test may be helpful, especially if the patient is at risk of steal. The radial artery is now commonly used as access for endovascular procedures and careful lookout for radial artery occlusion must be undertaken
- Preoperative ultrasound (vessel mapping) is helpful when:
  - No suitable veins are visualized on physical examination
  - There is a history of peripherally inserted central catheter (PICC) line insertion, IV drug abuse, or other vascular trauma

- There is a history of failed access
- Suspected central venous disease
- Mapping includes evaluation of bilateral cephalic and basilic veins for patency and diameter measurements and assessment of deep veins for outflow disease and of arteries including B-mode and Doppler evaluation
- The Kidney Disease Outcomes Quality Initiative (KDOQI) recommends a lifelong plan for access be developed which will be regularly reviewed and updated as necessary
  - Vessel identification and preservation
  - Access creation
  - Contingency plans for access dysfunction and succession or what to do when the access fails
- If the patient's veins are deemed not suitable by preoperative evaluation, then an AV graft should be placed
  - Grafts should be placed in chronic kidney disease (CKD) patients only if it is going to be used within 4–6 weeks
  - Grafts may develop intimal hyperplasia that results in dysfunction

Other Indications for Access Creation

- Failed or failing kidney transplant, transitioning from peritoneal dialysis (PD) because of recurrent infection, membrane failure or other reasons, failed or failing HD access, and presence of a tunneled central venous catheter (CVC) in those patients deemed suitable for AV access
- The use of a tunneled catheter should be avoided or shortened if at all possible
  - A catheter may be acceptable as sole access for the long term in patients with limited life expectancy, no feasible access sites, or where AV access would severely impair the patient's quality of life

Short-Term Use of Tunneled Catheters Is Appropriate When There Is:

- Injury or other limited access; difficulty occurs that is expected to resolve
- Need to initiate dialysis prior to maturation of AVF or healing of AV graft

- Short-term switch from PD to HD with expectation that patient will return to PD
- Temporary need for HD while waiting for a renal transplant to recover
- Need for dialysis before living-related kidney transplant can occur

Types of AV Access

- AVF is the preferred access, if it can be created, as it has fewer long-term complications such as thrombosis or infection and is less likely to require interventions to maintain function
- Careful evaluation must be undertaken prior to creating the fistula as a significant number fail to mature or require assistance in achieving functionality
  - The 2020 United States Renal Data System (USRDS) annual report found about 80% initiate dialysis with a tunneled catheter in 2018, relatively unchanged over the past decade, although 14.1% had maturing fistulas in addition. Of those patients who initiated HD in 2017 with a catheter, nearly 65% were using an AVF 18 months after HD initiation
- In the absence of suitable vessels, an alternative conduit is required. This is commonly an expanded polytetrafluoroethylene (ePTFE) graft, but may also include biological grafts such as the bovine carotid artery and other bioengineered grafts currently under investigation
- Early cannulation or "quick-stick" grafts allow safe use in the early postoperative period. Placement of this graft avoids use of a CVC
- The hemodialysis reliable outflow (HeRO) graft combines an ePTFE graft with a CVC, all subcutaneous. There is no venous anastomosis as the graft is connected directly to the catheter. This is intended for use in patients with central venous stenosis (CVS) or occlusion

Graft Configurations

- As the patient may require several access placements over the course of their lifetime, location of the first access is important because its failure may impact the feasibility of placing another access in that extremity
- If an AVF cannot be placed, creating a forearm loop graft may allow for placement of a subsequent upper-arm fistula if the outflow veins mature
- It is imperative that there is sufficient length of conduit superficial enough to easily cannulate to allow for adequate separation of needles and rotation of cannulation sites
  The access must be placed in an area easily exposed without discomfort due to patient's limited range of motion or other reasons.

One- Versus Two-Stage Basilic Vein Transposition

- Because of its depth and surrounding anatomy, the basilic vein usually requires transposition so that it can be easily cannulated
  - Creation of this type of fistula is accomplished in one or two stages
  - Advantages of the one-stage procedure include (1) the patient undergoes one surgery rather than two, which may significantly reduce the time that a catheter is in place and (2) dissection of the basilic vein, which may be lengthy, is accomplished before the vein is arterialized, possibly reducing blood loss
  - The main disadvantage, of course, is extensive surgery to create a fistula that may not mature
  - The basilic-brachial anastomosis is performed as the first step and the vein is superficialized only if the fistula has sufficiently matured

Fistula Versus Graft Trials

- Traditional teaching has been that AVFs are superior to prosthetic grafts for HD
  - Retrospective review of patients initiating dialysis with AVF (16%), arteriovenous graft (AVG) (3%), catheter plus fistula (7%), catheter plus graft (7%), and catheter only (52%)
  - In this study, temporizing catheter use was associated with higher mortality, higher infection, and lower patency of the access
  - AVF was associated with longer time of catheter-free dialysis, a better patency, and lower infection and lower mortality compared with prosthetic grafts
    - Many studies, however, may have been biased as they did not include the known significant rate of maturation failure (20%–60%) as a complication of AVF
    - Small number of randomized controlled trials (RCTs) evaluating fistula versus graft have indicated that grafts may be superior in sicker patients with poor vessels, which has led to the emphasis on careful preoperative analysis so that the "right" access is placed for each patient

Cannulation

- Maturation may be determined by physical examination at 4–6 weeks following creation
- The fistula should be visibly enlarged with a palpable thrill at the arterial anastomosis
- When the arm is raised above the level of the heart, a fistula with adequate venous outflow will flatten or collapse, depending on its location in the arm

- Pulse augmentation test is used to determine whether arterial inflow is adequate
- Duplex ultrasound evaluation may be obtained if the physical examination is unclear. Minimum duplex criteria for maturity include diameter of 4–5 mm and blood flow of 400–500 mL/min

ACCESS COMPLICATIONS AND TREATMENT

AV access complications may generally be divided into three categories:
- Thrombotic flow-related complications
- Nonthrombotic flow-related complications
  - Aneurysm or pseudoaneurysm
  - High-output heart failure
  - Steal syndrome
  - Ischemic myeloneuropathy
  - Noninfectious fluid collections
- Infectious complications

Thrombotic Flow-Related Complications

- Thrombosis is the most common reason for autogenous and prosthetic access failure
- Causes of thrombosis include
  - Poor venous conduit (<2.5 mm in diameter)
  - Venous stenosis (central or peripheral)
  - Myointimal hyperplasia at venous anastomosis in AVGs
  - Endothelial injury
  - Hypercoagulability
  Early access thrombosis should prompt investigation of arterial inflow, venous outflow, and technical failure at the anastomoses.
- Development of stenosis is the most common complication following access creation and can lead to AVF nonmaturation or AVF/AVG thrombosis
- Surveillance for access dysfunction is primarily based on physical examination by an experienced observer as treatment of stenosis in the absence of clinical findings does not improve access patency
- Clinical findings that suggest significant stenosis include
  - Reduced dialysis clearance
  - High venous or arterial pressures detected while on dialysis
  - Prolonged bleeding following removal of needles
  - Extremity edema
  - Paired thrill or pulsatility
  - Both AVF and AVG stenoses may be treated successfully with angioplasty alone. For better 6-month outcomes, placement of a self-expanding stent graft is suggested for
    - Recurrent venous anastomotic stenoses in AVG
    - In-stent restenosis for both AVG and AVF

- Treatment of a ruptured vein for either AVG or AVF
- Percutaneous thrombectomy can salvage the access in the short run, but long-term patency remains poor for both AVF and AVG
- Open surgical thrombectomy may be more favorable for recurrent lesions and where outcomes for endovascular treatments are poor, such as cephalic arch stenoses
- CVS threatens current and future accesses on that arm
  - Most common cause is a history CVC for dialysis and even pacer leads
  - Long duration of a catheter increases the risk of CVS but even catheters in place for less than a month can cause CVS
    - Presumed etiology is neointimal hyperplasia. CVS is also found in patients without a history of a CVC
  - Clinical symptomatology is the hallmark of diagnosis
    - Typical presentation is swelling, tenderness, and pain. Severe cases may cause cyanosis, or ulceration
  - Diagnosis and treatment include venogram with angioplasty and possibly stenting. Open surgical options include rib resection, venous turndown, and bypass

Nonthrombotic Flow-Related Complications: Aneurysm or Pseudoaneurysm

- An aneurysm is the pathological enlargement of the fistula due to flow characteristics, repetitive cannulation in the same area, and venous outflow obstruction leading to increased intraluminal pressure
- A pseudoaneurysm is a disruption of the wall of the graft or fistula, allowing blood to escape from the access
  - A fibrous capsule may form, creating the pseudoaneurysm sac. Incidence described in the literature has been highly variable from 5% to >60%
  - Pseudoaneurysms occur more frequently in AVGs comparison with AVFs
- Pseudoaneurysms and true aneurysms result in an increased risk of thrombosis, bleeding, and infection. The most dangerous complication is compromise of the overlying skin as exsanguination may occur with rupture
  - Urgent surgical intervention is required for
    - Rapid increase in size
    - Thinned shiny skin, especially if skin is adherent to the underlying access
    - Ulceration or eschar
    - Herald bleed
- Repair includes aneurysmorrhaphy or an interposition graft to replace the diseased segment
  - Assessment must be made of both arterial inflow and venous outflow vessels with corrections of any lesions identified

- Endovascular options included covered stent placement and concomitant diagnostic fistulogram to assess for other pathologies
- Extensive repair may require temporary catheter placement

Nonthrombotic Flow-Related Complications: High-Output Heart Failure

- Creation of an AV access can exacerbate heart failure due to progressive cardiac dilation
- High flow volumes (>2 L/min) and access flow to cardiac output ratio >30%–35% are consistent with high-output heart failure
- Treatment is to reduce flow to through the AV access. Persistently symptomatic patients will require access ligation

Nonthrombotic Flow-Related Complications: Steal

- Steal phenomenon is described as the radiologic findings of asymptomatic retrograde flow in the distal artery after access creation and can be present in a large percentage of patients (70%)
- Symptomatic dialysis access steal syndrome (DASS) is reported in 1%–4% of patients
- Risk factors for DASS include
  - Age older than 60 years
  - Female sex
  - Type 2 diabetes
  - Peripheral arterial disease
  - Coronary artery disease
  - Previous radial artery harvest
  - Multiple previous accesses
  - Previous DASS
  - Access based on the brachial artery
  Clinical symptoms and signs include
- Diminished or absent pulses which improve with access compression
- Dialysis-induced or exercise-induced ischemic hand pain
- Sensory changes
- Rest pain
- Weakness, motor loss, atrophy
- Ulceration, or gangrene

Classification of Steal

- **Stage I**: pale and/or cool hand without pain. Management is conservative
- **Stage II**: tolerable or intolerable pain during exercise or dialysis. Management is conservative and/or surgical

- **Stage III**: rest pain or loss of motor function, may be associated with small ulcers. Management is urgent surgical intervention with interruption of retrograde flow
- **Stage IV**: irreversible tissue loss, significant loss of function. Management is ligation and/or amputation
  Prevention strategies include
- Access creation based on careful preoperative assessment
- Operative strategies include
  - Use of radial or ulnar arteries, rather than the brachial
  - Small arteriotomies of no more than 4–6 mm in length
  - Use of a tapered graft (smaller end on arterial side) when using prosthetics
  - Preservation arterial collaterals
- Diagnosis includes noninvasive digit brachial index <0.6, absolute digital pressures <50 mm Hg, transcutaneous oxygen pressure <30 mm Hg, and pulse volume recordings (PVRs) with and without graft compression
  The primary objective for the management of DASS is to improve distal circulation while maintaining a functional access.
- **Percutaneous transluminal angioplasty (PTA)** of arterial inflow lesions
- **Distal revascularization and interval ligation (DRIL)** increases distal circulation by providing an additional channel, prevents retrograde flow by ligation of the brachial artery. A bypass, typically the greater saphenous vein, is created from artery at least 5–7 cm proximal from the anastomosis to a distal portion of the dominant artery
- **Proximalization of arterial inflow (PAI)** involves disconnecting the fistula close to the anastomosis followed by the creation of a new conduit with inflow from a proximal arterial site to the efferent outflow conduit distal to the ligation. The new conduit can be autologous or prosthetic
- **Revision using distal inflow (RUDI).** RUDI preserves inflow in the forearm vessel. The fistula is ligated at its origin with a new bypass, autologous vein or prosthetic, from the fistula to a distal forearm arterial source 2–3 cm from the bifurcation
- **Banding** reduces fistula size and increases resistance. This involves reducing the diameter of the fistula using plication, prosthetic bands, cuffs, or clips. The Miller technique involves placing a 4-mm balloon just beyond the arterial anastomosis and then percutaneous sutures around it. Banding can also be performed in AV accesses with high flows
- **Distal radial artery ligation/embolization (DRAL)** is performed specifically for patients with a radiocephalic fistula and a patent ulnar artery and palmar arch. This improves hand circulation by stopping the retrograde flow through the radial artery
- **Access ligation** is typically used for severe cases of DASS and leaves the patient without a functional access

Nonthrombotic Flow-Related Complications: Ischemic Myeloneuropathy

- Ischemic myeloneuropathy is a devastating complication that occurs in the immediate postoperative period after AV access creation
- It is described as arterial insufficiency involving a single extremity causing selective dysfunction of peripheral nerves
- Shunting of blood away from the distal extremity damages the distal peripheral nerve fibers with acute neurological symptoms, but not enough ischemia to damage muscle or skin
- Risk factors
  - Female sex
  - DM with peripheral neuropathy
  - PAD
- Presentation includes a warm hand, palpable radial pulse, or Dopplerable distal signal. Symptoms include pain, paresthesia, and/or numbness, motor weakness/paralysis in the distal upper extremity
- Treatment is immediate ligation of the AV access

Nonthrombotic Flow-Related Complications: Noninfectious Fluid Collections

- Noninfectious fluid collections include seromas, hematomas, and lymphoceles. A seroma is a collection of sterile, clear serum that is surrounded by a nonsecretory fibrous pseudocapsule. Surgical treatment is necessary when fluid collection
  - Interferes with cannulation
  - Compromises overlying skin
  - Continues to grow

Infectious Complications

- Infection is the second most frequent cause of death and loss of access
- Risk factors
  - Repeated cannulation
  - Poor hygiene
  - Age
  - Lower extremity access
  - Type II DM
- Infections occur more commonly in prosthetic access than autogenous access and even abandoned grafts may become infected
- *Staphylococcus aureus* and *S. epidermidis* are the predominating organisms, especially in upper-arm access, but Gram-negative organisms, and polymicrobial also occur
- Blood and other cultures must be obtained prior to initiating broad-spectrum antibiotics covering both Gram-negative and Gram-positive organisms
- Very limited access infection may be treated with antibiotics alone, but surgical excision is required for more advanced cases
- Prosthetic grafts are typically excised
- The access may be salvaged by placing an interposition graft if only a focal segment is infected. The remaining graft must be well incorporated within the soft tissue for this to be a successful strategy
- Anastomotic infection requires complete graft excision. Severe infections may require brachial artery ligation and arterial bypass with cryopreserved or autologous vein

SUGGESTED READINGS

Initiation of Hemodialysis/Type of AV Access

Lok CE, Huber TS, Lee T, et al. National Kidney Foundation. KDOQI Clinical Practice Guideline for Vascular Access: 2019 update. *Am J Kidney Dis.* 2020;75(4 suppl 2):S1-S164.

Santoro D, Benedetto F, Mondello P, et al. Vascular access for hemodialysis: current perspectives. *Int J Nephrol Renovasc Dis.* 2014;7: 281-294.

United States Renal Data System. *2020 USRDS Annual Data Report: Epidemiology of kidney disease in the United States.* National Institutes of Health, National Institute of Diabetes and Digestive and Kidney Diseases; 2020.

Wallace JR, Chaer RA, Dillavou ED. Report on the Hemodialysis Reliable Outflow (HeRO) experience in dialysis patients with central venous occlusions. *J Vasc Surg.* 2013;58(3):742-747.

Graft Configurations

Rooijens PP, Burgmans JP, Yo TI, et al. Autogenous radial-cephalic or prosthetic brachial-antecubital forearm loop AVF in patients with compromised vessels? A randomized, multicenter study of the patency of primary hemodialysis access. *J Vasc Surg.* 2005; 42:481-486.

Cannulation

Ferring M, Henderson J, Wilmink T. Accuracy of early postoperative clinical and ultrasound examination of arteriovenous fistulae to predict dialysis use. *J Vasc Access.* 2014;5:291-297.

Robbin ML, Chamberlain NE, Lockhart Me et al. Hemodialysis arteriovenous fistula maturity: US evaluation. *Radiology.* 2002;225:59-64.

AVF Versus AVG

Arhuidese IJ, Orandi JO, Nejim B, Malas M. Utilization, patency, and complications associated with vascular access for hemodialysis in the United States. *J Vasc Surg.* 2018;68(4):1166-1174.

Brown RS, Patibandia BK, Goldfarb-Rumyantzev AS. This survival benefit of "Fistula First, Catheter Last" in hemodialysis is primarily due to patient factors. *J Am Soc Nephrol.* 2017;28:645-652.

Cheung AK, Imrey PB, Alpers CE et al. Intimal hyperplasia, stenosis, and arteriovenous fistula maturation failure in the Hemodialysis Fistula Maturation Study. *J Am Soc Nephrol.* 2017;28(10):3005-3013.

Disbrow DE, Cull DL, Carsten CG III, Yang SK, Johnson BL, Keahey GP. Comparison of arteriovenous fistulas and arteriovenous grafts in patients with favorable vascular anatomy and equivalent access to healthcare: is reappraisal of the Fistula First initiative indicated? *J Am Coll Surg.* 2013;216:679-685.

Keuter XH, De Smet AA, Kessels AG, van der Sand PM, Welton RJ, Tordoir JH. A randomized multicenter study of the outcome of brachial-basilic arteriovenous fistula and prosthetic brachial-antecubital forearm loop as vascular access for hemodialysis. *J Vasc Surg.* 2008;47(2):395-401.

Lok CE, Sontrop JM, Tomlinson G, et al. cumulative patency of contemporary fistulas versus grafts (2000–2010). *Clin J Am Soc Nephrol.* 2013;8:810-818.

Roojiens PP, Burgmans JP, Yo TI et al. Autologous radial-cephalic or prosthetic brachial-antecubital forearm loop AVF in patients with compromised vessels? A randomized, multicenter study of the patency of primary hemodialysis access. *J Vasc Surg.* 2005;42(3):481-488; discussions 487.

Woo K, Ulloa J, Allon M, et al. Establishing patient-specific criteria for selecting the optimal upper extremity vascular access procedure. *J Vasc Surg.* 2017;65(4):1089-1103.e1081.

One- Versus Two-Stage Basilic Vein

Cooper J, Power AH, DeRose G, Forbes TL Dubois L. Similar failure and patency rates when comparing one- and two-stage basilic vein transposition. *J Vasc Surg.* 2015;61(3):809-816.

Sheta M, Hakmei J, London M, et al. One- versus two-stage transposed brachiobasilic arteriovenous fistulae: a review of the current state of the art. *J Vasc Access.* 2020;21(3):281-286.

Tan TW, Siracuse JJ, Brooke SB, et al. Comparison of one-stage and two-stage upper arm brachiobasilic arteriovenous fistula in the Vascular Quality Initiative. *J Vasc Surg.* 2019;69(4):1187-1195.e2.

Access Complications and Treatment

Inston N, Schanzer H, Widmer M, et al. Arteriovenous access ischemic steal (AVAIS) in haemodialysis: a consensus from the Charing Cross Vascular Access Masterclass 2016. *J Vasc Surg.* 2017;18(1):3-12.

Moore WS, Lawerence, P, Oderich, G. *Vascular and Endovascular Surgery: A Comprehensive Review.* Philadelphia PA, USA: Elsevier/Saunders; 2019:839-855.

Mudoni A, Cornacchiari M, Gallieni M, et al. Aneurysms and pseudoaneurysms in dialysis access. *Clin Kidney J.* 2015;8(4):363-367.

Sen I, Tripathi RK. Dialysis access associated steal syndromes. *Semin Vasc Surg.* 2016;29:212-226.

Sidawy AN, Perler BA. *Rutherford's Vascular Surgery and Endovascular Therapy.* 9th ed. Philadelphia PA, USA: Elsevier; 2019:2324-2348.

Vascular Trauma

JAIME BENARROCH-GAMPEL, MD, MS

EPIDEMIOLOGY OF VASCULAR TRAUMA

- 1%–2% of trauma patients present with associated vascular injuries.[1]
- Traumatic injuries remain the leading mortality cause for individuals <45 years old.[2]
- Male gender is more commonly associated with vascular injuries from penetrating mechanisms.
- Blunt vascular injuries have higher mortality rates compared with penetrating vascular injuries.[3]

TRAUMA PRINCIPLES

- Advanced Trauma Life Support (ATLS) protocol should be followed with any patient who presents after a trauma, including those with vascular injuries.
- Anatomy, exposure, and management principles are similar to those for elective vascular surgery.
- Diagnostic or hard signs of vascular injury include arterial/pulsatile bleeding, expanding hematoma, lack of pulses distal to the injury, or the presence of a thrill.
- Suggestive or soft signs of vascular injury include stable size hematoma, decreased pulse or pressure index, injury in close location to vascular structures, injury of associated structures (such as nerves or veins), or unexplained hypotension.
- The use of endovascular techniques was initially limited to the aorta (high morbidity and mortality with open interventions) or the distal carotid artery (where exposure was limited and difficult) but has now expanded to almost any vascular bed including techniques for hemorrhage control.[4]
- Conduits:
  - All open traumatic wounds are considered contaminated. The preferred conduit is autologous vein from a noninjured extremity. The great saphenous vein (GSV) is the most commonly used vein for repair.
    - Use of the ipsilateral GSV should be done only if there is no confirmed deep venous injury on that side.
  - A short-segment prosthetic graft (polytetrafluoroethylene or Dacron) may be considered to repair uncontaminated arterial injuries (likely from blunt trauma). Other areas where graft should be considered include the axillosubclavian arteries as well as the aortic bifurcation.
  - Although data are lacking, the use of rifampin-soaked Dacron grafts should be considered in infected fields.
- Use of shunts (Fig. 22.1)[5,6]:
  - Main indication to use shunts is in critically ill patients as part of a damage control strategy. The definite repair can be performed during the initial operation after the patient has been properly resuscitated or in postoperative period.
  - Additional indications include temporary distal perfusion as orthopedic injuries are repaired as well as during preparation for complex revascularization (such as an extraanatomic bypass).
  - The largest possible shunt should be placed in concordance with artery diameter.
  - The Argyle shunt is the most commonly used shunt. For larger vessels (aorta or iliacs) a small chest tube can be used for shunting.
  - The shunt should be 2–3 cm into each end of the artery. It should be secure to avoid intravascular migration or getting disconnected.
  - The benefit of heparin in the setting of a shunted artery has not been demonstrated.
- Use of heparin:
  - The use of heparin in vascular trauma remains controversial.
  - Recent data suggest that intraoperative anticoagulation during open arterial repair is not associated with decreased risk of repair failure or limb loss.[7]
  - Similarly, 2019 data have shown no benefit of intraoperative heparin during endovascular repair of blunt aortic injury.[8] Despite this, when deemed safe or if sheaths are feared to be occlusive, it may be used to avoid thrombotic complications.
  - The decision to use heparin should always be discussed with the trauma team in the setting of associated traumatic injuries at special risk for bleeding.

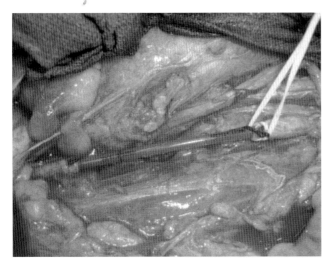

FIG. 22.1   **Use of Shunt in Vascular Trauma.**

TABLE 22.1   Injury Severity Based on Biffl (Denver Health) Classification[10]

Injury Grade	Description
I	Luminal irregularity or dissection with <25% luminal narrowing
II	Dissection or intramural hematoma with >25% luminal narrowing
III	Pseudoaneurysm
IV	Occlusion
V	Transection with free extravasation

CEREBROVASCULAR TRAUMA

- Neck zones:
  - Zone 1: below the cricoid cartilage
  - Zone 2: between the cricoid cartilage and the angle of the mandible. Most commonly affected zone
  - Zone 3: above the angle of the mandible
- Penetrating trauma
  - It is not uncommon to involve two zones of the neck.
  - Associated with esophageal and tracheal injuries.
  - In addition to hard and soft signs of vascular injury, the presence of Horner syndrome (sympathetic nerve plexus) or hoarseness (recurrent laryngeal nerve) is suspicious of vascular injury.
  - The Biffl classification (see later) should not be used to describe the characteristics of injuries from penetrating neck trauma.
  - Computed tomography angiography (CTA) is the preferred modality for the diagnosis of vascular injury in patients without signs of vascular or aerodigestive injury.
    - Previous literature recommended exploration for all neck injuries that had penetration of the platysma.
      - Led to 4%–50% negative explorations
- Blunt cerebrovascular trauma
  - Incidence of 1%–2% in the in-hospital trauma population.[9]
  - Occurs due to hyperextension/flexion and rotation of the neck or after direct neck trauma (especially with cervical fractures).
    - Motor vehicle collision, automobile versus pedestrian, chiropractors, "clothesline" mechanism, near-hanging, direct neck trauma etc.
  - Most common stroke mechanism is thrombus formation at the injured segment with consequent embolus. Stroke is more likely after carotid than vertebral artery injury.
  - Injury severity is based on the Biffl classification (Table 22.1).[10]

- Diagnostic is mainly with CTA. Most common screening indications are based on the Biffl (Denver Health)[11] and Miller (Memphis)[12] guidelines.
- Mainstay for treatment of blunt injuries is antithrombotic therapy. Either anticoagulation or antiplatelet agents can be used with similar results, but due to its safety profile, antiplatelet therapy such as aspirin is preferred as a first-line therapy.
  - Most trauma patients have other injuries with a contraindication to anticoagulation
    - Grade I injuries: 72% expected to completely heal
    - Grade II injuries: 33% heal, 33% stable, 33% progress to Pseudoaneurysm (PSA)
- Treatment options
  - Nonoperative management: occult and minor injuries (intimal flaps, non–flow-limiting dissections, and small pseudoaneurysm) can be managed with antithrombotic therapy and follow-up imaging. If there is worsening or enlargement of the lesion on follow-up imaging or symptoms of cerebral ischemia, an operative intervention should be considered.
  - Endovascular:
    - Covered stents are a valuable option to treat cerebrovascular injuries, especially in zones 1 or 3. They avoid the morbidity of a median sternotomy (zone 1) or difficult exposure (zone 3), but primarily for the carotid due to its size.
    - Coils can be used to treat pseudoaneurysms from the vertebral artery or for branches of the carotid artery.
    - Proximal control with balloon occlusion can be used in conjunction with open repair.
  - Open repair
    - All patients should have the chest in the operative field for proximal control if needed.
    - Proximal control is obtained on the chest (zone 1 injuries and proximal zone 2 injuries) or directly at the base of the neck (zone 2–3 injuries).
    - Exploration of the esophagus and trachea needs to be performed to rule out associated injuries.

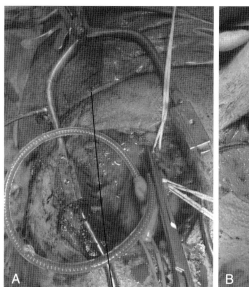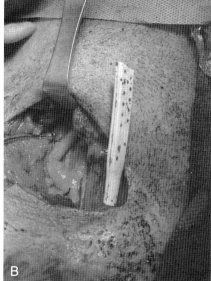

FIG. 22.2   (A and B) An interposition vein graft.

- Primary repair of the arterial injury can be performed in small lesions with clean borders that do not involve the full circumference of the vessel.
- An interposition vein graft is the modality of choice to repair these injuries given the risk for contamination and for smaller vessels, but prosthetic can be used if clean and larger (>~6mm) vessels (Fig. 22.2A and B).
- External carotid transposition requires ligation of the distal carotid artery with rotation of its stump to perform an anastomosis to the distal end of the internal carotid artery (ICA) can be used to manage proximal ICA injuries that preserve the bulb.
- Ligation should be reserved for patients in extremis or for those with injuries at the base of the skull that are not amenable to reconstruction.
  - Ligation of the ICA results in a 45% mortality and stroke (unlike chronic occlusions).
- Associated external carotid artery or venous injuries can be ligated with minimal clinical consequences.

THORACOABDOMINAL VASCULAR TRAUMA

- Diagnostic testing
  - Chest radiograph: present with associated hemothorax, widened mediastinum, obliteration of the aortic knob
  - CTA: screening modality of choice for thoracoabdominal aortic trauma
  - Others rarely used: transesophageal echocardiogram, magnetic resonance imaging, angiogram
- Thoracic aortic injury
  - Second most common cause of death in trauma patients after head trauma

- Majority of aortic-related deaths occurred before the opportunity for repair
- Blunt thoracic aortic injury classification range from intimal tear (Grade I), intramural hematoma (Grade II), pseudoaneurysm (Grade III), and free rupture (Grade IV) (Fig. 22.3)[13]
- Management:
  - Grade I–II: nonoperative management is recommended.

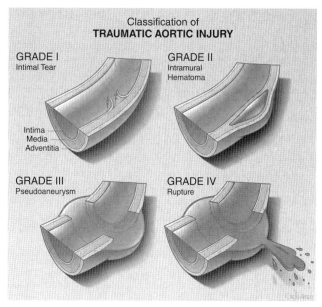

FIG. 22.3 **Classification of Traumatic Aortic Injury.** (Reprinted with permission from Azizzadeh A, Keyhani K, Miller CC 3rd, Coogan SM, Safi HJ, Estrera AL. Blunt traumatic aortic injury: initial experience with endovascular repair. *J Vasc Surg.* 2009;49(6):1403-1408.)

- Grade III: thoracic endovascular aortic repair (TEVAR) is the preferred technique for the management of these patients. While traditionally done within 24hrs, cases can be safely delayed to allow more emergent concerns (head, visceral etc) be addressed with no change in survival.[14,15]
  - Grade IV: immediate repair is indicated, preferably with TEVAR.
- TEVAR
  - Preferred technique for repair of thoracic aortic injuries.
  - Associated with decreased mortality when compared with open repair.[16]
  - *Resuscitation increases aortic diameter. Intravascular ultrasound should be used to confirm graft sizing.*
  - *Paraplegia is rare compared with other indications for TEVAR. Spinal drain is rarely used.*
  - Do *not* need standard 2-cm landing zone for traumatic aortic injury.
  - *Subclavian artery can be covered with limited concern.*
    - If arm ischemia, perform carotid-subclavian bypass.
  - Open repair of thoracic aorta
    - Decreased use in recent years
    - Can be done using distal aortic perfusion (distal cannula into the distal stump of the thoracic aorta) or using the clamp-and-sew technique
- Abdominal aortic injury:
  - Most commonly related to penetrating trauma.
  - Commonly associated with concomitant venous injuries.
  - A high index of suspicion for vascular injury should exist in patients with penetrating abdominal trauma and signs of hemorrhagic shock. These patients should be immediately taken to the operating room.
  - Patient with minor blunt injuries (intimal flaps, non–flow-limiting dissections) could be managed nonoperatively with image surveillance.
  - Resuscitative endovascular balloon occlusion (REBOA) should be considered in patients with abdominal trauma and signs of hemorrhagic shock.
  - Endovascular repair has limited utility in the management of abdominal aortic injuries due to penetrating trauma due to smaller aortas, but limbs and cuffs can occasionally be used for pseudoaneurysms or to temporize.
    - High risk of infecting graft when repaired open.
    - Open repair of the abdominal aorta is the most common technique (Fig. 22.4).
    - Supraceliac clamp should be considered for proximal control.
    - Exposure of the suprarenal aorta is obtained via the Mattox maneuver: left medial visceral rotation (incision lateral to the left colon and rotation of the stomach, spleen, pancreas, colon, and left kidney).
    - Exposure of the infrarenal aorta and iliac arteries is obtained via anterior exposure of the retroperitoneum.
    - Bowel injury with stool spillage increases the risk of graft infection. Using rifampin-soaked Dacron grafts and providing graft coverage (closing

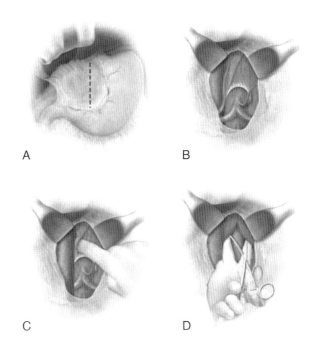

FIG. 22.4 Supraceliac exposure of the aorta. Enter lesser sac. Move esophagus to the left and divide the crus of the diaphragm and the medium arcuate ligament.

retroperitoneum, omental patch) should be strongly considered. Can also do extra-anatomic bypass and ligation if severely soiled.
- Other thoracolumbar injuries:
  - Subclavian artery injury:
    - Most commonly associated with penetrating trauma.
    - Best diagnosed with CTA.
    - Endovascular repair using covered stents is preferred for proximal injuries. Stent patency has been reported up to 84%.[17]
      - Cannot be used if covering the vertebral or left internal mammary artery (LIMA) in a coronary bypass graft (CABG) patient.
    - Double-access technique (from the common femoral artery and the radial/brachial artery) should be considered in patients with arteriovenous fistula to avoid misplacing the stent into the vein.
    - Open repair of the proximal subclavian artery requires extensive exposures: proximal right subclavian artery exposure is obtained via a median sternotomy with right cervical extension while left subclavian artery exposure is obtained via an anterior left thoracotomy.
  - Superior mesenteric artery (SMA)
    - Penetrating trauma is the most common mechanism of injury.
    - Most commonly identified during exploratory laparotomy in patients with penetrating abdominal trauma.
    - Exposure is obtained using left medial visceral rotation (as described earlier) for the suprapancreatic SMA and by direct dissection at the inferior border of the pancreas or by dissecting the root of the mesentery lateral to the ligament of Treitz.

- Management should be done by direct repair, interposition graft (preferably with vein due to the associated bowel injuries), or by ligation (for distal SMA if the bowel is necrotic). In critical patients, a damage control approach with shunting should be considered.
- Pseudoaneurysms can be explored if found in the mesentery and/or left alone if not expanding. Open repair, ligation or late coil embolization/stenting are acceptable.
- Distal ligation/embolization of SMA has higher risk of ischemia to the bowel, but acceptable in emergent conditions.
- Single, proximal ligation of celiac, SMA and IMA is usually well tolerated with intact collaterals.
- Autologous bypass is preferred over stenting when possible.
- Renovascular injuries
  - Most likely affect the left renal artery.
  - Clinical presentation is subtle.
  - After penetrating trauma, the diagnosis is mostly made intraoperatively.
  - Operative versus nonoperative management of renal injuries has been debated for years. Revascularization should be considered in patients where a renal artery injury leading to renal ischemia is identified within 1–3 hours.
  - Endovascular options include covered stents for the management of main renal artery injury and embolization for renal artery laceration, arteriovenous fistula, and pseudoaneurysm.
- Inferior vena cava (IVC) injuries[18]
  - Most commonly injured abdominal vessel.
  - Most common mechanism is penetrating trauma. It is usually fatal.
  - Exposure of injuries in the retrohepatic IVC segment should not be performed unless there is the presence of active hemorrhage that cannot be controlled with any form of tamponade.
  - Exposure of the perirenal IVC might require mobilization of the right kidney.

- Exposure of the common iliac vein confluence into the IVC area might require division of the right common iliac artery.
- Primary repair can be performed when the remnant lumen of the vessel is estimated to be at least 25%. Posterior wall wounds can be repaired via an anterior wound.
- Reconstruction with interposition grafts should be considered for patients with perirenal or suprarenal IVC injuries.
- *In critically ill patients with multiple injuries, ligation of the infrarenal IVC is the preferred management and can be very well tolerated in the long term.*

EXTREMITY VASCULAR TRAUMA

- Extremity vascular trauma is associated with lower mortality rates compared with truncal vascular injuries.[19]
- The mortality rate increases as the level of the injury becomes more proximal (i.e., higher mortality rate with common femoral artery injuries compared with popliteal injuries).[20]
- Often associated with bone fractures and nerve injuries.
- *Blunt trauma has higher rates of amputation.*[21]
- Most commonly injured artery in the lower extremity is the popliteal artery while in the upper extremity the radial/ulnar arteries are the most commonly injured.[20]
- Mangled extremity severity score (MESS) (Table 22.2)[22]
  - Developed in 1990 at Harborview Medical Center.
  - Factors used to calculate the score included skeletal/soft tissue damage, limb ischemia, patient's age, and presence of shock.
  - A score of 7 or higher is predictive of limb amputation.
- Diagnosis
  - Physical examination: presence of hard and/or soft signs of ischemia.
  - Normal pulse examination can be present in 5%–15% of patients with vascular injuries[23], especially when intimal irregularities are not occlusive (albeit unstable).

TABLE 22.2 **Mangled Extremity Severity Score (MESS)**[22]

Points	Skeletal/Soft Tissue	Ischemia[a]	Shock	Age
1	Low energy (stab, simple fracture, civilian GSW)	Pulse reduced or absent but perfusion normal	Transient hypotension (SBP <90 mm Hg)	30–50 years
2	Medium energy (open/multilevel fracture, dislocation, moderate crush)	Pulseless; paresthesias, diminished capillary refill	Persistent hypotension (SBP <90 mm Hg)	>50 years
3	High energy (shotgun, high-velocity GSW)	Cool, paralyzed, insensate, numb		
4	Very high energy (high-speed trauma with gross contamination)			

[a]Score doubled for ischemia >6 h.
GSW, Gunshot wound; *SBP*, systolic blood pressure.

- Ankle-brachial index (ABI) and brachial-brachial index (BBI) are most accurate for penetrating trauma. Although traditionally a threshold of 0.9 has been associated with the presence of arterial injury, recent data suggest an ABI ≤ 0.7 is more specific.[24]
- In cases where ABI/BBI are not accurate (older patients, diabetics), a difference of 0.1 between extremities is considered significant.
- In a trauma patient with suspected vascular injury, CTA is the imaging modality of choice with a sensitivity >95%[25] and can be performed at the same time as other computed tomography (CT) evaluations.
- Arteriography is used in patients who do not have preoperative image studies.
- Treatment
  - Patient with minor traumatic injuries (non–flow-limiting intimal defects, small pseudoaneurysms, distal arteriovenous fistulas) can be managed nonoperatively.
  - Patients with hard signs of vascular injury should be immediately taken to the operative room or interventional suite for repair.
  - Open repair remains the main technique for the management of peripheral vascular trauma.
    - Vascular control is obtained at a level proximal and distal to the injured vessel. Endovascular balloon occlusion can be used to obtain proximal control.
    - Proximal and distal embolectomy may need to be performed if thrombosed.
    - Debridement of devitalized tissue should be performed prior to vascular repair.
    - In patients with a focal arterial injury with <50% circumferential diameter and clean borders, primary repair or vein patch angioplasty with vein can be performed.
    - In case of a short injured segment, resection and end-to-end anastomosis can be performed. The vessel can be dissected proximally and distally to allow better mobilization and avoid tension between both ends.
    - In case of longer injured segments, an interposition graft should be performed, preferably with a contralateral great saphenous vein.
    - Ligation can be performed for single-vessel injury of a tibial or forearm vessel.
    - Fogarty catheters should be considered in cases where antegrade or retrograde bleeding from the nonaffected end of the artery is not adequate.
    - Securing soft tissue coverage is of paramount importance and should be obtained at the end of the repair.
  - Shunts are used in critically ill patients for damage control as well as to allow distal perfusion in combined vascular/orthopedic injuries during orthopedic stabilization prior to vascular repair.[26]
  - Combined vascular and orthopedic injuries have a high amputation rate and significant morbidity. In a recent multicenter study, temporary shunting followed by stabilization of the bony injury before definitive vascular repair seems to provide the best limb-salvage outcomes.[27]
- Fasciotomies
  - 40% of patients with lower extremity arterial injury receive a fasciotomy.
    - Fourfold reduction in eventual amputation and other complications
  - Four compartments to the lower extremity
    1. Anterior
    2. Lateral
    3. Superficial posterior
    4. Deep posterior
       - Vital that all four compartments be released
  - Compartment syndrome of the lower extremity following arterial trauma can lead to long-term functional impairment or limb loss (Fig. 22.5).

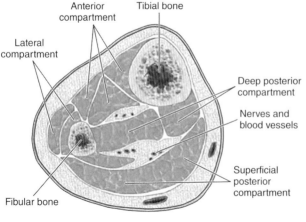

Cross-section through normal calf showing muscle compartments

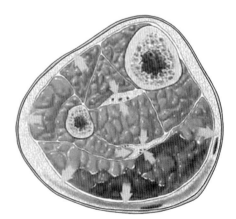

Compartment syndrome: Swelling of muscles causing compression of nerves and blood vessels

FIG. 22.5   **Compartment Syndrome.** (From Tomkins Z. CASE 3: A motor scooter rider with multiple closed fractures of the femur. In *Integrating Systems: Clinical Cases in Anatomy and Physiology*. Elsevier; 2021.)

- The most common compartment clinically affected is the anterior, and the most common nerve at risk is the peroneal nerve (motor and sensory). Ironically, its also the most commonly missed after attempted fasciotomy.
- Clinical markers for evolving compartment syndrome are: Pain in foot and leg at rest, pain with active or passive ankle motion, pain with palpation of anterior compartment, sensory loss over 1st web space and progressive weakness and paralysis of ankle motion.
- Predictors of compartment syndrome include prolonged ischemia (4–6 h), popliteal artery injury, associated venous injury, motor deficits, crush injuries and associated long-bone fractures.[28]

- Prophylactic fasciotomy should be strongly considered in the earlier scenarios.
  - Additional compartment pressure >30 mm Hg
- The ideal approach is the two-skin incision for the lower extremity or the two-skin three-compartment technique for the upper extremity distal to the elbow.
- Most common injured structure during fasciotomy is the deep peroneal nerve in the distal third of the leg. However, the common trunk and superficial (sensory) branches can be injured if the incision is made too close to fibular head.

REFERENCES

1. Mattox KL, Feliciano DV, Burch J, et al. Five thousand seven hundred sixty cardiovascular injuries in 4459 patients. Epidemiologic evolution 1958 to 1987. *Ann Surg.* 1989;209(6):698-705; discussion 706-697.
2. Eastridge BJ, Holcomb JB, Shackelford S. Outcomes of traumatic hemorrhagic shock and the epidemiology of preventable death from injury. *Transfusion.* 2019;59(S2):1423-1428.
3. Perkins ZB, De'Ath HD, Aylwin C, Brohi K, Walsh M, Tai NR. Epidemiology and outcome of vascular trauma at a British Major Trauma Centre. *Eur J Vasc Endovasc Surg.* 2012;44(2):203-209.
4. Reuben BC, Whitten MG, Sarfati M, Kraiss LW. Increasing use of endovascular therapy in acute arterial injuries: analysis of the National Trauma Data Bank. *J Vasc Surg.* 2007;46(6):1222-1226.
5. Feliciano DV. Pitfalls in the management of peripheral vascular injuries. *Trauma Surg Acute Care Open.* 2017;2(1):e000110.
6. Hornez E, Boddaert G, Ngabou UD, et al. Temporary vascular shunt for damage control of extremity vascular injury: a toolbox for trauma surgeons. *J Visc Surg.* 2015;152(6):363-368.
7. Humphries M, Blume MK, Rodriguez MC, DuBose JJ, Galante JM. Outcomes after anticoagulation for traumatic arterial injuries of the extremity. *JAMA Surg.* 2016;151(10):986-987.
8. Kenel-Pierre S, Ramos Duran E, Abi-Chaker A, et al. The role of heparin in endovascular repair of blunt thoracic aortic injury. *J Vasc Surg.* 2019;70(6):1809-1815.
9. Weber CD, Lefering R, Kobbe P, et al. Blunt cerebrovascular artery injury and stroke in severely injured patients: an international multicenter analysis. *World J Surg.* 2018;42(7):2043-2053.
10. Biffl WL, Moore EE, Offner PJ, Brega KE, Franciose RJ, Burch JM. Blunt carotid arterial injuries: implications of a new grading scale. *J Trauma.* 1999;47(5):845-853.
11. Burlew CC, Biffl WL, Moore EE, Barnett CC, Johnson JL, Bensard DD. Blunt cerebrovascular injuries: redefining screening criteria in the era of noninvasive diagnosis. *J Trauma Acute Care Surg.* 2012;72(2):330-335; discussion 336-337, quiz 539.
12. Miller PR, Fabian TC, Bee TK, et al. Blunt cerebrovascular injuries: diagnosis and treatment. *J Trauma.* 2001;51(2):279-285; discussion 285-276.
13. Azizzadeh A, Keyhani K, Miller CC III, Coogan SM, Safi HJ, Estrera AL. Blunt traumatic aortic injury: initial experience with endovascular repair. *J Vasc Surg.* 2009;49(6):1403-1408.
14. Smeds MR, Wright MP, Eidt JF, et al. Delayed management of Grade III blunt aortic injury: Series from a Level I trauma center. *J Trauma Acute Care Surg.* 2016;80(6):947-951.
15. Lee WA, Matsumura JS, Mitchell RS, et al. Endovascular repair of traumatic thoracic aortic injury: clinical practice guidelines of the Society for Vascular Surgery. *J Vasc Surg.* 2011;53(1):187-192.
16. DuBose JJ, Leake SS, Brenner M, et al. Contemporary management and outcomes of blunt thoracic aortic injury: a multicenter retrospective study. *J Trauma Acute Care Surg.* 2015;78(2):360-369.
17. DuBose JJ, Rajani R, Gilani R, et al. Endovascular management of axillo-subclavian arterial injury: a review of published experience. *Injury.* 2012;43(11):1785-1792.
18. Buckman RF, Pathak AS, Badellino MM, Bradley KM. Injuries of the inferior vena cava. *Surg Clin North Am.* 2001;81(6):1431-1447.
19. Kisat M, Morrison JJ, Hashmi ZG, Efron DT, Rasmussen TE, Haider AH. Epidemiology and outcomes of non-compressible torso hemorrhage. *J Surg Res.* 2013;184(1):414-421.
20. Kauvar DS, Sarfati MR, Kraiss LW. National trauma databank analysis of mortality and limb loss in isolated lower extremity vascular trauma. *J Vasc Surg.* 2011;53(6):1598-1603.
21. Liang NL, Alarcon LH, Jeyabalan G, Avgerinos ED, Makaroun MS, Chaer RA. Contemporary outcomes of civilian lower extremity arterial trauma. *J Vasc Surg.* 2016;64(3):731-736.
22. Johansen K, Daines M, Howey T, Helfet D, Hansen Jr ST. Objective criteria accurately predict amputation following lower extremity trauma. *J Trauma.* 1990;30(5):568-572; discussion 572-563.
23. Lebowitz C, Matzon JL. Arterial injury in the upper extremity: evaluation, strategies, and anticoagulation management. *Hand Clin.* 2018;34(1):85-95.
24. Hemingway J, Adjei E, Desikan S, et al. Re-evaluating the safety and effectiveness of the 0.9 ankle-brachial index threshold in penetrating lower extremity trauma. *J Vasc Surg.* 2020;72(4):1305-1311.e1.
25. Patterson BO, Holt PJ, Cleanthis M, et al. Imaging vascular trauma. *Br J Surg.* 2012;99(4):494-505.
26. Fox N, Rajani RR, Bokhari F, et al. Evaluation and management of penetrating lower extremity arterial trauma: an Eastern Association for the Surgery of Trauma practice management guideline. *J Trauma Acute Care Surg.* 2012;73(5 suppl 4):S315-S320.
27. Shahien AA, Sullivan M, Firoozabadi R, et al. Combined orthopaedic and vascular injuries with ischemia: a multicenter analysis. *J Orthop Trauma.* 2021;35(10):512-516.
28. Kluckner M, Gratl A, Gruber L, et al. Predictors for the need for fasciotomy after arterial vascular trauma of the lower extremity. *Injury.* 2021;52(8):2160-2165.

Vasculitis and Nonatherosclerotic Vascular Occlusive Disease

JACK S. BONTEKOE, MD, and JOHN E. RECTENWALD, MD, MS

VASCULITIS AND NONATHEROSCLEROTIC VASCULAR OCCLUSIVE DISEASE

Vasculitis

- Vasculitis is a group of inflammatory disorders of the arterial system that result in damage to normal vasculature and flow, resulting in end-organ and distal tissue ischemia and infarction.
- The vasculitides are divided into groups based on the size of the vessels involved, presence of immune complexes, organs affected, and the underlying disease pathophysiology (Table 23.1).
- Symptoms of each group of vasculitis are related to the size of vessels involved.
- Large-vessel vasculitis is more likely to present with symptoms such as limb claudication, bruits, asymmetric limb blood pressures, or absence of palpable pulses.
- Medium-vessel vasculitis may present with renal artery stenosis, coronary artery involvement, and skin involvement (digital gangrene, ulcers, livedo reticularis).
- Small-vessel vasculitis may present as purpura, renal disease at the level of the glomerulus, or alveolar hemorrhage.

LARGE-VESSEL VASCULITIS

Giant Cell Arteritis

Epidemiology
- Most common vasculitis in the elderly
- More common in white than in other racial groups
- Incidence increases with age (10 times more common in patients >80 years of age than those aged 50–60 years)

Etiology
- Unknown, yet speculated response to immunologic injury causes proliferation of myofibroblasts and thickening of arterial intima, leading to vessel narrowing and occlusion

Pathology
- Diffuse mononuclear cell infiltration or granulomatous inflammation with giant cells, leading to intimal fibrosis, destruction of internal elastic lamina, and vessel narrowing
- Arteries involved: most commonly carotid artery branches, aorta, main branches of the aorta

Signs/symptoms
- Classic presentation: elderly patient with new-onset headache and painless vision changes (diplopia, amaurosis fugax, blindness)
- Temporal tenderness, jaw claudication, fevers of unknown origin, arm claudication
- Physical examination demonstrates scalp tenderness, temporal artery tenderness, weak upper extremity pulses
  - Amaurosis fugax is a strong predictor of future blindness (precedes vision loss in 44% of patients)
- High association with polymyalgia rheumatica, a chronic syndrome involving stiffness and weakness of proximal joints (hips/shoulders), which is seen in 50%–75% of patients with giant cell arteritis (GCA)

Diagnostic evaluation
- The 1990 American College of Rheumatology criteria for diagnosis of giant cell arteritis requires at least three of the following five criteria to establish the diagnosis:
  - Age of disease onset >50 years of age
  - New-onset headache
  - Temporal artery abnormality (tenderness to palpation or decreased pulse in the absence of cervical atherosclerotic disease)
  - Elevated erythrocyte sedimentation rate (ESR)
  - Abnormal artery biopsy (mononuclear cell infiltration or granulomatous inflammation with multinucleated giant cells)

TABLE 23.1 List of Inflammatory Disorders of the Arterial System

Large-vessel	Giant cell arteritis Takayasu arteritis
Medium-vessel	Polyarteritis nodosa Kawasaki disease
Small-vessel • Immune complex–mediated	Anti–glomerular basement membrane disease Cryoglobulinemic vasculitis IgA vasculitis (Henoch-Schönlein purpura) Hypocomplementemic urticarial vasculitis (anti-C1q vasculitis)
• Antineutrophil cytoplasmic antibody–mediated (ANCA-associated pauci-immune)	Granulomatosis with polyangiitis (previously Wegener granulomatosis) Microscopic polyangiitis Eosinophilic granulomatosis with polyangiitis (previously Churg-Strauss syndrome)
Variable-vessel	Behçet disease Cogan syndrome
Single-organ vasculitis	Cutaneous leukocytoclastic vasculitis Cutaneous arteritis Primary CNS vasculitis (isolated angiitis of the CNS) Isolated aortitis Others
Vasculitis associated with systemic disease	Lupus vasculitis Rheumatoid vasculitis Sarcoid vasculitis Others
Vasculitis secondary to other etiology	Hepatitis C–associated cryoglobulinemic vasculitis Hepatitis B–associated vasculitis Syphilis-associated vasculitis Drug-associated immune complex vasculitis (hypersensitivity vasculitis) Cancer-associated vasculitis Others

CNS, central nervous system; *IgA,* immunoglobulin A.

- Gold standard to confirm diagnosis: temporal artery biopsy (2–3 cm in length)
- Ultrasound—"Halo" sign (noncompressible hypoechoic ring around the temporal artery lumen) is pathognomonic
- Laboratory results: nonspecific; elevated ESR, C-reactive protein (CRP)

Treatment
- Glucocorticoid therapy: oral prednisone initial dosing at 40–60 mg/day for 2–4 weeks followed by gradual taper and reevaluation
- Relapse: consider longer course of therapy, addition of methotrexate
- Impending vision loss: intravenous (IV) methylprednisolone (1000 mg/day × 3 days)
- All patients should receive aspirin 81 mg to reduce risk of arterial embolization

Complications
- Blindness (permanent vision loss by ischemic optic neuropathy occurs in 15%–20% of patients)

- Thoracic aortic aneurysm (TAA) (17-fold increased risk)
- Abdominal aortic aneurysm (AAA) (2.4-fold increased risk)

Role of the vascular surgeon
- Outcomes of surgical repair of AAA and TAA are similar to those without GCA
- Temporal artery biopsy to establish diagnosis

Takayasu Arteritis

Epidemiology
- Most commonly affects patients of East Asian descent
- 6–8 times more likely to occur in women than men
- Typically affects younger patients aged 20–40 years

Etiology
- Probable component of genetic predisposition as evidenced by the strong relationship to Asian ancestry

- Likely immune-mediated with associations to other autoimmune disorders, such as rheumatoid arthritis, systemic lupus erythematosus (SLE), inflammatory bowel disease (IBD)

Pathology

- Panarteritis involving all three vessel wall layers with skip lesions along the vessel segment
- Invasion of smooth muscle cells and fibroblasts with granulomatous inflammation causes intimal hyperplasia and adventitial fibrosis
- Acute intimal thickening may lead to end-organ ischemia, while chronic destruction of the elastic lamina leads to fibrosis and stenosis
- Stenotic disease more common than aneurysmal degeneration
- Arteries involved: subclavian (most common, 93%), common carotid (58%), abdominal aorta (47%)

Signs/symptoms

- Classic presentation: 30-year old female of Asian descent with absent pulses and hypertension
- Upper extremity claudication (62%), hypertension, inflammatory symptoms (carotidynia), cerebrovascular symptoms (syncope, transient ischemic attacks [TIAs], amaurosis fugax, visual disturbances), constitutional symptoms (fever, headache, myalgias, weight loss)
- Cardiac involvement: congestive heart failure (CHF), aortic regurgitation, myocarditis
- Pulmonary artery involvement (in contrast to GCA): chest pain, dyspnea, hemoptysis
- Examination may demonstrate diminished or absent pulses (53%–98%), hypertension, carotid bruits

Diagnostic evaluation

- The Rheumatology 1990 Criteria for the Classification of Takayasu Arteritis requires at least three of the following six criteria (sensitivity 90.5%, specificity 97.8%):
- Age of disease onset <40 years
- Claudication symptoms, especially in upper extremities
- Decreased brachial pulse in one or both arms
- Difference in systolic blood pressure >10 mm Hg between arms
- Bruit auscultated over subclavian or abdominal aorta
- Arteriographic abnormality showing narrowing or occlusion of the aorta, primary branches, large arteries in the extremities not due to arteriosclerosis or fibromuscular dysplasia (FMD)
- Imaging: computed tomography angiography (CTA) showing thickened arterial walls, skip lesions
- Laboratory results: anemia is common; elevated ESR, CRP

Treatment

- Glucocorticoid therapy induces remission in 60% of patients, yet most experience relapse of disease
- Self-limiting single–disease phase: 12%–20%
- Refractory therapy: anti–tumor necrosis factor (TNF), anti-interleukin (IL)-6 agents

Complications

- CHF is the most common cause of death

Role of vascular surgeon

- Generally reserved for management of symptomatic stenotic lesions
- Prioritize intervention when disease is in a quiescent state (12% restenosis rate compared with ~45% restenosis rate with intervention occurring in the active state)
- Surgical bypass to disease-free segments with continued corticosteroid therapy often results in excellent long-term survival rates

MEDIUM-VESSEL VASCULITIS

Polyarteritis Nodosum

Epidemiology

- Rare, affects 2–16 people per million
- 3:1 male/female predominance
- Peak incidence ~40 years of age

Pathogenesis

- Secondary to hepatitis B infection (mean time from presentation from hepatitis diagnosis: 7 months)
- Associated with other viral infections (most common vasculitis associated with hepatitis C and HIV), or as a paraneoplastic syndrome

Pathology

- Focal, transmural segments of fibrinoid necrosis with neutrophilic and lymphocytic infiltrates starting within the media, and progressing to intimal proliferation or aneurysmal dilatation
- Arteries involved: medium and small visceral segments, renal vessels

Signs/symptoms

- Classic presentation: middle-aged man with hepatitis B presenting with abdominal pain and skin lesions
- Usually presents with constitutional symptoms plus visceral end-organ dysfunction
- Cutaneous involvement: digital infarcts, palpable purpura, livedo reticularis, subcutaneous nodules
- Renal involvement (crescentic glomerulonephritis): hypertension, microscopic hematuria, or proteinuria
- Visceral/mesenteric involvement: may present as abdominal pain (major cause of morbidity)
- Note: polyarteritis nodosa (PAN) usually spares the lungs and upper respiratory tract, separating it from the antineutrophil cytoplasmic antibody (ANCA)-associated vasculitides

Diagnostic evaluation

- Arteriography: multiple saccular aneurysms and stenotic segments within the small and medium visceral vessels
- Laboratory results: positive hepatitis B serologies are common; ANCA testing should be negative

Treatment
- Steroid therapy can result in 5-year survival rates >80%, compared with 15% without
- Consider additional cyclophosphamide therapy in those with more severe PAN
- Visceral aneurysms may regress with proper medical treatment
- Initiate antiviral therapy in those with hepatitis B prior to starting immunosuppression

Complications
- Mortality is increased in those age >65 years, with renal insufficiency (creatinine >1.7 mg/dL), cardiomyopathy, or gastrointestinal involvement

Role of vascular surgeon
- Ruptured visceral artery aneurysms may be treated open or with coil embolization

Kawasaki Disease

Epidemiology
- Typically seen in children, with a peak incidence at 1 year of age; primary presentation is rare >age of 5 years
- More commonly affects boys than girls, and children of Japanese ancestry appear more susceptible
- Most common cause of acquired heart disease in children in the developed world

Etiology
- Multifactorial, likely immunologic due to evidence of altered immunity with a genetic component

Pathology
- The most serious manifestation is coronary arteritis leading to the development of coronary aneurysms
- Arteries involved: coronary, axillary, iliac

Signs/symptoms
- Classic presentation: 2-year-old boy with 1 week of high-grade fevers, conjunctivitis, chest pain
- See diagnostic criteria later

Diagnostic evaluation
- Clinical diagnostic criteria:
  - Prolonged high fever for >5 days
  - Conjunctival congestion
  - Changes in mucous membranes of the oral cavity
  - Peripheral edema or desquamation
  - Polymorphous exanthem
  - Acute nonsuppurative swelling of the cervical lymph nodes
- Echocardiography may show aneurysmal dilation of right, left, or anterior descending coronary arteries

Treatment
- Initial: high-dose aspirin and single-infusion immunoglobulin therapy
- Aspirin therapy is continued for 6–8 weeks after fever subsides

Complications
- Death from myocardial infarction or arrhythmia secondary to coronary artery aneurysm thrombosis

Role of vascular surgeon
- Aneurysm repair in noncoronary medium-sized vessels (iliac, axillary arteries)

SMALL-VESSEL VASCULITIS

Immune Complex–Mediated

Etiology
- Hypersensitivity vasculitis secondary to antigen exposure, leading to deposition of immune complexes within small arterial beds

Conditions
- Antiglomerular basement membrane (anti–glioblastoma multiforme [GBM]) disease
- Cryoglobulinemic vasculitis
- IgA vasculitis (Henoch-Schönlein purpura)
- Hypocomplementemic urticarial vasculitis (anti-C1q vasculitis)

Signs/symptoms
- Skin rash, fevers, evidence of end-organ dysfunction
- IgA vasculitis: child presenting with abdominal pain, bloody bowel movements, nephrotic syndrome

Treatment
- Steroids, potentially immunosuppression or plasmapheresis

Role of vascular surgeon
- Diagnosis and treatment referral

Antineutrophil Cytoplasmic Antibody (ANCA)-Associated Pauci-Immune

Etiology
- ANCAs: antibodies against specific proteins within neutrophil granules and lysosomal proteins in monocytes

Conditions
- Granulomatosis with polyangiitis (previously Wegener granulomatosis)
- Rare granulomatous vasculitis involving the respiratory tracts and kidney
- Upper and lower respiratory tracts: chronic sinusitis/purulent nasal drainage, epistaxis, chronic otitis media, pulmonary nodules, alveolar hemorrhage
- Kidney: necrotizing glomerulonephritis
- Microscopic polyangiitis
- Rapidly progressive necrotizing glomerulonephritis, diffuse alveolar hemorrhage, skin involvement (leukocytoclastic vasculitis)
- Eosinophilic granulomatosis with polyangiitis (previously Churg-Strauss syndrome)

- Patients may present with rhinitis, nasal polyposis, and adult-onset asthma that over years flares to a life-threatening systemic vasculitis with myocarditis, valvular insufficiency, gastroenteritis, alveolar hemorrhage

Treatment
- Steroids, potentially immunosuppression or plasmapheresis

Role of vascular surgeon
- Diagnosis and treatment referral

Nonatherosclerotic Vascular Occlusive Diseases

Thromboangiitis Obliterans (Buerger Disease) (PMID: 20421527)

Epidemiology:
- Predominately affects young male smokers <45 years
- More prevalent in the Middle East

Etiology
- Likely autoimmune secondary to tobacco exposure (possible causative relationship)

Pathology
- Non-necrotizing panvasculitis of small– and medium–vessels with highly cellular intraluminal thrombosis
- Note: internal elastic lamina remains intact (separate from atherosclerosis and vasculitis)
- Arteries involved: isolated lower extremities (50%), upper and lower extremities (30%–40%), isolated upper extremities (10%)

Signs/symptoms
- Classic presentation: mid–30-year-old male smoker with claudication and toe gangrene
- Intermittent claudication of upper or lower extremities progressing to ischemic rest pain, digital ulceration, and gangrene
- Superficial thrombophlebitis or Raynaud disease may present prior to claudication (~50% of patients)

Diagnostic evaluation
- Diagnostic criteria include:
  - Onset of distal extremity ischemic symptoms before 45 years of age
  - Exposure to tobacco
  - Absence of atherosclerotic risk factors, trauma, hypercoagulable or autoimmune disease, or embolic sources
  - No arterial disease proximal to popliteal arteries or brachial arteries
  - Either upper limb involvement of phlebitis migrans
  - Documented evidence of occlusive disease
- Arteriography: abrupt transition from normal vessel to focal segmental stenosis or occlusion in arteries distal to the brachial arteries in the upper extremities, or popliteal vessels in lower extremities bilaterally; corkscrew collaterals reconstitute distal segments
- Digital plethysmography: obstructive arterial waveforms of all digits bilaterally

Treatment
- Definitive therapy: tobacco cessation.
- Note: avoid nicotine replacement therapy as it may contribute to disease
- Management of tissue ischemia with local ulcer management (debridement, nail removal), amputation, or bypass
- Limited evidence for efficacy of calcium channel blockers, pentoxifylline; iloprost may be helpful in critical ischemia

Complications
- Relapse of disease is associated with resumed smoking
- Ischemic rest pain, tissue necrosis resulting in ulceration, infection
- Life expectancy is similar to controls likely due to lack of coronary artery involvement

Role of vascular surgeon
- Lower extremity amputation (upper extremity amputation is rare)
- May consider lower extremity bypass in those with distal targets, yet patency rates are suboptimal (30%–49% primary patency at 5 years)
- Revascularization is avoided

Fibromuscular Dysplasia (PMID: 21236620)

Epidemiology
- More commonly seen in females (9:1 female:male ratio)
- Most frequently occurs in women ages 20–60 years

Etiology
- Partially genetic, likely autosomal dominant with variable penetrance
- Renal artery FMD accounts for nearly 75% of FMD
- Extracranial cerebrovascular FMD commonly involves the internal carotid artery near the C1–C2 level

Pathology
- Classified into categories and subdivisions based on the arterial wall layer involved:
  - *Medial fibroplasia*: most common (80%–90% of FMD); alternating segments of thickened collagen deposits within the media followed by poststenotic dilations with thinned media, appears as a "string of beads"
  - *Intimal fibroplasia*: approximately 10%; focal concentric stenosis or long tubular lesions caused by intimal collagen deposits with fragmentation or duplication of the internal elastic lamina

Signs/symptoms
- Classic presentation: young female with new hypertension

- Renal artery FMD: new hypertension in young patient or poorly controlled hypertension; may be incidental finding or rarely presents as renal dysfunction from dissection or renal artery occlusion
- Extracranial cerebrovascular FMD: primarily asymptomatic or examination may show carotid bruit; if symptomatic, is more likely to present with nonspecific symptoms, such as dizziness, headache, pulsatile tinnitus, or audible "whooshing" sound, rather than specific neurologic symptoms of TIA, stroke, syncope, cranial nerve palsies
- Visceral and other arteries: typically incidental, can include the superior mesenteric or external iliac arteries. May present with ischemic symptoms secondary to arterial dissection or aneurysm

Diagnostic evaluation

- CTA imaging is most frequently used for initial evaluation or found incidentally
- Gold standard: contrast arteriography with "beads-on-a-string" morphology; intravascular ultrasound (IVUS) or measurement of pressure gradient is used to determine degree of stenosis
- Note: ultrasound is not accurate in determining stenosis due to the multiple segments of stenosis and dilation involved; no velocity criteria exist

Treatment

- Asymptomatic disease: routine monitoring, prophylactic aspirin 81 mg for primary stroke reduction in carotid or vertebral FMD
- Renovascular hypertension from renal artery FMD
- Angioplasty: new-onset hypertension in young patients, or chronic hypertension poorly controlled with medical management or evidence of declining renal function. Do *not* stent FMD patients
- Medical management with antihypertensives if blood pressure and renal function are controlled
- Cerebrovascular FMD:
- First line: percutaneous transluminal angioplasty (PTA) of symptomatic stenotic segments
- Primary open repair versus endovascular coiling reserved for aneurysmal disease

Complications

- Poorly controlled hypertension, renal infarction
- TIA or stroke
- Distal ischemia secondary to arterial dissections or thrombosis from aneurysmal segments

Role of vascular surgeon

- PTA: first line for symptomatic stenotic disease
- Endovascular stenting: reserved only for arterial dissections or complications of PTA
  - Note: renal artery stenting is avoided as FMD affects the mid to distal portions of the renal artery and in-stent restenosis complicates surgical repair
- Surgical revascularization: aneurysmal disease when no endovascular options are available, or failure of PTA

SUGGESTED READINGS

Moore WMS, Lawrence PF, Oderich GS. *Vascular and Endovascular Surgery: A Comprehensive Review*. 9th ed. Elsevier; 2019.

Olin JW, Sealove BA. Diagnosis, management, and future developments of fibromuscular dysplasia. *J Vasc Surg*. 2011;53(3):826-836. PMID: 21236620.

Piazza GP, Creager MA. Thromboangiitis obliterans. *Circulation*. 2010;121(16):1858-1861. PMID: 20421527.

Sidawy AN, Perler BA. *Rutherford's Vascular Surgery and Endovascular Therapy*. Philadelphia PA, USA: Elsevier Health Sciences; 2018.

Occlusive Venous Disease

ISABELLA KUO, MD

POSTTHROMBOTIC SYNDROME (PTS)

- Chronic sequelae of deep vein thrombosis (DVT)
- Symptoms (pain, heaviness, swelling, venous ulcers) worsen by standing and exercise
- Predictors of severity (severity of symptoms at 1 month, iliofemoral location, recurrent ipsilateral DVT, high body mass index [BMI], older age, female gender)
  Villalta score: measures severity of PTS using symptoms and clinical signs (Table 24.1)
- Prevention
  - Prevent deep venous thrombosis
  - Good quality early anticoagulation

ILIOFEMORAL DVT (IFDVT)

- Leads to ambulatory venous hypertension
- Risk factors
  - Virchow triad (venous stasis, endothelial injury, hypercoagulability)
  - Anatomy (iliac vein compression)
    - Most common cause—*May-Thurner syndrome* (left common iliac vein compressed by right common iliac artery)
      - Consider venous stenting
    - Consider more proximal disease when ultrasound demonstrates loss of phasicity in the common femoral vein
      - Ultrasound will show significant reflux with May-Thurner syndrome
      - Ultrasound will be flat-lined in the femoral with iliac occlusion

TABLE 24.1 **Villalta Score for Post Thrombotic Syndrome**

Symptoms/clinical signs	None	Mild	Moderate	Severe
Symptoms				
Pain	0 points	1 points	2 points	3 points
Cramps	0 points	1 points	2 points	3 points
Heaviness	0 points	1 points	2 points	3 points
Paresthesia	0 points	1 points	2 points	3 points
Pruritus	0 points	1 points	2 points	3 points
Clinical signs				
Pretibial edema	0 points	1 points	2 points	3 points
Skin induration	0 points	1 points	2 points	3 points
Hyperpigmentation	0 points	1 points	2 points	3 points
Redness	0 points	1 points	2 points	3 points
Venous ectasia	0 points	1 points	2 points	3 points
Pain on calf compression	0 points	1 points	2 points	3 points
Venous ulcer	Absent			Present

- Management
  - Anticoagulation
  - Venous thrombectomy
  - Catheter-directed thrombolysis (CDT)
    - Ultrasound-accelerated thrombolysis (EKOS EndoWave system)
  - Pharmacomechanical thrombolysis (PMT)
    - Rheolytic thrombectomy (AngioJet catheter [Boston Scientific])
    - Isolated segmental PMT (Trellis catheter)
  - Aspiration Thrombectomy
    - Penumbra CAT systems
    - JETi Thrombectomy System (Abbott)
  - Mechanical Extraction

- ClotTriever System (Inari Medical)
- Adjuncts: balloon angioplasty and stenting
- Trials
  - CaVenT study[1]: CDT + anticoagulation + compression superior to anticoagulation + compression alone in reducing PTS at 2 years
  - ATTRACT Study[2]: adding CDT to anticoagulation in proximal DVT did not reduce incidence of severe PTS, but did lower severity of PTS, swelling and pain; albeit higher risk of bleeding
- Treatment recommendations
  - Ninth edition of chest guidelines[3]—thrombolysis more beneficial in patients with:
    - IFDVT with symptoms <14 days
    - Good functional status
    - Life expectancy >1 year
    - Low risk of bleeding

IVC FILTER

- Inferior vena cava (IVC) filter does not treat existing DVT and pulmonary embolism (PE); therefore anticoagulate when possible
- Placement can be guided by fluoroscopy or intravascular ultrasound (IVUS)
- Absolute indications: presence of DVT or PE and
  - Bleeding complication from anticoagulation
  - Contraindication to anticoagulation
  - Failure of anticoagulation to prevent DVT or PE
- Relative indication: presence of DVT or PE and
  - Chronic PE with residual DVT and no cardiopulmonary reserve
  - Previous pulmonary thrombectomy for PE
  - Preexisting severe pulmonary hypertension or right heart failure
  - Free-floating iliocaval thrombus
  - Significant fall risk
- Contraindications to IVC filter placement
  - Chronically occluded IVC
  - Inability to access the IVC
  - Vena cava compression
  - No location in the IVC available for placement
- Complications
  - Access site hematoma or thrombosis
  - Filter migration
  - Filter fracture and embolization of fragments
  - Filter tine penetration into aorta, bowel or spine
  - Filter thrombosis

NONOPERATIVE TREATMENT OF CHRONIC VENOUS DISEASE

- Lifestyle modification (diet, exercise)
- Compression therapy (compression stockings, bandages, or pneumatic compression)

- Pharmacological therapy (diuretics, pentoxifylline, prostaglandins, phlebotropic agents)
- Local wound care

OPEN INTERVENTIONS FOR CHRONIC VENOUS OCCLUSIVE DISEASE

- Palma procedure: crossover saphenous vein transposition
  - Indication: symptomatic unilateral iliac vein obstruction
  - Need a normal contralateral iliofemoral venous system
  - Key steps of the procedure:
    - Expose common femoral vein on affected side
    - Dissect and mobilize contralateral great saphenous vein (GSV) up to the saphenofemoral junction on the UNAFFECTED side
    - Pull through a suprapubic tunnel
    - Perform an end-to-side anastomosis of GSV to the affected common femoral vein
    - Create arterio-venous fistula on the UNaffected side to increase patency
    - May consider placing the GSV through a reinforced prosthetic conduit.
  - Not recommended in morbidly obese patients due to compression
  - Patency: 70%–83% at 3–5 years
- Saphenopopliteal bypass
  - Indication: femoral or proximal popliteal vein obstruction
  - Use ipsilateral GSV or other suitable conduit
- Crossover femoral venous prosthetic bypass
  - Indications: symptomatic unilateral iliac vein obstruction if GSV is inadequate
  - Additional procedure: construction of a distal arteriovenous (AV) fistula on the affected side
  - Poor patency in general, so always do an AV fistula on the donor side

ENDOVASCULAR INTERVENTIONS FOR CHRONIC VENOUS OCCLUSIVE DISEASE

- Treatment of choice over open technique
- Venous stenting differs from arterial stenting
  - Balloon angioplasty not sufficient; therefore stent insertion mandatory
  - "Kissing" balloon technique in aortic bifurcation not necessary at confluence of common iliac veins
  - Need to use ultrasound guidance for access
  - IVUS is essential
    - Easy to undersize in the venous anatomy without IVUS.
  - Place stents into the IVC to avoid early restenosis
  - Large-diameter stents are recommended
  - Redilate stents after placement to avoid migration and ensure complete treatment of CIV

- OK to place stents across the inguinal ligament
  - Do not jail the deep femoral vein by placing stents past the femoral bifurcation
  - Avoid skip areas between two stents
- Management of bilateral iliac disease includes stenting Primary patency is the best when treating non-thrombotic indications (99%), followed by acute thrombosis (85%), followed by chronic PTS at 70% (PMID: 36642400). with double-barrel technique

ILIOCAVAL OBSTRUCTION

- Causes: May-Thurner syndrome, prior DVT, external compression from retroperitoneal fibrosis, tumors, aneurysms, trauma, radiation, congenital abnormalities
- Symptoms: leg swelling and venous claudication (exercise-induced pain in the thigh muscles)
- Diagnosis: duplex ultrasound, plethysmography, computed tomography (CT) or magnetic resonance imaging (MRI), contrast-enhanced phlebography
- Open treatment
  - Indication: failed conservative management or endovascular treatment
  - Short bypass preferred
  - Venous grafts
    - Autologous grafts have best patency (GSV, can be used as spiral or panel graft)
    - Expanded polytetrafluoroethylene (ePTFE)—best prosthetic replacement of large veins
      - Ringed PTFE will prevent external compression
  - Types of bypasses
    - Femoroiliac or Iliocaval bypass
      - Conduit: externally supported 10 mm to 14 mm PTFE
    - Inferior cavoatrial bypass
      - Conduit: externally supported 16 mm to 20 mm PTFE
    - IVC reconstruction
      - Indication: primary venous leiomyosarcoma, tumor invading the IVC
      - PTFE or bovine pericardial patch
  - Complications
    - DVT and PE
    - Early graft thrombosis
    - Perioperative bleeding
    - Graft infection
- Endovascular treatment
  - Apply principles of venous stenting
  - IVC filter—can be associated with vena cava stenosis
    - If stenosis is >50%, remove stent and/or stent across
  - Recanalization of occlusion can be done
- Hybrid treatment
  - For patients with femoral thrombosis and long iliac vein occlusion

- Open thrombectomy of common femoral vein with iliofemoral vein stenting
- Closure of femoral vein with GSV or bovine pericardial patch

SUPERIOR VENA CAVA (SVC) OBSTRUCTION

- Causes
  - Malignant: tumors of the lung and mediastinum
  - Benign: placement of intravenous (IV) catheters or pacemakers
- Superior vena cava (SVC) syndrome
  - Symptoms: wide range, but most commonly head and neck fullness worse with bending over and lying down
  - Physical findings: dilated neck veins and swelling of neck, face, and eyelids
- Treatment: open surgical (PMID: 29502774, 20371163)
  - Indication: patients with failed endovascular management or anatomy not suitable for endovascular technique
  - Conduits used for reconstruction from the IJ, innominate or subclavian veins to the right atrium
    - Femoral vein
    - Spiral saphenous vein graft
    - ePTFE
    - Cryopreserved graft
    - Caval patch possible when SVC is patent
  - Extraanatomic bypass with GSV from jugular vein to ipsilateral femoral vein; place GSV in externally supported PTFE to prevent compression
- Treatment: endovascular (PMID: 18241760)
  - Overview
    - Considered first-line therapy for SVC obstruction
    - Dual venous access (upper extremity and femoral) often needed
  - Treatment options
    - Thrombolysis
      - Catheter-directed
      - Pharmacomechanical
    - Balloon angioplasty and stenting
      - Balloon angioplasty as adjunct to stenting due to vessel wall recoil
      - Stents available
        - Gianturco Z-stent (Cook Medical, Inc.)—rigid self-expanding stainless steel stent (PMID: 33090095)
        - Palmaz stent (Cordis Corporation)—balloon expandable stent with high radial force, but at risk for migration
        - SMART stent (Cordis Corporation)—self-expanding stent, nitinol
        - Wallstent (Boston Scientific)—self-expanding stent, flexible and up to 24 mm in diameter available

- Stent grafts not often used because they can cover collaterals
- Care must be taken not to jail both sides

CENTRAL VENOUS OCCLUSION

- Causes: secondary to pacemakers, peripherally inserted central catheter (PICC) lines, central venous ports, hemodialysis catheters trauma, malignancy or thoracic outlet syndrome
- Higher rate with subclavian vein versus internal jugular vein catheters
- Increased incidence with left-sided catheters
- Hemodialysis patients
  - Most are asymptomatic until functioning ipsilateral AV access is constructed
    - Leads to venous hypertension
  - Signs and symptoms: chest and neck collateral veins; ipsilateral edema (arm, breast, face)
  - Central occlusion can decrease AV access blood flow and lead to thrombosis

- In some cases, collateral flow may be sufficient for patient to remain asymptomatic
- Treatment includes access ligation, endovascular therapy, open therapy
- Treatment options
  - Endovascular
    - Balloon angioplasty
    - Stenting
      - Recommended for >50% recoil after balloon angioplasty or recurrent stenosis within 3 months
      - Modes of failure: intimal hyperplasia
  - Open—depending on location of occlusion
  - Subclavian vein or axillary vein to right atrium bypass with PTFE
  - Extraanatomic bypass
    - Subclavian vein to ipsilateral internal jugular vein bypass
    - Internal jugular to internal jugular vein crossover
    - Ipsilateral internal jugular turndown
  - Axillary vein to external iliac vein bypass

REFERENCES

1. Enden T, Haig Y, Kløw NL, et al. Long-term outcome after additional catheter-directed thrombolysis versus standard treatment for acute iliofemoral deep vein thrombosis (the CaVenT study): a randomised controlled trial. *Lancet.* 2012;379(9810):31-38.
2. Vedantham S, Goldhaber SZ, Julian JA, et al. Pharmacomechanical catheter-directed thrombolysis for deep-vein thrombosis. *N Engl J Med.* 2017;377(23):2240-2252.
3. Kearon C, Akl EA, Anthony J Comerota AJ, et al. Antithrombotic therapy for VTE disease: antithrombotic therapy and prevention of thrombosis, 9th ed: American College of Chest Physicians Evidence-Based Clinical Practice Guidelines. *Chest.* 2012;141(suppl 2):e419S-e496S.
4. Espitia O, Douane F, Hersant J, et al. Venous Stent Network Investigators. Predictive Factors of Stent Patency in Iliofemoral Venous Diseases in a Multicentre Cohort Study. *Eur J Vasc Endovasc Surg.* 2023;65(4):564-572. PMID: 36642400.
5. Thulasidasan N, Morris R, Theodoulou I, et al. Medium-term outcomes after inferior vena cava reconstruction for acute and chronic deep vein thrombosis and retroperitoneal fibrosis. *J Vasc Surg Venous Lymphat Disord.* 2022;10(3):607-616. e2. PMID: 34508871.
6. Doty JR, Flores JH, Doty DB. Superior vena cava obstruction: bypass using spiral vein graft. *Ann Thorac Surg.* 1999;67(4):1111-1116. PMID: 10320259.
7. Femoral vein conduit reconstruction for SVC (video): https://www.sciencedirect.com/science/article/pii/S2468428723001302
8. Wik HS, Enden TR, Ghanima W, Engeseth M, Kahn SR, Sandset PM. Diagnostic scales for the post-thrombotic syndrome. *Thromb Res.* 2018;164:110-115. doi:10.1016/j.thromres.2017.10.022.

CHAPTER 25

Venous Insufficiency

JOEL HARDING, DO, and BRIGITTE SMITH, MD, MHPE, FACS, FSVS

EPIDEMIOLOGY OF VENOUS INSUFFICIENCY

- Frequency of chronic venous insufficiency (CVI) in the general population
  - Worldwide, CVI affects roughly 60% of the population.[1]
  - In Western countries, CVI affects roughly 17% of men and 40% of women.
- Venous ulceration from venous insufficiency
  - Seventy percent of ulcerations of the lower extremity are due to venous insufficiency.[2]
  - Venous ulceration, the most severe form of CVI, affects 2% of the US population.[3-5]
- Frequency of pathologies in patients with CVI
  - Superficial truncal insufficiency is frequently found in patients with CVI, ranging from 45% to 80%.[6,7]
  - In epidemiological studies the frequency of varicose veins fluctuated from 8% of the US population to as high as 32% to 40% in European studies.[8,9]
  - In patients with varicose veins, incompetent perforator vein frequency ranges from 44% to 63%.[10]
  - Telangiectasia is the most common form of venous disease and is reported to be present in up to 80% of the population in Western countries.[11]

ETIOLOGY OF VENOUS INSUFFICIENCY

- Venous hypertension (HTN) is the underlying cause of CVI.[12]

- Valvular insufficiency as a cause for venous HTN.
  - The direct cause of valvular insufficiency is not clearly understood, but one study showed that there are fewer valves in patients with CVI versus those without.[13] In addition to anatomical variants, estrogen may cause venous distention leading to valvular incompetence.[14]
- Venous obstruction can lead to venous HTN leading to CVI.
- Venous obstruction can be caused by pelvic masses, deep venous thrombosis, trauma, or iatrogenic injury.

FORMS OF VENOUS HYPERTENSION

Ambulatory Venous Hypertension

- In patients, as they walk they develop a gradient between the calf and thigh venous systems. The calf pump muscles cause fluctuations in venous pressure, but the thigh gradient is constant.
- In patients with venous HTN due to reflux, the reflux worsens during the relaxation cycle of calf pump muscles as there is an increased return of volume due to incompetent valves in the venous system.[15] This mechanism causes worsening of the refluxing system.

Hydrostatic Venous Hypertension

- Hydrostatic venous HTN is when the body is at rest and the only exertion of pressure on the venous system is gravitational. The level of hydrostatic pressure is measured at 0 mm Hg at the right atrium and increases to 90 mm Hg at the level of the ankles.
- Hydrostatic pressure causes venous engorgement but does not cause venous reflux as there is no gradient formed at the same hydrostatic level to cause flow.[16]

Endothelial Dysfunction as a Result of Venous Hypertension

- Long-standing venous HTN leads to inflammation causing extravasation of cytokines and endothelial dysfunction, manifesting in hyperpigmentation, ulceration, and pain.[17]

Risk Factors for Chronic Venous Insufficiency

- Family history, female sex, pregnancy, estrogen, prolonged standing and sitting postures, and obesity[18]

CLINICAL FEATURES OF VENOUS INSUFFICIENCY

- Clinical examination findings in CVI run the gamut of pain, itching, swelling, varicosities to skin staining and ulcerations of the lower extremities
- Lower extremity venous anatomy[19]
- Superficial veins (Fig. 25.1)
  - Great saphenous vein (GSV): accessory saphenous vein—runs lateral to the GSV. Circumflex vein—runs obliquely to the GSV
  - Small saphenous vein—a branch from the small saphenous is the posterior thigh circumflex vein (vein of Giacomini)
- Deep veins (Fig. 25.2)
  - Calf—includes the posterior tibial vein, peroneal vein, and anterior tibial vein, which confluence into the popliteal vein
- Thigh—includes the superficial femoral vein, deep femoral vein, and common femoral vein
- Perforating veins—insufficiency of these veins may lead to varicosities in the leg, even without reflux in the GSV
  - Medial leg perforators include: posterior tibial perforators and paratibial perforators
  - Medial thigh leg perforators include the perforating vein of the femoral canal
- Valves of the leg veins
  - GSV has on average 5 valves in the femoral segment and 3 in the crural segment.[20]
  - The deep femoral venous system has on average 2–6 valves and the popliteal system has 0–2 valves on average.[21]
  - The feet and the iliacs have no valves.[22]

Clinical Features of Lower Extremity Ulcers

- **Arterial Ulcerations**
  - Dry ulcer bed with minimal bleeding even with debridement

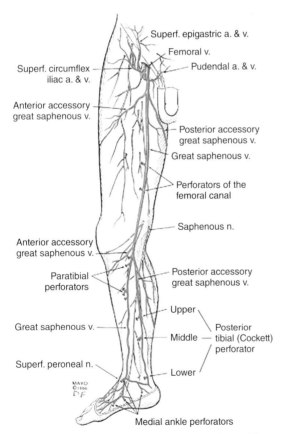

FIG. 25.1 Superficial Venous Anatomy. (From Mozes G, Gloviczki P. New discoveries in anatomy and new terminology of leg veins: clinical implications. *Vasc Endovasc Surg.* 2004;38:367-374.)

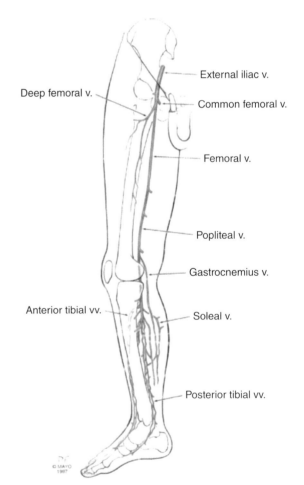

FIG. 25.2 Deep Venous Anatomy. (From Mozes G, Gloviczki P. New discoveries in anatomy and new terminology of leg veins: clinical implications. *Vasc Endovasc Surg.* 2004;38:367-374.)

- Usually distal on the extremity or tips of toes
- Absent pedal pulses
- **Venous Ulcerations**
  - Wet ulcer bed/weeping fluid
  - Lower extremity pitting edema
  - Primarily below the knee and on the medial aspect of the lower extremity
  - Associated with DVTs and varicose veins
- **Neuropathic Ulcerations**
  - Punched out lesions
  - Usually located at pressure points on the plantar aspect of the foot
  - Most commonly a/w diabetes or foot abnormalities (Charcot disease)
- See Box 25.1 from Society for Vascular Surgery (SVS) Guidelines for differential diagnosis for lower extremity ulcers.

Categorization of Clinical Findings

- See Table 25.1 for clinical, etiological, anatomical, and pathophysiological (CEAP) categories.

Venous Clinical Severity Score (VCSS)

- The Venous Severity Scoring (VSS) system was created in 2000 and is composed of three elements: Venous Disability Score (VDS), Venous Clinical Severity Score (VCSS), and Venous Segmental Disease Score.[23]
- The VSS was developed as a supplement to the CEAP scoring system as a tool that is more adaptable to tracking changes in clinical outcomes over a patient's clinical course, particularly those with severe venous disease (CEAP 4 through 6).[24]
- See Table 25.2 for revised VCSS.

BOX 25.1 Differential Diagnosis for Lower Extremity Ulcers

Vascular Disease
- Venous: postthrombotic syndrome, varicose veins, chronic venous reflux
- Arterial: peripheral arterial occlusive disease, hypertension, arteriovenous fistulas, arterial thrombosis, embolism, dysplasia, thromboangiitis obliterans, aneurysm
- Lymphatic: lymphedema
- Microangiopathy: type 2 diabetes, livedoid vasculopathy
- Vasculitis
- Hypertensive arteriolopathy

Neuropathic
- Peripheral neuropathy: type 2 diabetes, alcohol, medication, hereditary
- Central neuropathy: tabes dorsalis, myelodysplasia, syringomyelia, spina bifida, poliomyelitis, multiple sclerosis
- Metabolic
- Type 2 diabetes, gout, prolidase deficiency, Gaucher disease, amyloidosis, calciphylaxis, porphyria, hyperhomocysteinemia

Hematologic
- Sickle cell anemia, thalassemia, polycythemia vera, leukemia, thrombocythemia, lymphoma, myeloplastic disorders, disorders of coagulation factors (factors I–XIII), coagulation inhibitors (antithrombin III, activated protein C resistance, proteins C and S), or fibrinolysis factors (tissue plasminogen activator, plasminogen activator inhibitor, plasmin)

Autoimmune
- Rheumatoid arthritis, leukocytoclastic vasculitis, polyarteritis nodosa, Wegener granulomatosis, Churg-Strauss syndrome, systemic lupus erythematosus, Sjögren syndrome, scleroderma, Behçet disease, cryoglobulinemia

Exogenous
- Heat, cold, pressure, ionizing radiation, chemical, allergens, trauma

Neoplasia
- Basal cell carcinoma, squamous cell carcinoma (Marjolin ulcer), malignant melanoma, angiosarcoma, cutaneous lymphoma, papillomatosis cutis carcinoides, keratoacanthoma

Infection
- Bacterial: furuncles, ecthyma, mycobacterioses, syphilis, erysipelas, anthrax, diphtheria, chronic vegetative pyodermia, tropical ulcer
- Viral: herpes, variola virus, cytomegaly
- Fungal: sporotrichosis, histoplasmosis, blastomycosis, coccidioidomycosis
- Protozoal: leishmaniasis

Medication
- Hydroxyurea, leflunomide, methotrexate, halogens, coumarin, vaccinations, ergotamine, infiltration cytostatic agents

Genetic Defect
- Klinefelter syndrome, Felty syndrome, *TAP1* mutation, leukocyte adhesion deficiency, inherited hypercoagulable factors

Skin Disorder
- Pyoderma gangrenosum, necrobiosis lipoidica, sarcoidosis, perforating dermatosis, Langerhans cell histiocytosis, papulosis maligna atrophicans, bullous skin diseases

From O'Donnell TF Jr, Passman MA, Marston WA, et al. Management of venous leg ulcers: clinical practice guidelines of the Society for Vascular Surgery and the American Venous Forum. *J Vasc Surg.* 2014;60(suppl 2):3S-59S. Modified from Dissemond J, Korber A, Grabbe S. Differential diagnosis of leg ulcers. *J Dtsch Dermatol Ges.* 2006;4:627-634.

TABLE 25.1 Clinical, Etiological, Anatomical, and Pathophysiological (CEAP) Categories

Clinical Classification

C0	No visible or palpable signs of venous disease
C1	Telangiectases or reticular veins
C2	Varicose veins
C3	Edema
C4a	Pigmentation and/or eczema
C4b	Lipodermatosclerosis and/or atrophie blanche
C5	Healed venous ulcer
C6	Active venous ulcer
CS	Symptoms, including ache, pain, tightness, skin irritation, heaviness, muscle cramps, as well as other complaints attributable to venous dysfunction
CA	Asymptomatic

Etiologic Classification

Ec	Congenital
Ep	Primary
Es	Secondary (postthrombotic)
En	No venous etiology identified

Anatomic Classification

As	Superficial veins
Ap	Perforator veins
Ad	Deep veins
An	No venous location identified

Pathophysiologic Classification

Pr	Reflux
Po	Obstruction
Pr,o	Reflux and obstruction
Pn	No venous pathophysiology identifiable

From O'Donnell TF Jr, Passman MA, Marston WA, et al. Management of venous leg ulcers: clinical practice guidelines of the Society for Vascular Surgery and the American Venous Forum. *J Vasc Surg.* 2014;60(suppl 2):3S-59S. Modified from Eklöf B, Rutherford RB, Bergan JJ, et al. Revision of the CEAP classification for chronic venous disorders: consensus statement. *J Vasc Surg.* 2004;40: 1248-1252.

DIAGNOSTIC EVALUATION OF VENOUS INSUFFICIENCY

- Ultrasound is considered the most frequently used and studied form of venous interrogation to identify deep venous thrombosis and superficial venous reflux.[25,26] The current SVS Guidelines place venous duplex imaging in patients with a *leg ulcer* at a Grade-1 Level-B evidence.
- For patients with suspected venous disease, the SVS and American Venous Forum (AVF) recommend venous duplex of the deep and superficial system with a four-component examination: visualization of the vein, compressibility, venous flow, and augmentation (Grade-1 Level-A evidence).
- Fig. 25.3 shows venous ultrasound with augmentation, compression, and color flow.
- Fig. 25.4 shows GSV reflux.
- Reflux is defined as >500 ms of reflux in superficial veins, deep calf veins, deep femoral vein, and perforating veins and >1000 ms in common femoral veins, femoral veins, and popliteal veins.[27]
- Varicose veins are defined as >3 mm subcutaneous veins with a tortuous course on the lower extremity.[28]
- In 80% of limbs with cardiovascular disease (CVD), reflux is the offending cause, with 17% having isolated obstruction and only 2% with both reflux and obstruction.
- Patients with combined reflux and obstruction have the highest morbidity and mortality.[29]
- Venography, in light of duplex sonography, is reserved for a small subset of patients. Currently the SVS and AVF have combined venography, magnetic resonance venography (MRV), and computed tomography venography (CTV) as other imaging modalities that are reserved for pelvic congestion syndrome, nutcracker syndrome (NCS), May-Thurner syndrome, postthrombotic syndrome, and iliac venous obstruction and as a pre- or postoperative imaging modality.
- Venography is a diagnostic and interventional modality in patients with pelvic or abdominal reflux. Compared with transvaginal and transabdominal duplex ultrasonography, venography is a confirmatory study for pelvic and gondal reflux.
- Venography was considered the gold standard for imaging of venous obstruction prior to widespread usage of compressive ultrasound. It can still be considered in patients with clinical findings of a deep venous thrombosis and negative or inconclusive compressive ultrasound.[30]

TREATMENT OF VENOUS INSUFFICIENCY

Compression

- Considered first-line therapy in all cases of venous insufficiency.
- There are various forms of compression, from stockings to multilayered wraps. Stockings come in various stages of compression from 15 mm Hg to 40 mm Hg.

TABLE 25.2   **Table of Revised Venous Clinical Severity Scoring System**

Symptoms	None: 0	Mild: 1	Moderate: 2	Severe: 3
Pain or other discomfort (i.e., aching, heaviness, fatigue, soreness, burning)		Occasional pain or other discomfort (i.e., not restricting regular daily activities)	Daily pain or other discomfort (i.e., interfering with but not preventing regular daily activities)	Daily pain or discomfort (i.e., limits most regular daily activities)
Presumes venous origin Varicose veins "Varicose" veins must be >3 mm in diameter to qualify in the standing position		Few: scattered (i.e., isolated branch varicosities or clusters) Also includes corona phlebectatica (ankle flare)	Confined to calf or thigh	Involves calf and thigh
Venous edema Presumes venous origin		Limited to foot and ankle area	Extends above ankle but below knee	Extends to knee and above
Skin pigmentation Presumes venous origin	None or focal	Limited to perimalleolar area	Diffuse over lower third of calf	Wider distribution above lower third of calf
Inflammation More than just recent pigmentation (i.e., erythema, cellulitis, venous eczema, dermatitis)		Limited to perimalleolar area	Diffuse over lower third of calf	Wider distribution above lower third of calf
Induration Presumes venous origin of secondary skin and subcutaneous changes (i.e., chronic edema with fibrosis, hypodermitis). Includes white atrophy and lipodermatosclerosis		Limited to perimalleolar area	Diffuse over lower third of calf	Wider distribution above lower third of calf
Active ulcer number	0	1	2	>3
Active ulcer duration (longest active)	NA	<3 months	>3 months but <1 year	Not healed for >1 year
Active ulcer size (largest active)	NA	Diameter <2 cm	Diameter 2–6 cm	Diameter >6 cm
Use of compression therapy	0 Not used	1 Intermittent use of stockings	2 Wears stockings most days	3 Full compliance: stockings

From O'Donnell TF Jr, Passman MA, Marston WA, et al. Management of venous leg ulcers: clinical practice guidelines of the Society for Vascular Surgery and the American Venous Forum. *J Vasc Surg.* 2014;60(suppl 2):3S-59S. Modified from Vasquez MA, Rabe E, McLafferty RB, Shortell CK, Marston WA, Gillespie D, et al. Revision of the venous clinical severity score: venous outcomes consensus statement: special communication of the American Venous Forum Ad Hoc Outcomes Working Group. *J Vasc Surg.* 2010;52:1387-1396.

- Despite compression being first-line therapy, there is limited evidence that compression therapy is beneficial as the sole therapy for varicose veins, in the absence of healed or active ulcerations.[31] Regardless, many insurance companies require a minimum of 90 days of compression therapy prior to any suggested intervention.[32]
- Contraindication to compression therapy is arterial insufficiency with an arterial-brachial index (ABI) <0.5.[33]

Treatment for Truncal Vein Insufficiency

Surgical Intervention

- High ligation and venous stripping (HLS).
- Traditionally, HLS was the mainstay of treatment for venous insufficiency after failure of conservative therapy until the introduction of endovenous interventions.[34] There is comparable efficacy and outcomes compared with

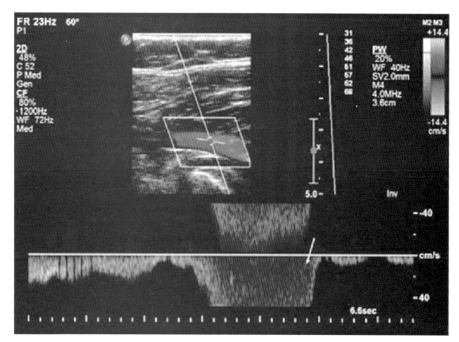

FIG. 25.3   Spectral Doppler waveform analysis of the lower limb veins. Spontaneous and respiratory phasic flow with a typical response to an augmentation maneuver and aliasing of the pulsed Doppler waveform (arrow). (Duplex ultrasound for evaluation of deep venous blood flow in fractured lower extremities - Scientific Figure on ResearchGate. Available from: https://www.researchgate.net/figure/Spectral-Doppler-waveform-analysis-of-the-lower-limb-veins-Spontaneous-and-respirophasic_fig2_316191326) [accessed 16 Aug, 2023].

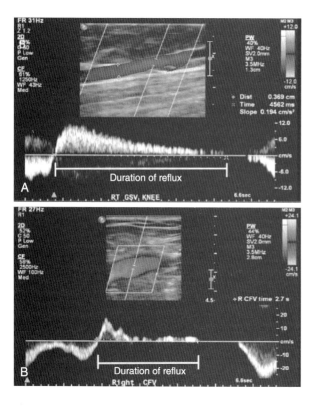

FIG. 25.4   Superficial and deep venous reflux. Notes: reflux is measured while imaging the vein in the transverse orientation. The proximal end of the vein is on the left side of the image. In the examination of the great saphenous vein, the vein is imaged in the transverse section with color Doppler ultrasound. The distal calf is rapidly compressed and released. The duration of flow reversal is measured beginning at the reversal of flow (A). Reflux in the deep system is assessed in a similar manner, except the patient is asked to perform a Valsalva maneuver to provoke reflux (B). (From *Ultrasound assessment of great saphenous vein insufficiency*—figure on ResearchGate. https://www.researchgate.net/figure/Superficial-and-deep-venous-reflux-Notes-Reflux-is-measured-while-imaging-the-vein-in_fig4_281426502. Accessed November 20, 2021.) (Journal of Vascular Diagnostics and Interventions 2015 3 25-31' Originally published by and used with permission from Dove Medical Press Ltd.)

TABLE 25.3 Randomized Clinical Trial Outcomes of Endovenous Treatment Versus High Ligation and Venous Stripping Outcomes and Complications

Method	Failure at 1 year (%)	Major complication (DVT, PE) (%)	Paresthesia (%)	Phlebitis (%)	Infection (%)
Stripping	4	1	5	5	1
Ultrasound-guided foam sclerotherapy	20	1	2	17	4
RFA	6	0	6	12	1
Laser	7	0	3	4	0

Endovenous intervention was found to be as effective as open surgical intervention; ultrasound-guided foam sclerotherapy had the highest failure rate and statistically significant rate of phlebitis.
DVT, Deep venous thrombosis; *PE,* pulmonary embolus; *RFA,* radiofrequency ablation.
Modified from Rasmussen LH, Lawaetz M, Bjoern L, et al. Randomized clinical trial comparing endovenous laser ablation, radiofrequency ablation, foam sclerotherapy and surgical stripping for great saphenous varicose veins. *Br J Surg.* 2011;98:1079.

endovenous ablation versus HLS, but with lower pain and early return to work with endovenous ablation.[35]
- Indication for HLS would be failed endovenous ablation or venous diameter is too large (>20 mm) or too small (<2 mm) for catheter-based treatment, or tortuosity of the GSV.[36]
- Avoidance of below-knee stripping is recommended due to the close proximity of the saphenous nerve.[37,38]

Endovenous Intervention

- Radiofrequency ablation (RFA)
  - Catheter placement into the saphenous vein under ultrasound with tumescence using lidocaine and saline to improve contact of the catheter with the vein wall and give anesthesia during the procedure. A series of ablations are made from the saphenofemoral junction (SFJ) down the leg.
- Laser ablation
  - Similar to RFA, a catheter is inserted under ultrasound into the GSV and advanced to the SFJ under ultrasound. Then tumescent is injected along the track of the vein for anesthetic and increasing venous wall apposition to the catheter. Then a series of ablations are made along the length of the vein down the leg.
- Sclerotherapy and sealant therapy
  - Polidocanol (sclerosant)
    - Trade names: Asclera, Varithena
    - Asclera—small reticular veins and spider veins
    - Varithena—foam therapy for GSV and larger veins
  - Sodium tetradecyl sulfate (sclerosant)
    - Trade names: Sotradecol
    - Sotradecol—sclerosant of uncomplicated varicose veins
  - Cyanoacrylate
    - Trade names: VenaSeal
    - Sealant that polymerizes intravascularly to close down veins

- See Table 25.3 for endovenous versus HLS randomized trial[39]

Treatment for Perforator Veins

- The SVS and AVF currently recommend treatment of "pathologic" perforating veins that includes those with an outward flow duration of 500 ms, with a diameter of 3.5 mm, located beneath a healed or open venous ulcer (CEAP class C5–C6)
- Subfascial endoscopic perforator ligation: insertion of ports below the saphenous fascia in the lower leg and ligating pathological perforators near healed or active ulcerations
- Sclerotherapy/sealant: injection of pathologic perforator veins under ultrasound guidance with sclerosant or sealant

Treatment of Varicose Veins

- Sclerotherapy: the SVS and AVF currently recommend foam or liquid sclerotherapy for varicose veins, spider veins, telangiectasia/spider veins
- Stab phlebectomies: reserved for concomitant GSV ablation or stripping, or for after failed sclerotherapy

Treatment of Venous Ulceration

- Compression, wound debridement, and treatment of superficial venous HTN with ablation, high ligation and stripping, or sclerotherapy.
- Rule out arterial insufficiency in any patient with non-healing lower extremity wounds. A simple ABI should be performed.

- If concomitant ulceration with an ABI <0.7, arterial perfusion should be improved.
- Image of treatment algorithm for mixed arterial venous ulcerations.

Treatment of Deep Venous Insufficiency

- Conservative treatment of deep venous insufficiency:
  - Exercise
  - Elevation
  - Elastic compression (the three E's)
- Deep venous reconstruction: for patients with lifestyle-limiting venous disease with deep venous reflux that have failed strict adherence to conservative management, valve transplantation or valve reconstruction has been described. It is recommended that prior to deep venous reconstruction, superficial reflux and pathological perforators have already been addressed.
- External valvuloplasty is done by placing sutures blindly into the valve to tighten the incompetent valves.
- Internal valvuloplasty involves making a venotomy with reconstruction of the valve directly.
- Autologous vein transplant can also be completed with placing an interposition graft into the affected venous segment.

CONTRAINDICATIONS TO TREATMENT OF VENOUS INSUFFICIENCY

- See Table 25.4 for relative contraindications to treatment of venous insufficiency.

TABLE 25.4   Relative Contraindication to Treatment of Venous Insufficiency

Acute deep venous thrombosis

Pregnancy

Arterial insufficiency

Arteriovenous fistula with venous reflux

Venous malformation with venous reflux

COMPLICATIONS OF VENOUS INSUFFICIENCY TREATMENT

- Thromboembolism—relatively low rate of thromboembolism in thermal endovenous ablation and foam sclerosis, <1%[40] (Table 25.5)
- Local complications from sclerotherapy
  - Skin necrosis can occur with extravasation of sclerosant and osmotic agents; this is a rare but devastating complication.
  - Hyperpigmentation, very common, occurs in 15%–20% and will typically resolve in 12 months,[41] can be treated in protracted cases with intense pulse light generator and radio waves.[42]
  - Allergic reaction has been documented in a handful of cases with sodium tetradecyl sulfate but is extremely rare.[43]

TABLE 25.5   Complication Rates of Surgical Stripping and Ligation Versus Catheter-based Ablations

Complication	Surgical Stripping and Ligation (%)	Endovenous Radiofrequency Ablation (%)	Endovenous Laser Ablation (%)
DVT/PE	0.7	0.5	0.4
Infection	2.0	1.0	0.7[a]
Paresthesia	6.7	7.8	3.3[b]
Superficial thrombophlebitis	2.9[c]	5.2%	5.5
Bruising	36.1	3.1[d]	34.5
Hematoma	13.5[e]	0.2	2.1
Skin burns	NA	0.7	0.7

[a]Lower rate of infection compared with surgical ligation and stripping.
[b]Lowest rate of paresthesia compared with RFA and HLS.
[c]Lower rates of SVT compared with RFA and EVLA.
[d]Lowest rate of bruising compared with HLS and EVLA.
[e]Highest rate of hematoma compared with EVLA and RFA.
DVT, Deep venous thrombosis; *EVLA,* endovenous laser ablation; *HLS,* high ligation and venous stripping; *PE,* pulmonary embolus; *RFA,* radiofrequency ablation; *SVT,* supraventricular tachycardia.
Modified from Dermody M, O'Donnell TF, Balk EM. Complications of endovenous ablation in randomized controlled trials. *J Vasc Surg Venous Lymphat Disord.* 2013;1(4):427-436.e1.

POSTOPERATIVE FOLLOW-UP AFTER VENOUS INSUFFICIENCY TREATMENT

- For endovenous thermal ablation to include laser ablation and radiofrequency ablation, a follow-up ultrasound within 1 week of treatment is recommended to identify and treat endothermal heat–induced thrombosis (EHIT)[44]
  - AVF EHIT (Table 25.6)
  - Treatment for EHIT[44] (Table 25.7)
- Compression therapy after venous treatment[45] (Table 25.8)
- Follow-up imaging after any venous intervention
- The AVF and SVS recommend follow-up imaging if there is recurrence of symptoms or recurrent varicose veins

TABLE 25.6   **American Venous Forum Endothermal Heat–Induced Thrombosis (EHIT) Definition**

EHIT Tier	Anatomical Location
EHIT I	Thrombus at the junction without protrusion into the common femoral vein
EHIT II	Thrombus protrusion into the common femoral vein with <50% of the lumen
EHIT III	Thrombus protrusion into the common femoral vein with >50% of the lumen
EHIT IV	Thrombus occluding the lumen of the common femoral vein that is contiguous with the treated great saphenous vein

TABLE 25.7   **Endothermal Heat–Induced Thrombosis Treatment**

EHIT Level	Treatment and Surveillance	Grade and Level of Evidence
EHIT I	No treatment or surveillance	Grade 2 Level C
EHIT II	No treatment with weekly surveillance duplex until thrombus resolves	Grade 2 Level C
EHIT III	Therapeutic anticoagulation with weekly surveillance until thrombus resolves	Grade 1 Level B
EHIT IV	Therapeutic anticoagulation in line with the CHEST guidelines	Grade 1 Level A

Modified from Kabnick LS, Sadek M, Bjarnason H, et al. Classification and treatment of endothermal heat-induced thrombosis: recommendations from the American Venous Forum and the Society for Vascular Surgery. *Phlebology*. 2021;36(1):8-25.

TABLE 25.8   **Compression Therapy After Venous Treatment**

Guideline	Recommendation	Grade and Level of Evidence
Compression after thermal ablation or vein stripping	Recommend use of compression after procedure	Grade 2 Level C
Dose of compression after thermal ablation or vein stripping	Recommend ≥20 mm Hg for compression	Grade 2 Level B
Duration after thermal ablation or vein stripping	Use clinical judgment	Best practice
Compression after sclerotherapy	Recommend immediate compression therapy after sclerotherapy to improve outcomes	Grade 2 Level C
Duration of compression after sclerotherapy	Use clinical judgment	Best practice
Compression after treatment with a venous ulcer	Recommend compression versus no compression	Grade 1 Level B

Modified from Lurie F, Lal BK, Antignani PL, et al. Compression therapy after invasive treatment of superficial veins of the lower extremities: clinical practice guidelines of the American Venous Forum, Society for Vascular Surgery, American College of Phlebology, Society for Vascular Medicine, and International Union of Phlebology. *J Vasc Surg Venous Lymphat Disord*. 2019;7(1):17-28.

INTRAABDOMINAL CAUSES OF VENOUS INSUFFICIENCY

- NCS—constellation of symptoms resulting from the compression of the left renal vein between the superior mesenteric artery and the aorta causing flank pain and hematuria.[46]
  - Duplex ultrasonography is typically first line and findings consistent with NCS are gonadal reflux as well as >5.0 ratio of velocities between the proximal and distal renal vein.[47]
  - Computed tomographic venography or MRV will show compression of the left renal vein, as well as a steep angle between the aorta and superior mesenteric artery that is <41 degrees, dilation of the left renal vein collaterals and pelvic collaterals.[48]
  - Venography allows for hemodynamic measurement of a venous gradient. There is a paucity of data on a numeric gradient that is confirmatory for NCS but previous literature has listed >3 mm Hg gradient as renal vein HTN. This, in correlation with sluggish flow from the left renal vein into the inferior vena cava (IVC) and dilated renal vein collaterals, points toward NCS.[49]

Treatment

- Open surgical repair revolves around improving outflow of the renal vein and decompressing the gradient

- Transposition of the renal vein inferiorly on the IVC with or without concomitant patchings or cuffing
- Transposition of the gonadal vein or using saphenous vein as a venous bypass[50]
- Image of surgical reconstruction (Fig. 25.5)
- Endovascular repair has been described, and can be achieved with high radial force stents that are oversized; however, data on long-term patency are limited and stents are susceptible to migration
- Endovascular repair should be relegated to patients who are poor open surgical candidates[51]

Pelvic Congestion Syndrome

- Syndrome characterized by chronic pelvic pain lasting more than 6 months that is noncyclic in premenopausal women with associated dysmenorrhea, dyspareunia, and varicosities of the pelvis or vulvar region.[52]
- Similar to NCS, pelvic congestion syndrome can be screened initially with duplex sonography. Identifying features are pelvic varicosities, venous dilation >6 mm, and retrograde flow in ovarian veins.[53]
- Venography is both a diagnostic and interventional modality. Diagnostic features are ovarian veins >10 mm, pelvic and uterine venous congestion, and retrograde filling of the left ovarian vein from the left renal vein.[54,55]
  - See Table 25.9 for ultrasound and venography findings of pelvic congestion syndrome.[53,56]

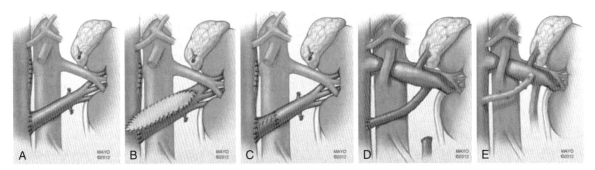

FIG. 25.5 Surgical reconstruction options for nutcracker syndrome. (A) Renal vein transposition. (B) Renal vein transposition with patch venoplasty. (C) Renal vein transposition with adjunct vein. (D) Gonadal vein transposition. (E) Saphenous vein bypass. (From Said SM, Gloviczki P, Kalra M, et al. Renal nutcracker syndrome: surgical options. *Semin Vasc Surg.* 2013;26:35-42.)

TABLE 25.9 **Ultrasound and Venography Findings of Pelvic Congestion Syndrome**

Ultrasound Findings of Pelvic Congestion Syndrome	Venography Findings in Pelvic Congestion Syndrome
Dilated left gonadal vein (>6 mm) with caudal flow	Renal vein reflux into >5 mm ovarian veins
Dilated arcuate veins (>5 mm) crossing the myometrium of the uterus	Contrast pooling into pelvic veins
Polycystic changes to the ovaries	Contrast crossing the pelvic midline
Pelvic varicoceles >5 mm	Thigh varicosities
Variable waveform during Valsalva maneuvers	Vulvar/perineal varicosities

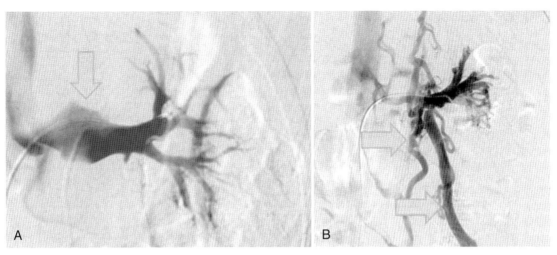

FIG. 25.6 Left renal vein (A) and dilated gonadal vein with multiple tributaries (B). (From Erben Y, Gloviczki P, Kalra M, et al. Treatment of nutcracker syndrome with open and endovascular interventions. *J Vasc Surg Venous Lymphat Disord.* 2015; 3[4]:389-396.)

- See Fig. 25.6 for image of left renal vein and gonadal vein with reflux and dilation on venography.
- Treatment is endovascular therapy with coil or sclerosant embolization of the ovarian veins.
- Treatment is technically successful >99% of the time with a low recurrence rate. The approach is either femoral or jugular venous access with cannulation of the left ovarian vein from the left renal vein or the right ovarian vein from the IVC directly.[57]
- In long-term follow-up, improvement of symptoms occurred in >80% of patients after embolization.[58,59]

May-Thurner Syndrome

- A compressive syndrome similar to NCS in that it involves compression of the left common iliac vein by the right common iliac artery, which may result in left leg swelling, and deep venous thrombosis of the left venous system.[60]
- Venous duplex is the first-line imaging for both identification of venous thrombosis and venous compression by the iliac artery.[61]

Treatment

- For both diagnostic and treatment purposes, venography allows for direct interrogation of the iliac vein with intravascular ultrasound to show real-time compression by the iliac artery.[62]
- If there is concomitant compression with acute iliofemoral deep venous thrombosis, lysis and mechanical thrombectomy can be performed as well.
- A self-expanding stent should be used for maximal radial force with proximal extension into the IVC to prevent migration.

REFERENCES

1. Rabe E, Guex JJ, Puskas A, Scuderi A, Fernandez Quesada F; VCP Coordinators. Epidemiology of chronic venous disorders in geographically diverse populations: results from the Vein Consult Program. *Int Angiol.* 2012;31(2):105-115.
2. Adam DJ, Naik J, Hartshorne T, Bello M, London NJ. The diagnosis and management of 689 chronic leg ulcers in a single-visit assessment clinic. *Eur J Vasc Endovasc Surg.* 2003;25(5): 462-468. doi:10.1053/ejvs.2002.1906.
3. Nussbaum SR, Carter MJ, Fife CE, et al. An economic evaluation of the impact, cost, and medicare policy implications of chronic nonhealing wounds. *Value Health.* 2018;21(1):27-32. doi:10.1016/j.jval.2017.07.007.
4. Hedayati N, Carson JG, Chi YW, Link D. Management of mixed arterial venous lower extremity ulceration: a review. *Vasc Med.* 2015;20(5):479-486. doi:10.1177/1358863X15594683.
5. Harding JP, Hedayati N. Challenges of treating mixed arterial-venous disease of lower extremities. *J Cardiovasc Surg (Torino).* 2021;62(5):435-446. doi:10.23736/S0021-9509.21.11901-9.
6. Coelho Neto F, de Oliveira RG, Gregório EP, Belczak SQ, de Araujo WJB. Saphenous reflux patterns in C2 patients: a record of 1196 ultrasound reports. *Phlebology.* 2020;35(6):409-415. doi:10.1177/0268355519889868.
7. Jain P, Savlania A, Behera A, Gorsi U. Distribution patterns of pathological venous reflux and risk factors in patients with skin

changes due to primary venous disease in North India. *Phlebology*. 2021;36(3):209-216. doi:10.1177/0268355520957193.

8. Eberhardt RT, Raffetto JD. Chronic venous insufficiency. *Circulation*. 2014;130(4):333-346. doi:10.1161/CIRCULATIONAHA.113.006898.

9. Evans CJ, Fowkes FG, Ruckley CV, Lee AJ. Prevalence of varicose veins and chronic venous insufficiency in men and women in the general population: Edinburgh Vein Study. *J Epidemiol Community Health*. 1999;53(3):149-153. doi:10.1136/jech.53.3.149.

10. Rutherford EE, Kianifard B, Cook SJ, Holdstock JM, Whiteley MS. Incompetent perforating veins are associated with recurrent varicose veins. *Eur J Vasc Endovasc Surg*. 2001;21(5):458-460. doi:10.1053/ejvs.2001.1347.

11. Beebe-Dimmer JL, Pfeifer JR, Engle JS, Schottenfeld D. The epidemiology of chronic venous insufficiency and varicose veins. *Ann Epidemiol*. 2005;15(3):175-184. doi:10.1016/j.annepidem.2004.05.015.

12. Raffetto JD, Mannello F. Pathophysiology of chronic venous disease. *Int Angiol*. 2014;33(3):212-221.

13. Sales CM, Rosenthal D, Petrillo KA, et al. The valvular apparatus in venous insufficiency: a problem of quantity? *Ann Vasc Surg*. 1998;12(2):153-155. doi:10.1007/s100169900133.

14. Ciardullo AV, Panico S, Bellati C, et al. High endogenous estradiol is associated with increased venous distensibility and clinical evidence of varicose veins in menopausal women. *J Vasc Surg*. 2000;32(3):544-549. doi:10.1067/mva.2000.107768.

15. Recek C. Calf pump activity influencing venous hemodynamics in the lower extremity. *Int J Angiol*. 2013;22(1):23-30. doi:10.1055/s-0033-1334092.

16. Arnoldi CC. Venous pressure in the leg of healthy human subjects at rest and during muscular exercise in the nearly erect position. *Acta Chir Scand*. 1965;130(6):570-583.

17. Chi YW, Raffetto JD. Venous leg ulceration pathophysiology and evidence based treatment. *Vasc Med*. 2015;20(2):168-181. doi:10.1177/1358863X14568677.

18. Raffetto JD, Khalil RA. Mechanisms of varicose vein formation: valve dysfunction and wall dilation. *Phlebology*. 2008;23(2):85-98. doi:10.1258/phleb.2007.007027.

19. Lee DK, Ahn KS, Kang CH, Cho SB. Ultrasonography of the lower extremity veins: anatomy and basic approach. *Ultrasonography*. 2017;36(2):120-130. doi:10.14366/usg.17001 28260355.

20. Czarniawska-Grzesińska M, Bruska M. Number of valves in superficial veins of the leg. *Folia Morphol (Warsz)*. 1999;58(3):233-237.

21. Moore HM, Gohel M, Davies AH. Number and location of venous valves within the popliteal and femoral veins: a review of the literature. *J Anat*. 2011;219(4):439-443. doi:10.1111/j.1469-7580.2011.01409.x.

22. Tretbar LL. Deep veins. *Dermatol Surg*. 1995;21(1):47-51. doi:10.1111/j.1524-4725.1995.tb00110.x.

23. Vasquez MA, Rabe E, McLafferty RB, et al. Revision of the venous clinical severity score: venous outcomes consensus statement: special communication of the American Venous Forum Ad Hoc Outcomes Working Group. *J Vasc Surg*. 2010;52(5):1387-1396. doi:10.1016/j.jvs.2010.06.161.

24. Rutherford RB, Padberg FT Jr, Comerota AJ, Kistner RL, Meissner MH, Moneta GL. Venous severity scoring: an adjunct to venous outcome assessment. *J Vasc Surg*. 2000;31(6):1307-1312. doi:10.1067/mva.2000.107094.

25. Malgor RD, Labropoulos N. Diagnosis and follow-up of varicose veins with duplex ultrasound: how and why? *Phlebology*. 2012;27(suppl 1):10-15. doi:10.1258/phleb.2011.012s05.

26. Garcia R, Labropoulos N. Duplex ultrasound for the diagnosis of acute and chronic venous diseases. *Surg Clin North Am*. 2018;98(2):201-218. doi:10.1016/j.suc.2017.11.007.

27. Labropoulos N, Tiongson J, Pryor L, et al. Definition of venous reflux in lower-extremity veins. *J Vasc Surg*. 2003;38(4):793-798. doi:10.1016/s0741-5214(03)00424-5.

28. Kistner RL, Eklof B. Classification and etiology of chronic venous disease. In: Gloviczki P, ed. *Handbook of Venous Disorders: Guidelines of the American Venous Forum*. 3rd ed. Hodder Arnold; 2009:37-46.

29. Labropoulos N, Waggoner T, Sammis W, Samali S, Pappas PJ. The effect of venous thrombus location and extent on the development of post-thrombotic signs and symptoms. *J Vasc Surg*. 2008;48(2):407-412. doi:10.1016/j.jvs.2008.03.016.

30. Rossi R, Agnelli G. Current role of venography in the diagnosis of deep-vein thrombosis. *Minerva Cardioangiol*. 1998;46(12):507-514.

31. Shingler S, Robertson L, Boghossian S, Stewart M. Compression stockings for the initial treatment of varicose veins in patients without venous ulceration. *Cochrane Database Syst Rev*. 2013;(12):CD008819. doi:10.1002/14651858.CD008819.pub3.

32. Calcagno D, Rossi JA. The impact of insurance company mandated compression stocking trial on rate of intervention in patients with symptomatic venous reflux disease. *Phlebology*. 2011;26(6):235-236. doi:10.1258/phleb.2010.010045.

33. Andriessen A, Apelqvist J, Mosti G, Partsch H, Gonska C, Abel M. Compression therapy for venous leg ulcers: risk factors for adverse events and complications, contraindications - a review of present guidelines. *J Eur Acad Dermatol Venereol*. 2017;31(9):1562-1568. doi:10.1111/jdv.14390.

34. Perrin, M. History of venous surgery. *Phlebolymphology*. 2011;18(3):123-129.

35. Rass K, Frings N, Glowacki P, et al. Comparable effectiveness of endovenous laser ablation and high ligation with stripping of the great saphenous vein: two-year results of a randomized clinical trial (RELACS study). *Arch Dermatol*. 2012;148(1):49-58. doi:10.1001/archdermatol.2011.272.

36. Joh JH, Kim WS, Jung IM, et al. Consensus for the treatment of varicose vein with radiofrequency ablation. *Vasc Specialist Int*. 2014;30(4):105-112. doi:10.5758/vsi.2014.30.4.105.

37. Morrison C, Dalsing MC. Signs and symptoms of saphenous nerve injury after greater saphenous vein stripping: prevalence, severity and relevance for modern practice. *J Vasc Surg*. 2003;38:886-890.

38. Sam RC, Silverman SH, Bradbury AW. Nerve injuries and varicose vein surgery. *Eur J Vasc Endovasc Surg*. 2004;27:113-120.

39. Rasmussen LH, Lawaetz M, Bjoern L, et al. Randomized clinical trial comparing endovenous laser ablation, radiofrequency ablation, foam sclerotherapy and surgical stripping for great saphenous varicose veins. *Br J Surg*. 2011;98:1079.

40. Dermody M, Schul MW, O'Donnell TF. Thromboembolic complications of endovenous thermal ablation and foam sclerotherapy in the treatment of great saphenous vein insufficiency. *Phlebology*. 2015;30(5):357-364. doi:10.1177/0268355514529948.

41. Reich-Schupke S, Weyer K, Altmeyer P, Stücker M. Treatment of varicose tributaries with sclerotherapy with polidocanol 0.5% foam. *Vasa*. 2010;39(2):169-174. doi:10.1024/0301-1526/a00002.

42. Mlosek RK, Woźniak W, Malinowska S, Migda B, Serafin-Król M, Miłek T. The removal of post-sclerotherapy pigmentation following sclerotherapy alone or in combination with

crossectomy. *Eur J Vasc Endovasc Surg.* 2012;43(1):100-105. doi:10.1016/j.ejvs.2011.10.005.

43. Watson JJ, Mansour MA. Cosmetic sclerotherapy. *J Vasc Surg Venous Lymphat Disord.* 2017;5(3):437-445. doi:10.1016/j.jvsv.2017.02.002.

44. Kabnick LS, Sadek M, Bjarnason H, et al. Classification and treatment of endothermal heat-induced thrombosis: Recommendations from the American Venous Forum and the Society for Vascular Surgery. *J Vasc Surg Venous Lymphat Disord.* 2021;9(1):6-22. doi:10.1016/j.jvsv.2020.06.008.

45. Lurie F, Lal BK, Antignani PL, et al. Compression therapy after invasive treatment of superficial veins of the lower extremities: clinical practice guidelines of the American Venous Forum, Society for Vascular Surgery, American College of Phlebology, Society for Vascular Medicine, and International Union of Phlebology. *J Vasc Surg Venous Lymphat Disord.* 2019;7(1):17-28. doi:10.1016/j.jvsv.2018.10.002.

46. Russo D, Minutolo R, Iaccarino V, Andreucci M, Capuano A, Savino FA. Gross hematuria of uncommon origin: the nutcracker syndrome. *Am J Kidney Dis.* 1998;32(3):E3.

47. Takebayashi S, Ueki T, Ikeda N, Fujikawa A. Diagnosis of the nutcracker syndrome with color Doppler sonography: correlation with flow patterns on retrograde left renal venography. *AJR Am J Roentgenol.* 1999;172(1):39-43.

48. Kim KW, Cho JY, Kim SH, et al. Diagnostic value of computed tomographic findings of nutcracker syndrome: correlation with renal venography and renocaval pressure gradients. *Eur J Radiol.* 2011;80(3):648-654.

49. Zerhouni EA, Siegelman SS, Walsh PC, White RI. Elevated pressure in the left renal vein in patients with varicocele: preliminary observations. *J Urol.* 1980;123(4):512-513.

50. Erben Y, Gloviczki P, Kalra M, et al. Treatment of nutcracker syndrome with open and endovascular interventions. *J Vasc Surg Venous Lymphat Disord.* 2015;3(4):389-396. doi:10.1016/j.jvsv.2015.04.003.

51. Quevedo HC, Arain SA, Abi Rafeh N. Systematic review of endovascular therapy for nutcracker syndrome and case presentation. *Cardiovasc Revasc Med.* 2014;15(5):305-307.

52. Brown CL, Rizer M, Alexander R, Sharpe EE III, Rochon PJ. Pelvic congestion syndrome: systematic review of treatment success. *Semin Intervent Radiol.* 2018;35(1):35-40. doi:10.1055/s-0038-1636519.

53. Park SJ, Lim JW, Ko YT, et al. Diagnosis of pelvic congestion syndrome using transabdominal and transvaginal sonography. *AJR Am J Roentgenol.* 2004;182(3):683-688. doi:10.2214/ajr.182.3.1820683.

54. Geier B, Barbera L, Mumme A, et al. Reflux patterns in the ovarian and hypogastric veins in patients with varicose veins and signs of pelvic venous incompetence. *Chir Ital.* 2007;59(4):481-488.

55. Phillips D, Deipolyi AR, Hesketh RL, Midia M, Oklu R. Pelvic congestion syndrome: etiology of pain, diagnosis, and clinical management. *J Vasc Interv Radiol.* 2014;25(5):725-733. doi:10.1016/j.jvir.2014.01.030.

56. Durham JD, Machan L. Pelvic congestion syndrome. *Semin Intervent Radiol.* 2013;30(4):372-380. doi:10.1055/s-0033-1359731.

57. Ignacio EA, Dua R, Sarin S, et al. Pelvic congestion syndrome: diagnosis and treatment. *Semin Intervent Radiol.* 2008;25(4):361-368. doi:10.1055/s-0028-1102998.

58. Venbrux AC, Chang AH, Kim HS, et al. Pelvic congestion syndrome (pelvic venous incompetence): impact of ovarian and internal iliac vein embolotherapy on menstrual cycle and chronic pelvic pain. *J Vasc Interv Radiol.* 2002;13(2 Pt 1):171-178. doi:10.1016/s1051-0443(07)61935-6.

59. Kwon SH, Oh JH, Ko KR, Park HC, Huh JY. Transcatheter ovarian vein embolization using coils for the treatment of pelvic congestion syndrome. *Cardiovasc Intervent Radiol.* 2007;30(4):655-661. doi:10.1007/s00270-007-9040-7.

60. Mousa AY, AbuRahma AF. May-Thurner syndrome: update and review. *Ann Vasc Surg.* 2013;27(7):984-995. doi:10.1016/j.avsg.2013.05.001.

61. Suwanabol PA, Tefera G, Schwarze ML. Syndromes associated with the deep veins: phlegmasia cerulea dolens, May-Thurner syndrome, and nutcracker syndrome. *Perspect Vasc Surg Endovasc Ther.* 2010;22(4):223-230.

62. Ahmed HK, Hagspiel KD. Intravascular ultrasonographic findings in May-Thurner syndrome (iliac vein compression syndrome). *J Ultrasound Med.* 2001;20(3):251-256.

CHAPTER 26

Vascular Diseases in the Young

ARASH FEREYDOONI, MD, MHS, GUILLERMO A. ESCOBAR, MD, and MICHAEL D. SGROI, MD

POPLITEAL ENTRAPMENT SYNDROME (PAES)

Pathophysiology

- Extrinsic compression of the popliteal artery during active plantar flexion.
- In normal anatomical position, the medial head of gastrocnemius inserts onto the superior and posterior surface of the medial femoral condyle.[1]
- PAES results from either an abnormal course of the popliteal vessels or an aberrant attachment of the *medial gastrocnemius muscle* or plantaris muscle over the normally positioned vessels.
- PAES can result in progressive fibrosis, rarely occlusion or aneurysmal degeneration.[1]
- Embryologically, the gastrocnemius splits from one proximal head to two, and the medial head migrates laterally. At the same time, the sciatic artery degrades and the popliteal artery forms with the superficial femoral artery (SFA) extending down to the tibialis. Mistiming is thought to occur in PAES.

There are six types of PAES (Fig. 26.1):

Type I   Normal anatomical position of the medial head of gastrocnemius, but the popliteal artery is not straight; it loops around it medially to reach the central popliteal space.
Type II Abnormal, more lateral attachment of the medial head of the gastrocnemius onto the femoral metaphysis encroaches on the popliteal artery.

Type III A tendinous or muscular accessory slip arises from embryologic remnants of the gastrocnemius muscle.
Type IV The popliteal artery is deep and ventral to the popliteus muscle, causing compression. This is the only variant in which the nerve is not involved.[2]
Type V   Compression involving the popliteal vein, as primary etiology (vein alone) or associated with concomitant artery entrapment.
Type VI Functional entrapment. No clear anatomical abnormality. Believed to be from hypertrophy of muscle or its lateral attachment. Functional testing reveals occlusion of popliteal artery flow.[3]

Epidemiology and Clinical Presentation

- Described by Stuart in 1879.
- Predominant in young active adults, with nearly half of patients aged 21–40 years and 30% aged 20 years or younger.[1]
- Historically, males > females (8–9:1).[4] May be historically related to more athletic activities in males.
- Symptoms: pain, paresthesia, and numbness after strenuous physical activity (usually after running/rowing) and are completely reversed with rest.
- Rarely, claudication may also be paradoxical: pain after cessation of activity (reperfusion?) or activity-improving symptoms.

There are six classes of symptom severity, with classes 1 and 2 more common than others.[5]

Class 0	Asymptomatic
Class 1	Pain, paresthesia, and cold foot after physical activity
Class 2	Claudication while walking (>100 ft)
Class 3	Claudication while walking (<100 ft)
Class 4	Rest pain
Class 5	Necrosis

Diagnosis

- Pulses almost always are palpable at rest, but disappear with active plantarflexion *against resistance*, or sometimes with passive dorsiflexion.

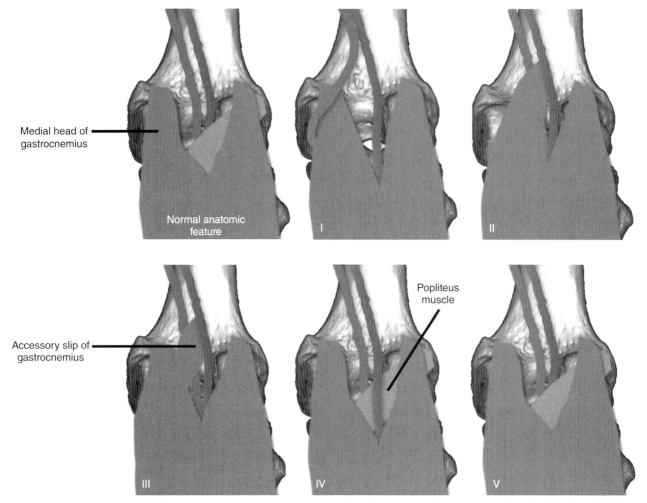

Medial head of gastrocnemius

Normal anatomic feature

I

II

Accessory slip of gastrocnemius

III

Popliteus muscle

IV

V

FIG. 26.1   The popliteal artery is running medial to the medial head of the gastrocnemius muscle, which has a normal insertion. The arterial detour is more medial *(I)*. The insertion of the medial head of the gastrocnemius muscle is higher and more lateral *(II)*. There is an accessory slip of the medial head of the gastrocnemius muscle that inserts into the intercondylar region and compresses the popliteal artery *(III)*. The popliteal artery is compressed when passing under the popliteal muscle *(IV)*. The popliteal vein is caught by the same muscular or fibrous entrapment *(V)*. (From Lejay A, Delay C, Georg Y, et al. Five year outcomes of surgical treatment for popliteal artery entrapment syndrome. *Eur J Vasc Endovasc Surg.* 2016;51(4):557-64.)

- In popliteal artery occlusion, pulses are absent.
- Ankle-brachial indices (ABIs) are normal at rest, but exercise ABIs drop (usually require running until symptoms appear to see drop).
- Duplex ultrasound during calf muscle contraction shows compression of the popliteal artery and elevated velocities with elevated diastolic flow upon rest.
- Computed tomography angiography (CTA) and magnetic resonance angiography (MRA) *may* delineate aberrant muscle arrangement and/or vascular abnormalities, better with imaging at rest and stress.[2,6]
- Angiography with provocative maneuvers against significant resistance during active plantar flexion will discover equivocal cases.

Management

- Posterior approach to the popliteal space with simple myotomy and release in otherwise normal vessels. Medial approach will not allow adequate freeing up of the popliteal space.
- Aneurysmal or diseased arteries may require repair or revascularization.
- *Stenting is contraindicated.*
  - Thrombolysis followed by surgical decompression and/or arterial reconstruction may be used for acute occlusion.
- Medial approach may be considered for PAES types I and II or when a bypass is planned starting from SFA or ending onto tibial branches.

- Rare disadvantages of posterior approach are for bypasses: limited access to the saphenous vein and difficult to reach tibial outflow targets.[7]

Outcomes and Follow-up

- Improvement in approximately 80% of patients and 5-year patency rate of 84% after surgical management.[7]
- In the case of extensive lesions upstream or downstream from the popliteal artery, outcomes are significantly worse.[7]
- Long-term follow-up involves clinical examination and duplex ultrasonography 1 month after the surgery and every 6 months thereafter.[7]

CYSTIC ADVENTITIAL DISEASE

Pathophysiology

- Rare disorder in which cysts form from mucinous accumulation within vessel adventitia. These cysts are lined with a cuboidal epithelial layer and contain myxoid material rich in hyaluronic acid.[8]
  - Most commonly in the popliteal artery.
- Enlarging cysts can gradually compress the arterial lumen, resulting in functional occlusion without thrombus.

The exact etiology of cystic adventitial disease remains unknown, but there are four proposed theories:
1. Developmental: mesenchymal mucus-secreting cells are implanted in the adventitia of the vessel during development.
2. Traumatic: chronic bending at the knee leads to chronic cystic degeneration.
3. Synovial: cyst origin arises from an articular branch connecting the affected vessel to the knee joint, allowing tracking of synovial fluid.
4. Developmental: cystic adventitial disease is part of a larger systemic disorder.

Epidemiology and Clinical Presentation

Cystic adventitial disease is encountered predominantly in middle-aged men, with an average male to female ratio of 15:1 and an incidence of 1:1200 in patients with claudication.[9]
- Presentation: short-distance unilateral claudication that develops relatively suddenly over weeks to months and requires prolonged recovery from ischemic symptoms.[10]
- These patients typically lack any risk factors associated with atherosclerotic vascular disease.[10]

Diagnosis

- ABI testing does not allow cystic adventitial disease to be distinguished from other stenotic diseases.[11]
- On duplex ultrasound, a thin, echogenic, pulsating line may be seen, separating the lumen of the vessel and the cyst, representing the tunica intima and media.[12]
- CTA and MRA are more useful for evaluating the relationship between the cysts and vessels or the surrounding structures, detecting communication between a cyst and an adjacent joint, and ruling out other alternative etiologies such as popliteal aneurysm or PAES.[10,13]
- On angiography, pathognomonic characteristics such as the hourglass sign (concentric compression) or scimitar sign (eccentric compression) are best appreciated on lateral projections.[14]

Management

- The treatment options typically include percutaneous cyst aspiration or resectional (adventitial "stripping" and/or resection of artery with interposition graft or medial bypass).[15,16]
- Aspiration is reserved for simple cysts or those who decline operative intervention.
  - Cyst recurrence—as high as 30% in 15 months.[12]
- Excision of adventitia has best long-term relief and reduced need for reintervention.[17]
- Complete resection and reconstruction with bypass or interposition (using great saphenous vein [GSV] can be done through a posterior approach).
- Extrinsic compression may cause fibrosis and thrombus formation in the popliteal artery, necessitating reconstruction with a bypass.[10]
- *No role for endovascular treatment.*

Outcomes and Follow-up

- After ~70 days 90% of patients report symptom relief with resection of adventitia.[17]

PERSISTENT SCIATIC ARTERY

Pathophysiology

- The sciatic artery is the major supplier of blood flow to the lower limbs from the aorta during the embryonic period. The sciatic normally devolves except for the inferior/superior gluteal, popliteal, and peroneal arteries. It is replaced in the thigh by the SFA.
- The persistent sciatic artery (PSA) is the continuation of the internal iliac artery all the way to the popliteal and

tibial vessels, often accompanied by variable development of the femoral arteries.[18,19]

The Pillet classification of PSA is based on the partial or total absence of the femoral axis[20]:

Type I   A complete PSA with a normal femoral artery
Type II   A complete PSA with an incomplete femoral axis
Type III An incomplete superior PSA
Type IV   An incomplete inferior PSA
Type V   PSA originating from the median sacral artery

- The most commonly reported variant of sciatic artery is type II (incomplete or absent femoral).[19]

Epidemiology and Clinical Presentation

- The estimated incidence of PSA is 0.03%–0.06%.[18]
- Asymptomatic in 40% of cases.[21]
- PSA is bilateral in 25% of patients.[21]
- The most common complication of PSA is aneurysmal degeneration (25%–58%), which may present with a pulsatile gluteal mass, local thrombosis, or distal embolization.[18,19,22]
  - Chronic compression of the PSA from the sacrospinal ligament and the frequent flexion of the hip joint may be responsible for aneurysm formation.[19]

- Sciatic nerve compression from PSA aneurysm can also cause numbness of the lower limbs.

Diagnostic

- *Classic* presentation (Type II): palpable popliteal pulse and pedal pulses *without* a femoral pulse, or a fluctuating pulsatile mass in the greater trochanter region should lead to the suspicion of a PSA. *Another presentation may include acute limb ischemia from embolism (from a peri-gluteal aneurysm) or spontaneous thrombosis of the aneurysm and the PSA.*[22]
- Usually, CT or MRA is necessary. The gold standard diagnostic test is angiography. Findings of an enlarged internal iliac artery diameter on CT or angiography should raise the suspicion of PSA (Fig. 26.2).[23]

Management

- Asymptomatic patients do not require surgical intervention and close surveillance to monitor for aneurysmal degeneration is adequate.
- There is no defined size threshold for repair of PSA aneurysms, but its exclusion is fundamental, given the high risk of complications.

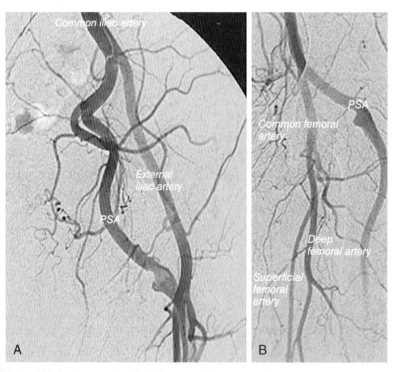

FIG. 26.2   (A) Angiography of a 53-year-old woman who presented with severe claudication pain. Images at the iliac level show a type II persistent sciatic artery *(PSA)* in combination with a small aneurysm. (B) Images at femoral level show a hypoplastic superficial femoral artery. Distally, the popliteal artery is occluded. (From van Hooft IM, Zeebregts CJ, van Sterkenburg SMM, de Vries WR, Reijnen MMPJ. The persistent sciatic artery. *Eur J Vasc Endovasc Surg.* 2009;37(5):585-591.)

- If the femoral axis is complete, PSA may be ligated or embolized. Open ligation or excision carries the risk of sciatic nerve damage. When SFA is absent or incomplete and PSA has long occlusion, surgical bypass, in the form of femoropopliteal/tibial bypass or PSA-popliteal/tibial bypass, is the treatment of choice.[18,21,23]

Outcomes and Follow-up

- Total exclusion of the PSA aneurysm can be assessed on 6-month follow-up with CTA and patency of bypass assessed earlier with duplex ultrasound.[22,23]

ILIAC ARTERY ENDOFIBROSIS

Pathophysiology

- Subintimal fibrosis and nonatherosclerotic stenosis/occlusion in the external > common iliac artery.
- Likely due to mechanical loading, lengthening, and kinking of the external iliac artery.[24]
  - Repeated injury by the enlarged psoas muscle pushing up on the iliac artery, which is "pinned" proximally at the aorta, and distally at the tight inguinal ligament.[24]
- Commonly occurs in young endurance athletes, *especially cyclists* or rowers.

Clinical Presentation

- Commonly exercise-induced leg weakness, thigh > calf pain (and numbness of feet), and resolution of symptoms within 5 minutes of cessation of exercise.[25]

Diagnostic

- Exercise (ideally on stationary bike) *to effort*, with pre- and postexercise ABI.
  A pressure drop of >20 mm Hg in both legs in a patient (even if unilateral symptoms) is considered positive.[25]
- CTA/MRA may *not* show stenosis!
- *Angiography may also be falsely negative unless oblique views obtained (intravascular ultrasound [IVUS] may be needed).*

Management

- Cessation of exercise prevents progression but will not regress (most do not quit)[26]
- Surgical approach:
  - Ideally endarterectomy and primary repair ± vein patch
  - May need interposition grafting (vein or prosthetic)
  - Inguinal ligament "release" is controversial
  - Endovascular intervention *is contraindicated*[25]

Follow-Up and Outcomes

- During the postoperative period, cessation of sports for at least 6–8 weeks +/− daily aspirin.
- Annual surveillance with noninvasive imaging is recommended. Symptomatic stenosis or aneurysmal disease subsequent to patch angioplasty (>3.0 cm) should be repaired surgically.

MIDDLE AORTIC SYNDROME

Pathophysiology

- Middle aortic syndrome (MAS) is a rare disease characterized by the stenosis of distal thoracic or abdominal aorta and/or visceral branches.[27–29]
- The etiologies include most commonly congenital, Takayasu arteritis, neurofibromatosis, and Williams syndrome.[30,31] *Neurofibromatosis* type 1 *is the most common disorder associated with abdominal aortic coarctation* (with classis café-au-lait skin spots).[30,31]
- Intimal fibroplasia is the most common histological finding in aortas.[32]

Epidemiology and Clinical Presentation

- MAS comprises 0.5%–2.0% of aortic coarctations.[30]
- The most common findings in young MAS are *renovascular hypertension*, chronic mesenteric, and lower extremity claudication/hypotrophy.
- The stenosis or occlusion in the distal thoracic or abdominal aorta is best diagnosed on CTA.[28]

Management

- Surgical treatment is indicated for treatment of refractory hypertension and/or claudication.[30]
- Depending on the location and extent of aortic lesion, surgical treatment may involve thoracoabdominal bypass or aortic patch angioplasty (*both best for YOUNG children/growing aorta*) or interposition aortic graft (full-grown aorta).[28,33]
- Dacron or polytetrafluoroethylene (PTFE) can be used for aortic bypass, as well as the branches *in adults*.
- *In children* reimplantation of visceral branches to aorta or aortic graft is ideal. *Internal iliac artery is best for visceral bypass* >> prosthetic > vein to allow for growth and to minimize aneurysmal changes. Can cure hypertension.[34]
- Angioplasty/stenting of visceral branches is generally contraindicated in MAS. It can lead to dissection/thrombosis/disruption, associated with nephrectomy/emergency surgery and complicates otherwise-simple open repair. Reported, but *not* first line.[34–37]
- Antiplatelet agent postreconstruction.

Follow-Up and Outcomes

- The patency and integrity of revascularization should be assessed by CTA at 1, 6, and 12 months after the operation and annually.
- The most common cause of death in patients with MAS is congestive heart failure (CHF) (untreated coarctation and hypertension). Survival rate 20 years after surgery is ~75%.[38]

THORACIC AORTIC COARCTATION

Pathophysiology

- Aortic coarctation is narrowing of the thoracic aorta, typically at the insertion of the ductus arteriosus or just distal to it.
- Focal coarctation is often associated with other congenital heart defects, including bicuspid aortic valve (60%), aortic arch anomalies (18%), ventricular septal defect (13%), mitral valve abnormalities (8%), and subaortic stenosis (6%).[39]

Epidemiology and Clinical Presentation

- Aortic coarctation accounts for 6%–8% of all congenital heart disease and occurs with an incidence of 3–4 cases out of 10,000 live births with a male predominance of 2:1.[40]
- There is also a high prevalence of aortic coarctation in Turner, DiGeorge, and Noonan syndromes.[41]
- Long term, the increased afterload from obstruction of flow due to coarctation leads to significant hypertension in the aorta and proximal branch vessels and may lead to systemic ventricular dysfunction, aneurysm formation, and premature atherosclerosis.
- Pulse wave propagation is slowed distal to the coarctation, thereby delaying and diminishing femoral pulse relative to radial pulse.
- Most pediatric patients are asymptomatic, but in severe cases or later in life, they can present with severe hypertension causing headaches, epistaxis, heart failure, or aortic dissection.[40]

Diagnosis

- Extremity blood pressures should be measured to assess for weak or absent femoral pulses, but this may be misleadingly lower than expected in the setting of significant collateral formation.
- Other physical examination findings include prominent and nondisplaced apical impulse and systolic or continuous murmur radiating to scapula or thorax from collaterals.[40]

- Chest x-rays may show cardiomegaly, sans serif E reverse 3 sign from dilated left subclavian artery and poststenotic dilation distal to coarctation, rib notching from collaterals, and dilated ascending aorta if associated bicuspid aortic valve.[40]
- The best tool for assessment of the lesion morphology is CTA and cardiac MRI.

Management

Significant coarctation is defined as[42]:
- Resting peak-to-peak gradient >20 mm Hg across the stenosis in the catheterization laboratory or by echocardiography *or*
- Resting peak-to-peak gradient >10 mm Hg or mean Doppler systolic gradient >10 mm Hg in the presence of decreased left ventricular systolic function, aortic insufficiency, or collateral flow
- Unrepaired significant aortic coarctation portends poor prognosis. Without repair, the mean age of death is 34 years and the common causes of death may be congestive heart failure, aortic rupture, bacterial endocarditis, or intracranial hemorrhage.[43] Thus, repair of significant coarctation is necessary. Open surgical techniques include[40]: Types of thoracic aortic coarctation treatment

1. Resection and end-to-end anastomosis
2. Patch angioplasty, involving division of ductal tissue by an incision across the coarctation
3. Subclavian flap angioplasty: the left subclavian artery is ligated and divided. A longitudinal incision from the proximal left subclavian artery is made and extended beyond the coarctation. The subclavian flap is turned down and enlarges this area
4. Resection with extended end-to-end anastomosis. The coarcted segment is broadly resected and an oblique anastomosis is made between the undersurface of the transverse arch and the proximal descending aorta

- In patients who are not surgical candidates, endovascular therapy may be considered.
  - Due to the high elastic recoil of coarctation, balloon angioplasty carries a significant rate of recoarctation (15%) and aneurysmal degeneration from intimal and medial tears (24%–35%).[40,42]
  - The Coarctation of the Aorta Stent Trial (COAST) showed that, in children and young adults, stenting required repeat stent dilation in 13% of cases with no need for surgical intervention.[44] Stent fractures were found in 21% of patients, but none were clinically significant.[44]

Follow-Up and Outcomes

- The survival rates for open operative repair of coarctation are 93%, 86%, and 74% at 10, 20, and 30 years after primary repair, respectively, which are significantly lower than age- and sex-matched controls.[45]

- The most common cause of late death is coronary artery disease, followed by sudden death, heart failure, cerebrovascular accident, and ruptured aortic aneurysm.[45]
- The rate of aneurysm formation is 3%–20%, with older age at the time of repair, patch angioplasty technique, and bicuspid aortic valve as risk factors.[46–48]
- Rate of freedom from reintervention is 97%, 92%, and 89% at 10, 20, and 30 years with older age and end-to-end anastomosis technique independently associated with lower rate of reintervention.[45] The most common reason for any cardiac reintervention is aortic valve surgery.[45]

PEDIATRIC RENAL ARTERY STENOSIS

Pathophysiology, Epidemiology, and Clinical Presentation

- Renal artery stenosis (RAS) is an uncommon cause of renin-mediated hypertension in children.
- Genetic and inflammatory diseases affecting the vasculature account for 15% of RAS cases.[49] Some cases are associated with MAS (see earlier) and also exhibit medial fibroplasia (Fig. 26.3).
- Pediatric RAS is often associated with stenosis of the celiac or superior mesenteric artery in 50% of RAS cases and the abdominal aorta in 70% of RAS cases.[50]
- Renal artery lesions are often bilateral (54%) and frequently ostial (66%).[51]

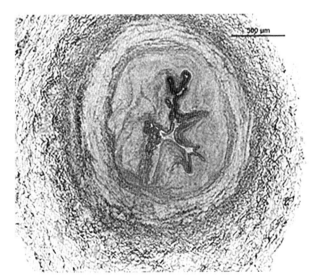

FIG. 26.3 Stenosis Due to Excessive Intimal Fibroplasia With Sparse Media (Movat stain, original magnification ×40). (From Coleman DM, Eliason JL, Stanley JC. Arterial reconstructions for pediatric splanchnic artery occlusive disease. *J Vasc Surg.* 2018;68(4):1062-1070.)

Diagnosis and Management

- Refractory hypertension unresponsive to optimal drug therapy is the basis for surgical intervention. The mean age at the time of surgical intervention is 9–10 years.[51]

Endovascular Management

- The current practice guidelines in high-volume tertiary pediatric centers consider renal artery angioplasty for mid, distal, and segmental renal stenoses that appear multifocal, weblike, or beaded by angiography or with IVUS.[51] Angioplasty is also preferred for recurrent stenosis at anastomosis sites. Renal and aortic stenting should be avoided in pediatric patients and used only for salvage cases.[51]

Open Management

- Primary reimplantation is favored for ostial or proximal main RAS and open surgical revascularization for single and focal stenoses of the mid, distal, or segmental renal arteries.
- In situ reconstruction is favored to preserve important collaterals and to limit intraoperative warm ischemia.
- Ex vivo reconstruction is rarely utilized and performed only in those with complex lesions or aneurysms along with multiple existing segmental arteries.[51] Reimplantation onto the aorta of the normal renal artery, beyond its stenosis, is preferred.[51]
- *In pediatric patients, anastomosis is preferably done with interrupted sutures to permit future diameter growth.*[51]
- The hypogastric artery is favored as a conduit. Patches and grafts are sized sufficiently large enough so as not to become constrictive as the patient grows.[34] Vein grafts are avoided due to high risk of aneurysmal degeneration. Vein grafts inside "cuffs" or prosthetic is last resort.[51]

Follow-Up and Outcomes

- Postoperative monitoring of blood pressure and renal function, annual duplex to monitor renal size/mass and velocities; annual ABI and echocardiography to evaluate development of CHF.[51]
- Up to 20% of patient require reintervention.[51] Children undergoing remedial operations were less likely (33%) to be cured of hypertension.
- Hypertension benefit (cured or improved) in more than 80% of treated patients.[51]

CHRONIC COMPARTMENT SYNDROME

Pathophysiology

- Chronic compartment syndrome (CCS) is caused by an increase in intracompartment pressure during exercise and is commonly seen in young athletes.[52]

- The pathophysiology is not well known, but it has been attributed to exercise-induced increase in blood flow, causing the stiff osteofascial compartments to expand while there is little capacity to accommodate the increase in volume.[53]

Epidemiology and Clinical Presentation

- Estimates of incidence in patients with chronic exercise-induced lower leg pain are 14%–27%, with equal prevalence in men and women.[54,55]
- Symptoms are pain, tightness, cramping, weakness, and paresthesia during exertion, which disappear with activity cessation.[53] CCS does not cause any permanent damage to tissues within the compartment.
- Critical to ensure this is not popliteal entrapment.

Diagnosis

- Physical examination of patients suffering from CCS is often normal with no neurovascular deficit, since symptoms appear only during exercise.

- The diagnosis is confirmed by intracranial pressure (ICP) measurement after symptoms are provoked with a standardized treadmill test[56]:
  - Preexercise pressure ≥15 mm Hg
  - 1-minute postexercise pressure ≥30 mm Hg or
  - 5-minute postexercise pressure ≥20 mm Hg

Management

- CCS is usually treated conservatively at first with physical rehabilitation and preexercise deep tissue massages. Regulating exercise has been shown to alleviate symptoms, which may not be feasible for professional athletes.
- For patients who fail conservative management, fasciotomy may be offered, which can be open[57] or endoscopic.[58,59]

Follow-Up and Outcomes

- Symptom relief after fasciotomy ranges from 48% to 94%.[52]
- Complications included hematoma (2.7%–22.5%), nerve injury (2%–18.6%), deep venous thrombosis (2.7%), and symptom recurrence (0.7%–8.4%).[52]
- ~10% may need revision fasciotomy.[52]

REFERENCES

1. Cavallaro A. Popliteal artery entrapment. In: Cavallaro A, ed. *Aneurysms of the Popliteal Artery*. Cham: Springer Nature Switzerland AG 2021:73-88.
2. López Garcia D, Arranz MA, Tagarro S, Camarero SR, Gonzalez ME, Gimeno MG. Bilateral popliteal aneurysm as a result of vascular type IV entrapment in a young patient: a report of an exceptional case. *J Vasc Surg*. 2007;46(5):1047-1050.
3. Bouhoutsos J, Daskalakis E. Muscular abnormalities affecting the popliteal vessels. *Br J Surg*. 1981;68(7):501-506.
4. di Marzo L, Cavallaro A, Sciacca V, Mingoli A, Stipa S. Natural history of entrapment of the popliteal artery. *J Am Coll Surg*. 1994;178(6):553-556.
5. Insua JA, Young JR, Humphries AW. Popliteal artery entrapment syndrome. *Arch Surg*. 1970;101(6):771-775.
6. Zhong H, Liu C, Shao G. Computed tomographic angiography and digital subtraction angiography findings in popliteal artery entrapment syndrome. *J Comput Assist Tomogr*. 2010;34(2):254-259.
7. Lejay A, Delay C, Georg Y, et al. Five year outcomes of surgical treatment for popliteal artery entrapment syndrome. *Eur J Vasc Endovasc Surg*. 2016;51(4):557-564.
8. Flanigan DP, Burnham SJ, Goodreau JJ, Bergan JJ. Summary of cases of adventitial cystic disease of the popliteal artery. *Ann Surg*. 1979;189(2):165-175.
9. Miller A, Salenius JP, Sacks BA, Gupta SK, Shoukimas GM. Noninvasive vascular imaging in the diagnosis and treatment of adventitial cystic disease of the popliteal artery. *J Vasc Surg*. 1997;26(4):715-720.
10. Jeong S, Kwon TW, Han Y, Cho YP. Effectiveness of surgical treatment with complete cyst excision for cystic adventitial disease of the popliteal artery. *Ann Vasc Surg*. 2021;72:261-269.
11. Elias DA, White LM, Rubenstein JD, Christakis M, Merchant N. Clinical evaluation and MR imaging features of popliteal artery entrapment and cystic adventitial disease. *Am J Roentgenol*. 2003;180(3):627-632.
12. Li S, King BN, Velasco N, Kumar Y, Gupta N. Cystic adventitial disease-case series and review of literature. *Ann Transl Med*. 2017;5(16):327.
13. Ortmann J, Widmer MK, Gretener S, et al. Cystic adventitial degeneration: ectopic ganglia from adjacent joint capsules. *Vasa*. 2009;38(4):374-377.
14. Tomasian A, Lai C, Finn JP, Gelabert H, Krishnam MS. Cystic adventitial disease of the popliteal artery: features on 3T cardiovascular magnetic resonance. *J Cardiovasc Magn Reson*. 2008;10(1):38.
15. Desy NM, Spinner RJ. The etiology and management of cystic adventitial disease. *J Vasc Surg*. 2014;60(1):235-245.e11.
16. Jibiki M, Miyata T, Shigematsu H. Cystic adventitial disease of the popliteal artery with spontaneous regression. *J Vasc Surg Cases Innov Tech*. 2018;4(2):136-139.
17. Motaganahalli RL, Smeds MR, Harlander-Locke MP, et al. A multi-institutional experience in adventitial cystic disease. *J Vasc Surg*. 2017;65(1):157-161.
18. van Hooft IM, Zeebregts CJ, van Sterkenburg SMM, de Vries WR, Reijnen MMPJ. The persistent sciatic artery. *Eur J Vasc Endovasc Surg*. 2009;37(5):585-591.

19. Brantley SK, Rigdon EE, Raju S. Persistent sciatic artery: embryology, pathology, and treatment. *J Vasc Surg*. 1993;18(2): 242-248.

20. Pillet J, Albaret P, Toulemonde JL, Cronier P, Raimbeau G, Chevalier JM. [Ischio-popliteal artery trunk, persistence of the axial artery]. Article in French) *Bull Assoc Anat (Nancy)*. 1980;64(184): 97-110.

21. Yamamoto H, Yamamoto F, Ishibashi K, et al. Intermediate and long-term outcomes after treating symptomatic persistent sciatic artery using different techniques. *Ann Vasc Surg*. 2011;25(6):837.e9-15.

22. Santaolalla V, Bernabe MH, Hipola Ulecia JM, et al. Persistent sciatic artery. *Ann Vasc Surg*. 2010;24(5):691.e7-10.

23. Ahn S, Min SK, Min SI, et al. Treatment strategy for persistent sciatic artery and novel classification reflecting anatomic status. *Eur J Vasc Endovasc Surg*. 2016;52(3):360-369.

24. Schep G, Bender MH, van de Tempel G, Wijn PF, de Vries WR, Eikelboom BC. Detection and treatment of claudication due to functional iliac obstruction in top endurance athletes: a prospective study. *Lancet*. 2002;359(9305):466-473.

25. INSITE Collaborators (INternational Study group for Identification and Treatment of Endofibrosis). Diagnosis and management of iliac artery endofibrosis: results of a Delphi Consensus Study. *Eur JVasc Endovasc Surg*. 2016;52(1):90-98.

26. Hinchliffe RJ. Iliac artery endofibrosis. *Eur J Vasc Endovasc Surg*. 2016;52(1):1-2.

27. Stanley JC, Criado E, Eliason JL, Upchurch GR, Berguer R, Rectenwald JE. Abdominal aortic coarctation: surgical treatment of 53 patients with a thoracoabdominal bypass, patch aortoplasty, or interposition aortoaortic graft. *J Vasc Surg*. 2008;48(5):1073-1082.

28. Kim SM, Jung IM, Han A, et al. Surgical treatment of middle aortic syndrome with Takayasu arteritis or midaortic dysplastic syndrome. *Eur J Vasc Endovasc Surg*. 2015;50(2):206-212.

29. Panayiotopoulos YP, Tyrrell MR, Koffman G, Reidy JF, Haycock GB, Taylor PR. Mid-aortic syndrome presenting in childhood. *Br J Surg*. 2005;83(2):235-240.

30. Connolly JE, Wilson SE, Lawrence PL, Fujitani RM. Middle aortic syndrome: distal thoracic and abdominal coarctation, a disorder with multiple etiologies. *J Am Coll Surg*. 2002;194(6): 774-781.

31. Delis KT, Gloviczki P. Middle aortic syndrome: from presentation to contemporary open surgical and endovascular treatment. *Perspect Vasc Surg Endovasc Ther*. 2005;17(3): 187-203.

32. Heider A, Gordon D, Coleman DM, Eliason JL, Ganesh SK, Stanley JC. Histologic and morphologic character of pediatric abdominal aortic developmental coarctation and hypoplasia. *J Vasc Surg*. 2022;76(2):556-563.e4.

33. Coleman DM, Eliason JL, Ohye RG, Stanley JC. Long-segment thoracoabdominal aortic occlusions in childhood. *J Vasc Surg*. 2012;56(2):482-485.

34. Coleman DM, Eliason JL, Stanley JC. Arterial reconstructions for pediatric splanchnic artery occlusive disease. *J Vasc Surg*. 2018;68(4):1062-1070.

35. Eliason JL, Coleman DM, Criado E, et al. Remedial operations for failed endovascular therapy of 32 renal artery stenoses in 24 children. *Pediatr Nephrol*. 2016;31(5):809-817.

36. Trimarchi S, Tolva VS, Grassi V, Frigiola A, Carminati M, Rampoldi V. Descending thoracic and abdominal aortic coarctation in the young: surgical treatment after percutaneous approaches failure. *J Vasc Surg*. 2008;47(4):865-867.

37. Carr John A. The results of catheter-based therapy compared with surgical repair of adult aortic coarctation. *J Am Coll Cardiol*. 2006;47(6):1101-1107.

38. Miyata T, Sato O, Koyama H, Shigematsu H, Tada Y. Long-term survival after surgical treatment of patients with Takayasu's arteritis. *Circulation*. 2003;108(12):1474-1480.

39. Teo LLS, Cannell T, Babu-Narayan SV, Hughes M, Mohiaddin RH. Prevalence of associated cardiovascular abnormalities in 500 patients with aortic coarctation referred for cardiovascular magnetic resonance imaging to a tertiary center. *Pediatr Cardiol*. 2011;32(8):1120-1127.

40. Kim YY, Andrade L, Cook SC. Aortic coarctation. *Cardiol Clin*. 2020;38(3):337-351.

41. Bayer ML, Frommelt PC, Blei F, et al. Congenital cardiac, aortic arch, and vascular bed anomalies in PHACE syndrome (from the International PHACE Syndrome Registry). *Am J Cardiol*. 2013;112(12):1948-1952.

42. Stout KK, Daniels CJ, Aboulhosn JA, et al. 2018 AHA/ACC guideline for the management of adults with congenital heart disease: executive summary: a report of the American College of Cardiology/American Heart Association Task Force on Clinical Practice Guidelines. *J Am Coll Cardiol*. 2019;73(12): 1494-563.

43. Campbell M. Natural history of coarctation of the aorta. *Br Heart J*. 1970;32(5):633-640.

44. Taggart NW, Minahan M, Cabalka AK, Cetta F, Usmani K, Ringel RE. Immediate outcomes of covered stent placement for treatment or prevention of aortic wall injury associated with coarctation of the aorta (COAST II). *JACC Cardiovasc Interv*. 2016;9(5):484-493.

45. Brown ML, Burkhart HM, Connolly HM, et al. Coarctation of the aorta: lifelong surveillance is mandatory following surgical repair. *J Am Coll Cardiol*. 2013;62(11):1020-1025.

46. Jenkins NP, Ward C. Coarctation of the aorta: natural history and outcome after surgical treatment. *QJM*. 1999;92(7):365-371.

47. Oliver JM, Alonso-Gonzalez R, Gonzalez AE, et al. Risk of aortic root or ascending aorta complications in patients with bicuspid aortic valve with and without coarctation of the aorta. *Am J Cardiol*. 2009;104(7):1001-1006.

48. Oliver JM, Gallego P, Gonzalez A, Aroca A, Bret M, Mesa JM. Risk factors for aortic complications in adults with coarctation of the aorta. *J Am Coll Cardiol*. 2004;44(8):1641-1647.

49. Porras D, Stein DR, Ferguson MA, et al. Midaortic syndrome: 30 years of experience with medical, endovascular and surgical management. *Pediatr Nephrol*. 2013;28(10):2023-2033.

50. Rumman RK, Matsuda-Abedini M, Langlois V, et al. Management and outcomes of childhood renal artery stenosis and middle aortic syndrome. *Am J Hypertens*. 2018;31(6):687-695.

51. Coleman DM, Eliason JL, Beaulieu R, et al. Surgical management of pediatric renin-mediated hypertension secondary to renal artery occlusive disease and abdominal aortic coarctation. *J Vasc Surg*. 2020;72(6):2035-2046.e1.

52. Ding A, Machin M, Onida S, Davies AH. A systematic review of fasciotomy in chronic exertional compartment syndrome. *J Vasc Surg*. 2020;72(5):1802-1812.

53. Dunn JC, Waterman BR. Chronic exertional compartment syndrome of the leg in the military. *Clin Sports Med*. 2014;33(4):693-705.

54. Bong MR, Polatsch DB, Jazrawi LM, Rokito AS. Chronic exertional compartment syndrome: diagnosis and management. *Bull Hosp Jt Dis.* 2005;62:77.

55. Hutchinson MR, Ireland ML. Common compartment syndromes in athletes. *Sports Med.* 1994;17(3):200-208.

56. Pedowitz RA, Hargens AR, Mubarak SJ, Gershuni DH. Modified criteria for the objective diagnosis of chronic compartment syndrome of the leg. *Am J Sports Med.* 1990;18(1):35-40.

57. Dai AZ, Zacchilli M, Jejurikar N, Pham H, Jazrawi L. Open 4-compartment fasciotomy for chronic exertional compartment syndrome of the leg. *Arthrosc Tech.* 2017;6(6):e2191-e2201.

58. Croutzet P, Chassat R, Masmejean EH. Mini-invasive surgery for chronic exertional compartment syndrome of the forearm: a new technique. *Tech Hand Up Extrem Surg.* 2009;13(3):137-140.

59. Pozzi A, Pivato G, Kask K, Susini F, Pegoli L. Single portal endoscopic treatment for chronic exertional compartment syndrome of the forearm. *Tech Hand Up Extrem Surg.* 2014; 18(3):153-156.

CHAPTER 27

Vascular Malformations and Infantile Vascular Tumors

ANUDEEP YEKULA, MBBS, and NAIEM NASSIRI, MD

INTRODUCTION

- During early embryogenesis, primitive blood vessels are derived from mesoderm by coalescing of endothelial precursor cells after stimulation with vascular endothelial growth factor (VEGF).[1]
- After the primitive capillary network forms, vessels differentiate into networks of arteries, veins, and lymphatics under the direction of the molecular determinants, ephrin type-B receptor 4 (ephrin B-4) ephrin-B2, and VEGF-R3, respectively.[1]
- Vascular anomalies encompass a broad clinical spectrum ranging from lesions of cosmetic concern to life-threatening conditions.
- Two broad types of vascular anomalies—hemangiomas and vascular malformations.[2]
  - Hemangiomas are found to be generally benign neoplasms of endothelial cells; vascular malformations are congenital lesions caused by developmental errors during angiogenesis.

CLASSIFICATION

- The term "hemangioma" or derivatives thereof continues to be generalized in reference to anomalous vascular lesions.
- Using consistent and proper nomenclature is critical in the management of vascular anomalies as misnomers and improper terminology have clinical implications and consequences.[3]
- The International Society for Study of Vascular Anomalies (ISSVA) classification categorizes vascular anomalies broadly into two major categories which include:
  - Vascular tumors (mainly hemangiomas) and
  - Vascular malformations

- Vascular malformations are then subcategorized based on their hemodynamics and flow properties into:
  - High-flow malformations which include:
    - Arteriovenous malformations (AVMs) and
    - Arteriovenous fistulae (AVF)
  - Low-flow malformations which include:
    - Capillary malformations (CMs)
    - Venous malformations (VMs), and
    - Lymphatic malformations (LMs)
    - Combined or mixed malformations which can include combinations thereof.
- Vascular malformations can occur as simple, isolated lesions or in combination with other malformations.
- Combined malformations are more commonly encountered as part of a syndrome.
  - Klippel-Trenaunay syndrome, Congenital Lipomatous Overgrowth, Vascular malformations, Epidermal nevus, Skeletal deformities (CLOVES) syndrome, Proteus syndrome, Parkes-Weber syndrome, etc.
- Thanks to advancements in DNA sequencing, it is now recognized that the vast majority of vascular malformations are caused sporadically by somatic mosaic gene mutations.[4]
- Two major signaling pathways:
  - RAS/MAPK/ERK pathway is typically involved in high-flow malformations
  - PI3K/AKT/mTOR pathway is typically involved in low-flow malformations and associated syndromes.

HEMANGIOMAS

Pathophysiology and Clinical Presentation

- Hemangiomas are generally benign vascular tumors of infancy with an endothelial cell origin.
- The most common subtype is the classic infantile hemangioma (IH), which is not a congenital entity and usually appears within the first 2 months of life.
  - It features an erythematous, warm, compressible, hyperemic tumor, nodule, or plaque with various unpredictable patterns of distribution, though it is most commonly an isolated entity.

- Undergoes an initial proliferation phase until approximately 12 months of age.
  - This is followed by a gradual involution phase which can last until adolescence.
  - Lastly, there is a prolonged and protracted involuted phase which involves remodeling of the remnant residual tissue.
- Other rarer and more aggressive endothelial neoplasms include kaposiform hemangioendothelioma (KHE) and tufted angioma.
  - Entities associated with a serious consumptive coagulopathy termed Kasabach-Merritt phenomenon.

Kasabach-Merritt Phenomenon

Diagnostics

- Diagnosis of IH is clinically based on characteristic onset, features, and clinical behavior.
- Duplex ultrasound and handheld Doppler can be helpful clinical adjuncts demonstrating well-vascularized, high-flow, low-resistance signals.
- If more than three distinct lesions are identified, the diagnosis of hemangiomatosis is made, which warrants imaging investigation—mainly magnetic resonance imaging (MRI)—for cerebral and visceral IHs.[5]

Treatment

- Treatment of inconspicuous IH without proximity to critical organs is mainly supportive and observational, as they will eventually involute without significant clinical consequences.
- Cosmetically conspicuous lesions and/or those jeopardizing development and function of critical organs warrant further treatment.
  - The mainstay of treatment of IHs is oral propranolol—a nonselective, adrenergic receptor blocker—which is continued until the proliferation phase comes to an end at about 12 months of age.[6]
  - Topical timolol has also been used for more superficial and less bulky lesions.

VASCULAR MALFORMATIONS

High-Flow AVMs and AVFs

Pathophysiology and Clinical Presentation

- AVMs and AVFs represent pathologic connections between arteries and veins upstream of capillary level (Fig. 27.1A).
- They can occur as isolated lesions or as part of broader syndromes such as Parkes-Weber syndrome or hereditary hemorrhagic telangiectasia (HHT) syndrome.[7]
- The shunting of the blood away from capillaries prematurely into draining veins can cause venous hypertension,

distal steal phenomena, and rarely cardiopulmonary overload.[8] Two broad angioarchitectural subtypes exist and include:
- AVFs featuring direct arteriovenous connections, and
- AVMs, which classically feature an intervening nidus—a convoluted, high-flow, low-resistance conglomerate of poorly differentiated vessels that have neither an arterial nor a venous designation.

Diagnostics

- Contrast-enhanced MRI including T2, fat-suppressed series, is the gold-standard, noninvasive imaging modality for imaging of vascular malformations.
- Selective angiography is the invasive imaging modality of choice for delineation of feeding arteries and draining veins (Fig. 27.1B).

Treatment

- The cornerstone of treatment for AVMs is nidus penetration and elimination.
  - Anything short of eradicating the nidus—such as surgical ligation or coil embolization of feeding vessels—is a futile and harmful endeavor.
  - Nidal penetration is best achieved superselectively using a coaxial, microcatheter-based platform. Most commonly achieved via an antegrade, transarterial route, retrograde transvenous nidal access is also described.[9]
  - Direct percutaneous nidal access can also be performed under road map guidance with direct stick embolization (DSE) (Fig. 27.1C–D).[7]
    - The choice of embolic material depends on the vessel size and flow characteristics.
  - Occlusive polymerizing agents:
    - n-Butyl cyanoacrylate (NBCA) glue which is mixed with ethiodol to slow glue polymerization time and provide radiopacity
    - Ethylene vinyl alcohol copolymer (Onyx) which is mixed with the solvent dimethyl sulfoxide (DMSO)
  - Nonpolymerizing, protein-denaturing agents:
    - Absolute ethanol—due to high toxicity profile of the agent (e.g., skin sloughing, nerve injury, cardiac arrhythmias, central cardiopulmonary toxicity, and death), it should only be used with extreme caution and by experienced hands only.
- In addition to these more traditional options, we have recently shown the feasibility of superselective AVM nidal penetration and embolization using platinum-based, high-density packing coils.[10]
- Lastly, for the treatment of AVFs with more direct arteriovenous connections, proximal occluding devices such as coils, plugs, and detachable balloons are appropriate.[4,11]

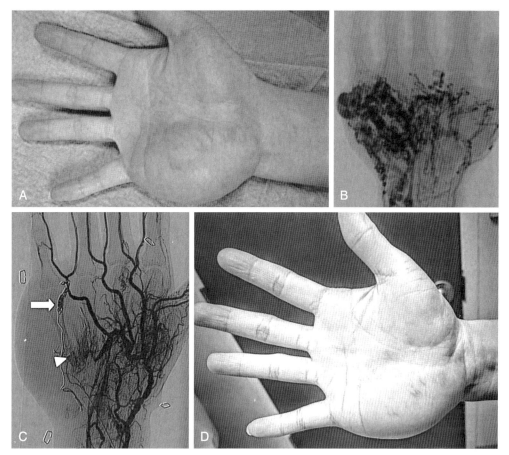

FIG. 27.1 (A) Localized high-flow arteriovenous malformation of the right hypothenar region. (B) Arteriogram showing prominent palmar arch nidus located along the ulnar aspect of the hand and fed by a radial-dominant palmar arch with decreased distal digital flow and prompt venous outflow filling. (C) Transvenous coil embolization of venous drainage was performed *(arrow)*, deposited in nidus venous drainage tract. This was followed by transarterial and direct stick nidus embolization using Onyx *(arrowhead)*. There is significant improvement in digital flow with no evidence of nontarget embolization. (D) Follow-up examination shows markedly reduced bulge at the hypothenar eminence. (Reproduced with permission from Nassiri N, Cirillo-Penn NC, Thomas J. Evaluation and management of congenital peripheral arteriovenous malformations. *J. Vasc. Surg.* 2015;62:1667-1676.)

Low-Flow Lymphatic Malformations

Pathophysiology and Clinical Presentation

- LMs are lymph-filled spaces containing serous or chylous fluid.
- LMs are particularly at risk for bleeding and infection (Fig. 27.2A).[11] There are three morphologic types:
  - Macrocystic (>2 cm)
  - Microcystic (<2 cm)
  - Mixed—combined macro- and microcystic
- LMs tend to be lesions of childhood and infancy and have a predilection for the head and neck (50%), followed by the trunk and extremities (40%) and the viscera (10%).[4]

- LMs can be sporadic or part of a broader syndrome such as CLOVES and Klippel-Trenaunay syndrome (KTS). They are commonly associated with somatic activating mutations in *PIK3CA*.[12,13]

Diagnostics

- Along with the clinical diagnosis, duplex ultrasound imaging and contrast-enhanced MRI are useful in assessing the anatomy and morphology of LMs.
  - Ultrasound features include an avascular, hypoechoic, cystic structure with or without fluid-fluid levels.[4]

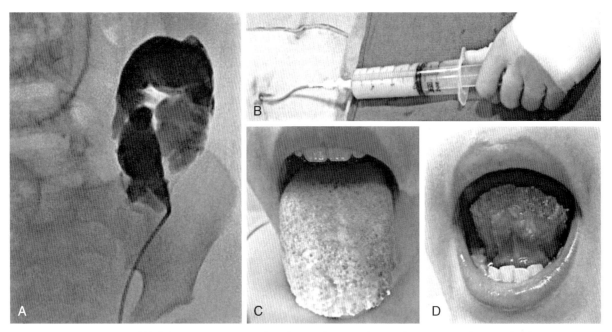

FIG. 27.2   (A) Direct stick access into large, intraperitoneal, macrocystic lymphatic malformation with lymphangiography demonstrating outline, extent, and contour of the malformation following percutaneous drainage of serous content. (B)–(D) demonstrate difficult to drain microcystic lymphatic malformation of the tongue. (Reproduced with permission from Nassiri N, Thomas J, Cirillo-Penn NC. Evaluation and management of peripheral venous and lymphatic malformations. *J Vasc Surg Venous Lymphat Disord.* 2016;4:257-265.)

- MRI is the gold-standard imaging modality and features a T2 isointense-to-hyperintense cystic lesion with characteristic rim enhancement.

Treatment

- Once discovered, treatment of LMs is indicated as these lesions are at high risk of secondary infection, hemorrhage, or rapid expansion with mass effect on adjacent organs.
- First-line treatment is direct percutaneous access of the LM cyst with transcatheter drainage to obtain maximum wall collapse.
- This is followed by injection of a sclerosant into remnant to cause an inflammatory reaction, leading to fibrosis of the cystic space (Fig. 27.2B).[13,14]
- Commonly used sclerosing agents are:
  - Doxycycline, with antiendothelial growth factor and antimetalloproteinase properties, often the first-line agent of choice for peripheral LMs[15,16]
  - Bleomycin, an antineoplastic agent with cumulative dose restrictions owing to the rare risk of pulmonary fibrosis
  - Ethanol, which is highly effective but toxic as previously discussed, and
  - Sodium tetradecyl sulfate (STS), a detergent-like compound acting as an anionic surfactant

- The main cause of recurrence is usually inadequate drainage of the cystic cavity.[17] For lesions refractory to the first endovascular intervention, multiple staged treatments using more aggressive sclerosants such as bleomycin and ethanol, laser photocoagulation, or surgical excision may be necessary.[18,19]
- Surgical excision of macrocystic LMs carries a high risk of cystic wall violation and leakage of content, infection, and recurrence (40%–50%).[17]
- In general, macrocystic LMs are much more effectively treated by direct percutaneous drainage and sclerotherapy (response rates of >80% with single session) than microcystic and mixed LMs (response rates of up to 50%) (Fig. 27.2C–D).[16]
  - Microcystic lesions usually require multiple sessions or adjunctive procedures.[20]

Low-Flow Venous Malformations

Pathophysiology and Clinical Presentation

- VMs are the most common vascular malformation, comprising >75% of all lesions.
- Distorted low-flow vessels often appear as a bluish/purple, soft, compressible venous cluster predominantly in the skin and mucosa (Fig. 27.3).[21]

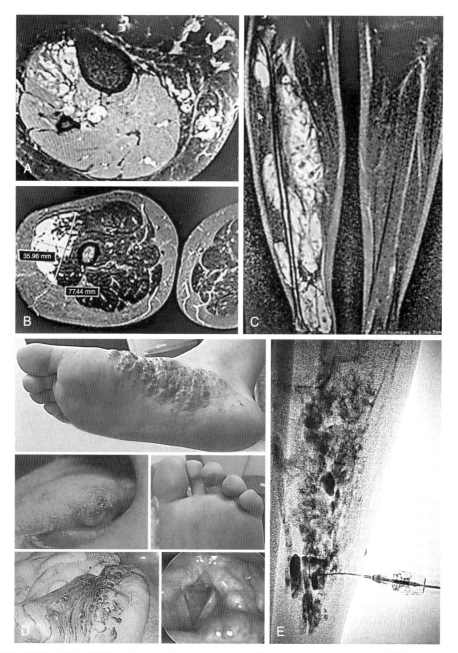

FIG. 27.3 (A)–(C) Contrast-enhanced magnetic resonance imaging (MRI) demonstrating hallmark hyperintense features of low-flow venous malformations of the subcutaneous and intramuscular tissues on T2 fat-suppressed series. (D) Characteristic clinical features of low-flow venous malformations throughout various body parts including the viscerae and mucosa. (E) Direct stick embolization of a superficial extremity venous malformation. (Reproduced with permission from Nassiri N, Thomas J, Cirillo-Penn NC. Evaluation and management of peripheral venous and lymphatic malformations. *J Vasc Surg Venous Lymphat Disord.* 2016;4:257-265.)

- VMs are not proliferative lesions, but they do grow in size with age, and, unlike hemangiomas, they never spontaneously regress.[22]
- VMs often remain asymptomatic until triggered by an injury, thrombosis, or hormonal fluctuations during puberty, menses, and pregnancy.

The common symptoms of VMs are pain, swelling, and disfigurement.[21]

- Can be part of broader syndromes
  - KTS, CLOVES, Proteus, blue rubber bleb nevus, Maffucci, and glomuvenous malformation syndromes, etc.

Diagnosis

- Duplex ultrasound and contrast-enhanced MRI are the imaging modalities of choice.[17,23]
  - VMs appear as dilated, tortuous channels with a faint, venous pattern flow and occasional phleboliths.
  - Contrast-enhanced MRI is the gold-standard imaging modality for VMs with characteristic T2 hyperintense lesions on fat-suppressed series (Fig. 27.3A–C).[17]
  - Hematologic evaluation at the time of diagnosis with fibrinogen and D-dimer is important to assess for the presence of localized intravascular coagulopathy (LIC), which may progress to disseminated intravascular coagulopathy (DIC) if left untreated.[24,25]

Treatment

Indications for treatment include pain, functional impairments, cosmetic disfigurement, hematologic derangements, and associated psychosocial complications (Fig. 27.3D).

- The mainstay of treatment for VMs is DSE (Fig. 27.3E).[14]
  - Ultrasound-guided, percutaneous needle access of the malformation lumen with intraluminal venography to ascertain the angioarchitecture of the VM including its draining system and connection patterns with the systemic circulation.
  - Direct infusion of a sclerosant of choice.
    - Ethanol is by far the most potent embolic agent, with technical success rates of >90% and extremely rare recurrence rates.[23,26] However, its toxic adverse effect profile has limited its use, particularly in the pediatric population.[27,28]
- Surgical resection may be considered for focal, isolated lesions or refractory lesions or as an adjunctive modality to sclerotherapy.[29]

Mixed Vascular Malformations Associated With Other Syndromes

Pathophysiology and Clinical Presentation

- The most common syndrome associated with the presence of VM is KTS.[30]
- KTS is a capillary-lymphatic-venous malformation and is typically diagnosed at birth and features the clinical triad of CMs, bony and/or soft tissue extremity asymmetry, and underlying lymphatic-venous malformations.[31]
- Unlike Parkes-Weber syndrome, KTS has no arteriovenous shunting.
- Another overgrowth syndrome with similar features is CLOVES as defined by clinical features of congenital lipomatous overgrowth, vascular malformations, epidermal nevi, and skeletal deformities.
  - Rather than being distinct clinical entities, KTS and CLOVES belong to the *PIK3CA*-related Overgrowth

Syndrome (PROS) spectrum and represent various features along a range of phenotypes caused by *PIK3CA* genetic mutation.[30,32]

- There are two major patterns of venous pathology associated with KTS and other related overgrowth syndromes—venous malformations and venous hypertension associated with the congenitally incompetent lateral marginal vein (LMV):
  1. The VMs of KTS are consistent with the previously described sporadic VMs, which feature isolated, cavernous clusters of anomalous veins spread throughout various soft tissue planes of the affected extremity.
  2. The congenitally incompetent LMV is present in <20% of KTS patients. It can be present in isolation or coexist with acquired incompetence of the saphenous system.
- Anomalous marginal veins of the trunk and extremities in KTS and CLOVES are a major source of venous hypertension-related morbidity and potentially lethal thromboembolic events.[33,34] Therefore, their treatment is always warranted.
- LMV tends to arise near the lateral aspect of the foot, malleolus, or knee and courses cephalad along the lateral aspect of the lower limb.

Diagnostics

- Patients with syndromic low-flow vascular malformation require an initial screening contrast-enhanced MRI to look for and characterize underlying vascular malformations in the affected body part.
- Dedicated duplex ultrasound studies are necessary to verify MRI findings, analyze flow patterns, confirm an intact deep venous system, rule out deep vein thrombosis, and interrogate for reflux in the saphenous system and/or LMV when present.[35]

Treatment

- If saphenous reflux is identified in the presence of an intact deep venous system, traditional endoluminal ablative measures are recommended.[33]
- If an LMV is identified, regardless of the severity of symptoms, compression therapy should be initiated.
  - These congenital incompetent venous structures are best treated by coil embolization of the venous outflow tract, followed by transcatheter sclerosant delivery from proximal to distal, along the main venous trunk, or STS-based mechanicochemical ablation (MOCA) of the main trunk.[36,37]
- Once all incompetent veins have been addressed, DSE of any coexisting clusters of VM can be performed in as many sessions as necessary.
- Persistently refractory veins may require more traditional surgical bulk excision. Stab phlebectomy for

excision of persistent varicosities following ablation of culprit vein can be performed.

- Oral rapamycin has begun to play a growingly more prominent role as an essential adjunctive modality in the treatment of PROS, particularly in patients with organ- and/or life-threatening conditions refractory to other measures.

- Syndromes featuring high-flow AVMs and fistulas include Parkes-Weber and Rendu-Osler-Weber syndromes.
  - These require AVM and AVF embolization as the mainstay of treatment as previously described along with supportive measures to address other coexisting hematologic and soft tissue deformities.

REFERENCES

1. Wolf K, Hu H, Isaji T, Dardik A. Molecular identity of arteries, veins, and lymphatics. *J Vasc Surg.* 2019;69:253-262.
2. Mulliken JB, Glowacki J. Hemangiomas and vascular malformations in infants and children: a classification based on endothelial characteristics. *Plast Reconstr Surg.* 1982;69:412-422.
3. Hassanein AH, Mulliken JB, Fishman SJ, Greene AK. Evaluation of terminology for vascular anomalies in current literature. *Plast Reconstr Surg.* 2011;127:347-351.
4. Nassiri N, Cirillo-Penn NC, Thomas J. Evaluation and management of congenital peripheral arteriovenous malformations. *J Vasc Surg.* 2015;62:1667-1676.
5. Moukaddam H, Pollak J, Haims AH. MRI characteristics and classification of peripheral vascular malformations and tumors. *Skeletal Radiol.* 2009;38:535-547.
6. Hasan M, Rahman M, Hoque S, Zahid Hossain AKM, Khondker L. Propranolol for hemangiomas. *Pediatr Surg Int.* 2013;29:257-262.
7. Nassiri N, Cirillo-Penn NC, Crystal DT. Direct stick embolization of extremity arteriovenous malformations with ethylene vinyl alcohol copolymer. *J Vasc Surg.* 2017;65:1223-1228.
8. Wassef M, Blei F, Adams D, et al. Vascular anomalies classification: recommendations from the *International Society* for the *Study* of *Vascular Anomalies. Pediatrics.* 2015;136:e203-e214.
9. Nassiri N, Thomas J, Rahimi S. Fibrodysplastic implications for transvenous embolization of a high-flow pelvic arteriovenous malformation in Osler-Weber-Rendu syndrome. *J Vasc Surg Cases.* 2015;1:16-19.
10. Bellamkonda KS, Fereydooni A, Trott K, Lee Y, Mehra S, Nassiri N. Superselective intranidal delivery of platinum-based high-density packing coils for treatment of arteriovenous malformations. *J Vasc Surg Cases Innov Tech.* 2021;7:230-234.
11. Nassiri N, Dudiy Y, Carroccio A, Rosen RJ. Transarterial treatment of congenital renal arteriovenous fistulas. *J Vasc Surg.* 2013;58:1310-1315.
12. Boscolo E, Coma S, Luks VL, et al. AKT hyper-phosphorylation associated with PI3K mutations in lymphatic endothelial cells from a patient with lymphatic malformation. *Angiogenesis.* 2015;18:151-162.
13. Osborn AJ, Dickie P, Neilson DE, et al. Activating PIK3CA alleles and lymphangiogenic phenotype of lymphatic endothelial cells isolated from lymphatic malformations. *Hum Mol Genet.* 2015;24:926-938.
14. Nassiri N, Thomas J, Cirillo-Penn NC. Evaluation and management of peripheral venous and lymphatic malformations. *J Vasc Surg Venous Lymphat Disord.* 2016;4:257-265.
15. Chaudry G, Burrows PE, Padua HM, Dillon BJ, Fishman SJ, Alomari AI. Sclerotherapy of abdominal lymphatic malformations with doxycycline. *J Vasc Interv Radiol.* 2011;22:1431-1435.
16. Burrows PE, Mitri RK, Alomari A, et al. Percutaneous sclerotherapy of lymphatic malformations with doxycycline. *Lymphat Res Biol.* 2008;6:209-216.
17. Burrows PE. Endovascular treatment of slow-flow vascular malformations. *Tech Vasc. Interv Radiol.* 2013;16:12-21.
18. Lee BB, Do YS, Byun HS, Choo IW, Kim DI, Huh SH. Advanced management of venous malformation with ethanol sclerotherapy: mid-term results. *J Vasc Surg.* 2003;37:533-538.
19. Lee BB, Kim DI, Huh S, et al. New experiences with absolute ethanol sclerotherapy in the management of a complex form of congenital venous malformation. *J Vasc Surg.* 2001;33(4):764-772.
20. Raveh E, Waner M, Kornreich L, et al. [The current approach to hemangiomas and vascular malformations of the head and neck]. Article in Hebrew. *Harefuah.* 2002;141:783-7888, 859, 858.
21. Will Y, Eric McDuffie J, Olaharski AJ, Jeffy BD. *Drug Discovery Toxicology: From Target Assessment to Translational Biomarkers.* Hoboken, NJ: John Wiley & Sons; 2016.
22. Boon LM, Ballieux F, Vikkula M. Pathogenesis of vascular anomalies. *Clin Plast Surg.* 2011;38:7-19.
23. Burrows PE, Mason KP. Percutaneous treatment of low flow vascular malformations. *J Vasc Interv Radiol.* 2004;15:431-445.
24. Blei F. Medical and genetic aspects of vascular anomalies. *Tech Vasc Interv Radiol.* 2013;16:2-11.
25. Lee BB, Baumgartner I, Berlien P, et al. Diagnosis and treatment of venous malformations. Consensus document of the International Union of Phlebology (IUP): updated 2013. *Int Angiol.* 2015;34:97-149.
26. Alomari A, Dubois J. Interventional management of vascular malformations. *Tech Vasc Interv Radiol.* 2011;14:22-31.
27. Wong GA, Armstrong DC, Robertson JM. Cardiovascular collapse during ethanol sclerotherapy in a pediatric patient. *Pediatr Anaesth.* 2006;16:343-346.
28. Barranco-Pons R, Burrows PE, Landrigan-Ossar M, Trenor CC III, Alomari AI. Gross hemoglobinuria and oliguria are common transient complications of sclerotherapy for venous malformations: review of 475 procedures. *AJR Am J Roentgenol.* 2012;199:691-694.
29. Dompmartin A, Vikkula M, Boon LM. Venous malformation: update on aetiopathogenesis, diagnosis and management. *Phlebology.* 2010;25:224-235.
30. Fereydooni A, Dardik A, Nassiri N. Molecular changes associated with vascular malformations. *J Vasc Surg.* 2019;70:314-326.e1.
31. Jacob AG, Driscoll DJ, Shaughnessy WJ, Stanson AW, Clay RP, Gloviczki P. Klippel-Trénaunay syndrome: spectrum and management. *Mayo Clin Proc.* 1998;73:28-36.
32. Vahidnezhad H, Youssefian L, Uitto J. Klippel-Trenaunay syndrome belongs to the PIK3CA-related overgrowth spectrum (PROS). *Exp Dermatol.* 2016;25:17-19.

33. Fereydooni A, Nassiri N. Evaluation and management of the lateral marginal vein in Klippel-Trénaunay and other PIK3CA-related overgrowth syndromes. *J Vasc Surg Venous Lymphat Disord.* 2020;8:482-493.

34. Alomari AI, Burrows PE, Lee EY, Hedequist DJ, Mulliken JB, Fishman SJ. CLOVES syndrome with thoracic and central phlebectasia: increased risk of pulmonary embolism. *J Thorac Cardiovasc Surg.* 2010;140:459-463.

35. Kim YW, Lee BB, Cho JH, Do YS, Kim DI, Kim ES. Haemodynamic and clinical assessment of lateral marginal vein excision in patients with a predominantly venous malformation of the lower extremity. *Eur J Vasc Endovasc Surg.* 2007;33:122-127.

36. Lim Y, Lim Y, Fereydooni A, et al. Mechanochemical and surgical ablation of an anomalous upper extremity marginal vein in CLOVES syndrome identifies PIK3CA as the culprit gene mutation. *J Vasc Surg Cases Innov Tech.* 2020;6:438-442.

37. Nassiri N, Crystal D, Huntress LA, Murphy S. Transcatheter embolization of persistent embryonic veins in venous malformation syndromes. *J Vasc Surg Venous Lymphat Disord.* 2017;5:749-755.

Index

Note: page numbers followed by 'b' represent boxes; by 'f' represent figures; by 't' represent tables.

Antineutrophil cytoplasmic antibody (ANCA)-associated pauci-immune, 170–171
Antiplatelets, 14
    for asymptomatic and symptomatic disease, 91
    for peripheral arterial disease, 2
    pharmacology of, 22–23
Antithrombin III (AT III), 12
Antithrombotic therapy, for peripheral arterial disease, 2
Aorta
    arch types of, 52, 52b, 52f
    shaggy, 83
    zones of, 52, 52b, 52f
Aortic arch branching, variations of, 56, 58f
Aortic dissection, 45–50
    acute presentation of, 46
    adjunctive procedures for, 48–49
    anatomic classification systems of, 46
    classification by clinical status, 46, 46t
    epidemiology of, 45
    follow-up for, 49
    indications for intervention in, 47–48
    initial evaluation and diagnosis of, 46f, 47
    initial management of, 47
    malperfusion and, 47, 47f
    pathophysiology of, 45, 46f
    risk factors of, 45
        genetic/congenital, 45
        medical/acquired, 45
        modifiable, 45
    temporal classification of, 45
    type A, 47
    type B
        chronic, 49
        complicated, 47–48
        endovascular interventions for, 48, 48f
        medical management of, 7
Aortic endografts, infected, 69, 80
Aortic neck angulation, for EVAR, 74t
Aortic neck diameter, for EVAR, 74t
Aortic neck length, for EVAR, 74t
Aortoenteric fistula, abdominal aortic aneurysm with, 67–68
Aortofemoral bypass (AFB), for aortoiliac occlusive disease, 84, 85t
Aortoiliac occlusive disease (AIOD), 83–88
    aneurysmal disease and, 85
    diagnostic evaluation of, 83–84
    endovascular repair for, 84–85, 85t
    epidemiology of, 83
    etiology of, 83
    follow-up for, 86
    nonoperative intervention for, 84
    open reconstruction for, 84
    postoperative complications of, 85–86
    signs/symptoms of, 83
    treatment of, 84–85
Apixaban, 14
Apnea test, 42
Ardeparin, 13
ARDS see Acute respiratory distress syndrome
Argatroban, 13, 20
Arrhythmias, 38–39
ARSCA see Aberrant right subclavian artery
Arterial duplex ultrasound, for chronic PAD, 120
Arterial embolism, acute mesenteric ischemia due to, 147–148
Arterial stenting, for chronic venous occlusive disease, 174–175
Arterial thoracic outlet syndrome (aTOS), 106–107
Arterial wall, anatomy of, 45
Arteriography, for aortoiliac occlusive disease, 84
Arteriovenous fistula (AVF)
    access to, types of, 154
    high-flow, 202, 203f
Arteriovenous malformations (AVMs), high-flow, 202, 203f
Ascending pharyngeal artery branches, carotid body tumors and, 98
Aspiration catheters, 114b

Aspirin, 14, 22
    for asymptomatic and symptomatic disease, 91
    for peripheral arterial disease, 2
ASTRAL trial, 143
Asymptomatic Carotid Atherosclerosis Study (ACAS), 90
Asymptomatic Carotid Surgery Trial (ACST), 90
Atherosclerosis, 142
Atherosclerotic carotid artery disease
    asymptomatic and symptomatic, surgical management for, 91
    carotid endarterectomy for, 91–93, 92t
    epidemiology and pathophysiology of, 89
    imaging for, 89–90
    seminal clinical trials in, 90
aTOS see Arterial thoracic outlet syndrome
Atrial kick, 37
Atropine, 23
AVF see Arteriovenous fistula
AVMs see Arteriovenous malformations
Axillofemoral bypass, for aortoiliac occlusive disease, 84

B
Ballard, for TAAA, 54
Balloon-expandable stent, for aortoiliac occlusive disease, 84, 85t
Banding, for dialysis access steal syndrome, 156
BASIL trial see Bypass versus Angioplasty in Severe Ischemia of the Leg trial
Basilic vein transposition, one- versus two-stage, 154
Below-knee amputation (BKA), 123, 133
Berlin criteria, 36
Best Endovascular versus Surgical Therapy in patients with Critical Limb Ischemia trial (BEST-CLI trial), 124
Best medical therapy (BMT), for asymptomatic and symptomatic disease, 90–91
BEST-CLI trial see Best Endovascular versus Surgical Therapy in patients with Critical Limb Ischemia trial
Beta-blockers, for heart failure, 39
Biffl classification, 160t
Bivalirudin, 13, 20
BKA see Below-knee amputation
Bleomycin, for low-flow lymphatic malformations, 204
Blunt cerebrovascular trauma, 160
Blunt thoracic aortic injury, TEVAR for, 55
BMT see Best medical therapy
Brachial plexus, 103
Brachial-brachial index (BBI), 164
Bradyarrhythmias, 38
Brain death, 42–43
Broad spectrum antibiotics, 147
Bronchoalveolar lavage, for ARDS, 36
Buerger disease, 171
Bypass versus Angioplasty in Severe Ischemia of the Leg trial (BASIL trial), 123–124

C
CAA see Celiac artery aneurysm
Calcium, imbalances, 40–41
Calcium channel blocker, 7
Cannulation, in vascular access, 154–155
Cardiac arrest
    postoperative, 38
    in trauma, 38
Cardiac output, 37–39
Cardiac tamponade, 31
Cardiogenic shock, 32
Carotid artery dissection, management of, 98
Carotid artery stenting (CAS), carotid endarterectomy versus, 95–96
Carotid body tumors (CBTs), 98
Carotid endarterectomy (CEA), 91–93, 92t
    carotid artery stenting versus, 95–96
    cerebral hyperperfusion after, 94–95
    eversion endarterectomy, 93f
    neuromonitoring during, 93–94
    with patch angioplasty, 92f
    restenosis after, 96–97
    shunts for, 93f, 94–95
    stroke after, 94, 94f